NUTRITION
AND
DIET MODIFICATIONS

THIRD EDITION

NUTRITION AND DIET MODIFICATIONS

THIRD EDITION

BY CAROLYNN E. TOWNSEND

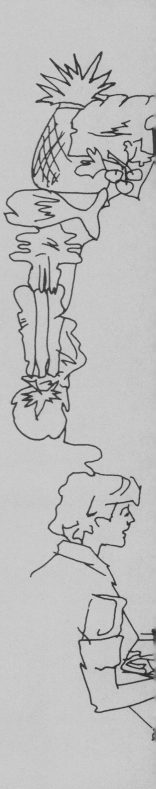

DELMAR PUBLISHERS
COPYRIGHT © 1980
BY LITTON EDUCATIONAL PUBLISHING, INC.

10 9 8 7 6 5 4 3 2 1

LIBRARY OF CONGRESS CATALOG CARD NUMBER: 78-74166
ISBN: 0-8273-1324-1

Printed in the United States of America
Published Simultaneously in Canada by
Delmar Publishers, A Division of
Van Nostrand Reinhold, Ltd.

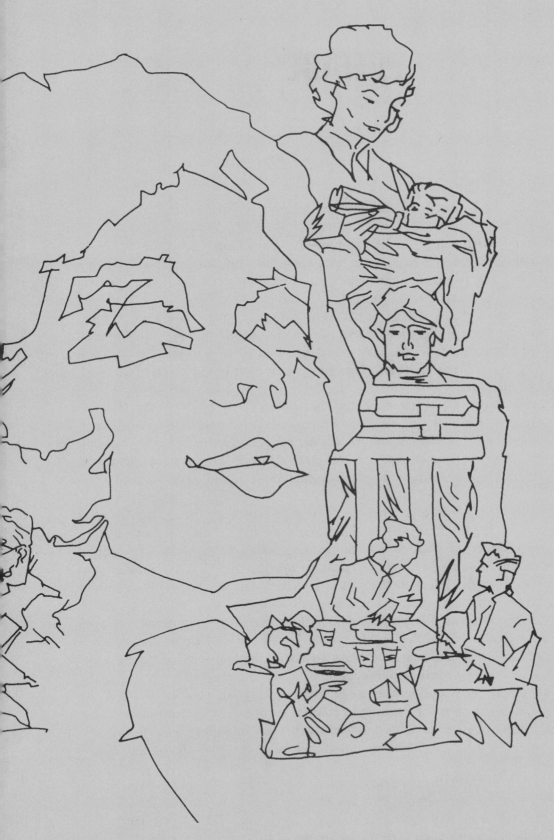

DELMAR PUBLISHERS • ALBANY, NEW YORK 12205
A DIVISION OF LITTON EDUCATIONAL PUBLISHING, INC.

PREFACE

Nutrition and Diet Modifications is a time-saving teaching aid written especially for students requiring basic instruction in, and application of, fundamental nutrition and diet therapy. It is planned to meet the needs of the person just entering the field and also to serve as the basic text for those desiring a refresher course.

Section 1 deals with the science of basic nutrition. It explains how the body prepares food for use through digestion, absorption, and metabolism. Because a knowledge of each of the nutrients is necessary in order to plan good nutrition, the chemical composition, function in the body, and food sources for each of the six essential nutrients have been included.

Planning nutritious meals based on the Basic Four food groups is the focus of section 2. Cultural, regional, and religious influences on eating habits are discussed. Tables on energy needs for various ages; recommended daily dietary allowances; additives; charts on retail cuts of meat and the best method for cooking each cut have been included in this section. Information on purchasing food, grading, labeling and packaging is also included.

Section 3 covers the use of kitchen equipment, how to recognize signs of spoiled food, and ways to reduce food related illnesses. An extensive glossary of cookery terms has been included in order to help the student understand recipes. This section also deals with the metric system as it relates to nutrition. Charts showing how to convert from the English system to the metric system and from the metric system to the English system give the student a working knowledge of the metric system. A chart on metric equivalents of common household measures gives a quick reference for metric equivalents. This chapter on metric is valuable in helping the students gradually adapt to the metric system. Ways to adapt the family menu to meet the requirements of a special diet are also discussed.

The nutritional needs during pregnancy and lactation for the mother, and the diet and preparation of food for the infant comprise section 4. The importance of the nourishment the infant receives in utero as well as that received during the first year of life and its relationship to the future mental and physical development of the child is discussed.

In the fourth section, the student is introduced to diet therapy and the role it plays in health maintenance. Foods that are allowed on the various therapeutic diets and sample menus for each are included to give the student a clear understanding of each diet. The final chapter deals with the technique of tube feeding a patient.

The Appendix contains several tables pertinent to nutrition. Of particular importance and usefulness in planning menus is the U.S.D.A.'s table of "Nutritive Values of the Edible Part of Food." An extensive bibliography has also been included to provide for further reading and research.

Carolynn Townsend, the author of this text, graduated cum laude from Gustavus Adolphus College in St. Peter, Minnesota with a B.A. in Home Economics and Education. She participated in SPAN (Student Project for Amity Among Nations) through the University of Minnesota. This project culminated in an 89-page report of a field study on food habits of British youth. Mrs. Townsend has had many years experience teaching home economics to high school students.

Other books in Delmar's nursing series include:

Ferris / *Body Structures and Functions,* text and slides

Anderson and Shapiro / *Obstetrics for the Nurse*

Noonan / *Emotional Adjustment to Illness*

Caldwell and Hegner / *Geriatrics: A Study of Maturity*

Hornemann / *Basic Nursing Procedures*

Huber, Spatz, and Coviello / *Homemaker-Home Health Aide*

A current catalog including prices of all Delmar educational publications is available upon request. Please write to:

Catalog Department
Delmar Publishers
50 Wolf Road
Albany, New York 12205

Or call Toll Free: (800) 354-9815

CONTENTS

SECTION 1 BASIC NUTRITION
Text Page

Chapter 1 Introduction to Nutrition 1
Chapter 2 The Body's Use of Food 8
Chapter 3 Carbohydrates and Fats. 19
Chapter 4 Proteins. 30
Chapter 5 Minerals. 38
Chapter 6 Vitamins 48

Section Evaluation 59

SECTION 2 MEAL PLANNING

Chapter 7 The Basic Four Food Groups 62
Chapter 8 Planning Appetizing Meals. 72
Chapter 9 Developing Good Eating Habits. 78
Chapter 10 Evaluating and Preserving Food Quality 85
Chapter 11 Purchasing Food 103

Section Evaluation 113

SECTION 3 MEAL PREPARATION

Chapter 12 Using Kitchen Equipment Efficiently 115
Chapter 13 Preventing Food-Related Illness 122
Chapter 14 Reading Recipes 129
Chapter 15 Measuring and Weighing Ingredients 137
Chapter 16 Preparing the Patient's Meal 145

Section Evaluation 150

SECTION 4 FOOD FOR MOTHER AND BABY

Chapter 17 Diet During Pregnancy and Lactation 152
Chapter 18 Diet During Infancy 158

Section Evaluation 165

SECTION 5 SPECIAL DIETS

Chapter 19   Introduction to Diet Therapy   167
Chapter 20   Liquid Diets   172
Chapter 21   The Soft Diet   177
Chapter 22   The Light Diet.   181
Chapter 23   The Bland Diet   185
Chapter 24   Diets Modified in Residue Content   188
Chapter 25   High and Low Calorie Diets.   194
Chapter 26   The Diabetic Diet   201
Chapter 27   Fat Controlled Diets   206
Chapter 28   Protein Diets.   212
Chapter 29   Sodium Restricted Diets   216
Chapter 30   Allergy Diets.   222
Chapter 31   Tube Feeding   227

Section Evaluation   233

Appendix   236
Bibliography   284
Acknowledgments.   287
Index.   288

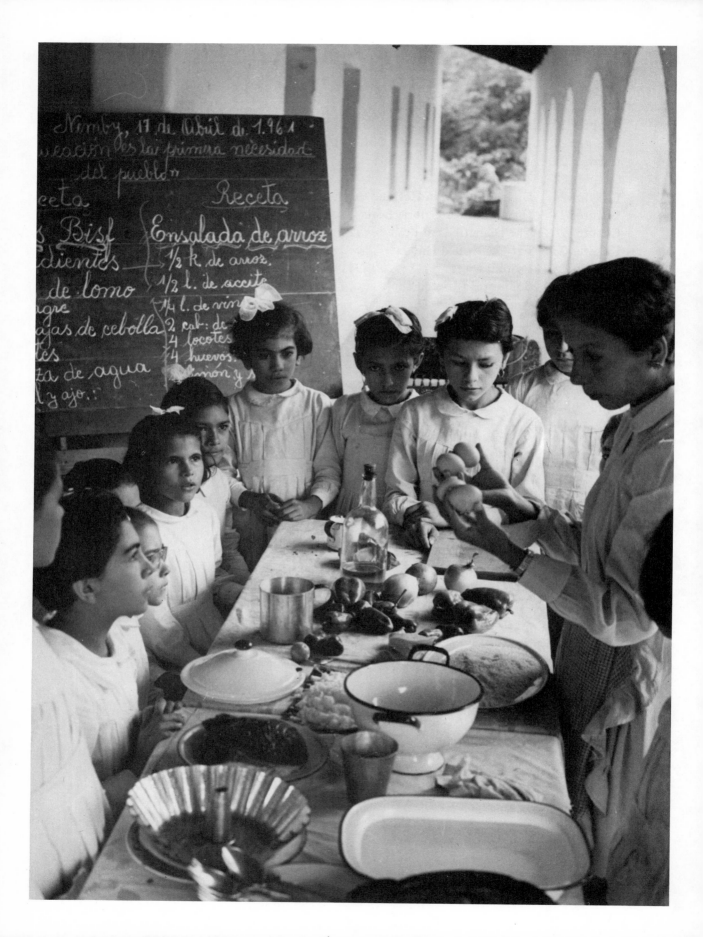

Section 1
BASIC NUTRITION

Chapter 1
Introduction to Nutrition

OBJECTIVES

After studying this chapter, the student should be able to:

- List the essential nutrients and identify their primary functions.
- Identify physical characteristics affected by nutrition.
- Identify ways in which malnutrition affects the body.
- Identify at least four hollow calorie foods.

Most people enjoy food. Although they eat primarily because they are hungry, they also find eating pleasant because of the memories it may invoke, the social climate it promotes and because the taste of the food is pleasing to them. Unfortunately, many people make their food selections only on the basis of taste and are not aware of the way the body uses the foods they like to eat.

There is an old saying, "You are what you eat." This statement has great significance when the results of good or poor nutrition are considered. *Nutrition* is the result of those processes whereby the body takes in and uses food for growth, development and the maintenance of health. Nutrition helps determine the height and weight of an individual. Nutrition also may affect the body's ability to resist disease, the length of one's life, and the state of one's physical and mental well-being.

Good nutrition enhances one's appearance. People with good nutrition usually have shiny hair, clear skin, clear eyes, erect *posture* (body position), alert expressions, and firm flesh on well-developed bone structures. Good nutrition aids emotional adjustments, provides *stamina* (one's resistance to fatigue or illness), and promotes a healthy appetite. It also helps establish regular sleep and elimination habits.

ESSENTIAL NUTRIENTS

A *nutrient* is a chemical substance found in food, that supplies the body with needed nourishment. (To *nourish* is to provide necessary foods.) In order for the body to be well-nourished, foods containing various nutrients should be eaten regularly. The essential nutrients are:

- Carbohydrates
- Fats

- Proteins
- Minerals
- Vitamins
- Water

A nutrient must accomplish at least one of three functions:

- Supply heat and energy to the body
- Build and repair body tissues
- Regulate body processes

Carbohydrates and fats primarily furnish heat and energy. Proteins are used mainly to build and repair body tissues with the help of vitamins and minerals. Proteins also provide energy when carbohydrate and fat reserves are low. Vitamins, minerals and water help regulate the various body processes such as circulation, respiration, digestion and elimination.

Water comprises about 58 percent of body weight and is found in all body tissues. Water aids in the breakdown of food. It makes up most of the *blood plasma* (fluid part of the blood) which carries food to all parts of the body and removes wastes. Water helps the body tissues absorb food. Food which is not used becomes waste and is excreted. Water helps move the waste through the body and prevents constipation. Because of its importance in maintaining body processes, the average person needs to drink the *equivalent* (equal amount) of six to eight glasses of water each day.

MALNUTRITION

Malnutrition is a condition that results when the cells do not receive an adequate supply of the essential nutrients because of poor diet or poor utilization of food. Sometimes it occurs because people do not or cannot eat enough of the foods that provide the essential nutrients to satisfy body needs. Other times people may eat full, well-balanced diets, but suffer from diseases which prevent

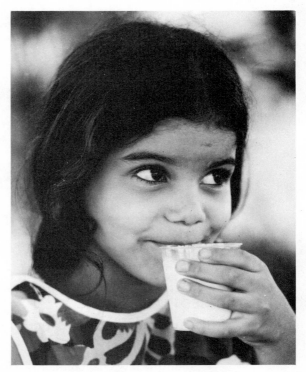

Fig. 1-1. A child's appearance is enhanced when she is well-nourished. (*Courtesy of the United Nations/ Guthrie*)

normal usage of the nutrients. Treatments such as drug therapy or surgery sometimes create changes that prevent food from being used normally.

Some characteristics of people suffering from malnutrition are: dull, lifeless hair; greasy pimpled facial skin; dull eyes; slumped posture; fatigue and depression shown in spiritless expressions and behavior. Malnourished persons may be underweight or overweight and skeletal growth may be stunted. Resistance to disease is reduced and recovery is slower than in healthy people. Appetite may be poor or excessive, resulting in underweight or overweight. Sleep may be affected because malnutrition influences the nervous system, just as it affects all body systems. Irritability and nervousness may result. Constipation is common. The attention span is reduced. Mental retardation,

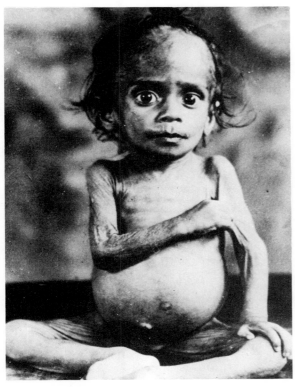 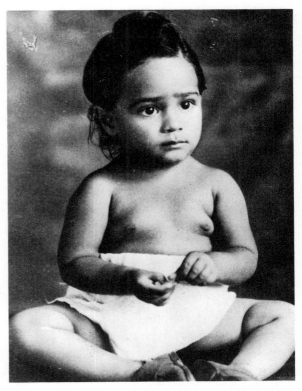

A. Signs of severe malnutrition (swollen abdomen, sagging skin, and sunken eyes) are easily seen in this two-year-old girl.

B. After 10 months of diet therapy, improvements in nutritional status are evident.

Fig. 1-2 A proper diet can produce great improvement, even after severe malnutrition. *(Courtesy of World Health Organization)*

disease, and even death can result from severe malnutrition.

A disease which directly results from a lack of a certain nutrient is called a *deficiency disease.* Beriberi is an example of a deficiency disease. Beriberi affects the nervous system, causing weakness, paralysis, and sometimes death. It is due to a lack of a vitamin (thiamine) in the diet.

Iron deficiency is a common form of malnutrition in the United States, particularly among women of childbearing age. *Iron* is a mineral component of the blood and, therefore, is lost during each menstrual period. In addition, there is an increased need for iron during pregnancy.

Persons most prone to malnutrition are infants, preschool children, adolescents, the elderly, and pregnant women (especially if they are adolescents). If mothers do not know about proper nutrition, their children will suffer. Infants and preschool children depend on their mothers' selection of foods. Preschool children may face an additional hazard as they are usually particular about what they eat.

Adolescents may eat often, but at unusual hours. They may miss regularly scheduled meals, become hungry, and satisfy this hunger with snacks of hollow calorie foods such as potato chips, cakes, sodas and candy. *Hollow calorie foods* provide large amounts of sugar, fat, and calories, but very limited amounts of proteins, vitamins and minerals. Adolescents are subject to *peer pressure;* that is, they are influenced by the opinions of their friends. If friends favor the hollow calorie foods, it is difficult for an adolescent to differ with them. Crash diets, which unfortunately are so common among adolescents, sometimes result in a form of malnutrition. This condition occurs because certain essential nutrients are eliminated from the diet.

Pregnancy increases a woman's appetite and the need for certain nutrients, especially proteins, minerals and vitamins. Pregnancy during adolescence requires extreme care in food selection. The young mother-to-be requires a diet that provides sufficient nutrients for the developing fetus, as well as for her own still-growing body.

The elderly are often alone and unwell. Their living conditions are not always conducive to forming a healthy appetite. Part of the joy of eating is sharing one's food in pleasant company. Lack of companionship or illness can make eating unpleasant and difficult.

THE STUDY OF NUTRITION

A detailed study of nutrition and its relationship to body functions, general health and specific illnesses is essential for the nurse or homemaker. Patients, family members, and friends frequently ask questions regarding nutrition. An understanding of nutrition is useful when helping others whose eating habits require improvement.

Sometimes patients undergo *diet therapy,* which means that their medical treatment in-

cludes eating prescribed foods in specified amounts. The nurse must be able to check a patient's tray quickly to see that it actually contains the correct foods for the diet prescribed.

Patients frequently have questions and complaints about a diet which is new to them. Explanations should be made clearly and simply. Anyone who plans or prepares meals should be able to apply the principles of nutrition. They should have knowledge of the value of sound nutrition.

Parents need to have a good, basic knowledge of nutrition for the sake of their personal health, the health of their children and in order to instruct the children in proper dietary habits. Greater knowledge about nutrition would help eliminate many health problems caused by malnutrition.

SUMMARY

Nutrition is the process by which the body uses food for growth, development and the maintenance of health. Signs of good nutrition include shiny hair, clear skin and eyes, erect posture, a well-developed body, an alert expression, a pleasant disposition, a healthy appetite, and regular habits of sleep and elimination. Nutrition helps determine a person's height, weight, resistance to disease and length of life.

To be well-nourished, one must eat foods which supply heat and energy, build and repair body tissue, and regulate body functions. To accomplish these functions, foods must contain the six essential nutrients: carbohydrates, fats, proteins, minerals, vitamins and water.

DISCUSSION TOPICS
1. Why is eating pleasant?
2. What is the relationship of nutrition and heredity to each of the following?
   - the development of physique
   - the ability to resist disease
   - the lifespan

3. How does nutritional status affect personality?

4. What health habits, in addition to good nutrition, contribute to making a person healthy?

5. What are the six essential nutrients? What are their three basic functions?

6. Of what value is water to the body?

7. Why are women prone to iron deficiency?

8. Why are some foods called hollow calorie foods? Give examples of these foods.

9. If anyone in the class has been on a crash diet to lose weight, discuss its effects on the individual.

10. What is meant by the saying, "You are what you eat?"

SUGGESTED ACTIVITIES

a. List ten signs of good nutrition and ten signs of poor nutrition.

b. Write an essay discussing personal nutrition. List possible improvements.

c. List the foods you have eaten in the past 24 hours. Underline the hollow calorie foods.

d. Using a biology textbook as your source, describe one or more of the following body processes: circulation, respiration, elimination.

e. Write a brief description of how you feel at the end of a day when you know you have not eaten wisely.

WORD STUDY

appetite	equivalent	obesity
beriberi	fats	peer pressure
blood plasma	hollow calorie foods	posture
carbohydrate	iron	protein
constipation	malnutrition	respiration
deficiency	mental retardation	skeletal
deficiency disease	mineral	stamina
diet therapy	nourish	stunted
digestion	nutrient	vitamin
elimination	nutrition	water

REVIEW

A. Multiple choice. Select the *letter* which precedes the best answer.

1. The result of those processes whereby the body takes in and uses food for growth, development, and maintenance of health is called
   a. respiration
   b. diet therapy
   c. nutrition
   d. digestion

2. Nutrition is important in helping to determine a person's
   a. height and weight
   b. ability to resist disease
   c. physical and mental well-being
   d. all of the above

3. In order to nourish the body adequately, one must
   a. keep warm at all times
   b. eat the essential nutrients
   c. sleep 10 hours each night
   d. resist all disease

4. Nutrients used primarily to provide heat and energy to the body are
   a. water, vitamins and minerals
   b. carbohydrates and fats
   c. none of these
   d. all of these

5. Nutrients used mainly to build and repair body tissues are
   a. proteins, minerals, and vitamins
   b. carbohydrates and fats
   c. water and fats
   d. iron and fats

6. Foods such as potato chips, cakes, sodas, and candy are called
   a. dietetic foods
   b. essential nutrient foods
   c. hollow calorie foods
   d. nutritious foods

7. An inadequate supply of essential nutrients in the diet may result in
   a. stamina
   b. malnutrition
   c. indigestion
   d. diabetes

8. Beriberi is caused by lack of a
   a. protein
   b. carbohydrate
   c. vitamin
   d. fat

9. The nutrient which comprises about 58 percent of the body weight is
   a. protein
   b. vitamin A
   c. carbohydrate
   d. water

10. In the United States, a common form of malnutrition is
    a. iron deficiency
    b. lactation
    c. scurvy
    d. diabetes

B. Match the term listed in column I with its definition in column II.

Column I

_____ 1. posture
_____ 2. stamina
_____ 3. nutrients
_____ 4. blood plasma
_____ 5. protein
_____ 6. beriberi
_____ 7. peer pressure
_____ 8. diet therapy
_____ 9. iron
_____ 10. swollen abdomen

Column II

a. body position
b. physical change that may be due to malnutrition.
c. deficiency disease caused by lack of thiamine
d. deficiency disease caused by lack of iron
e. fluid part of blood
f. one's resistance to fatigue or illness
g. chemical substances found in food and essential for nourishing the body
h. influence by the opinions of friends
i. mineral that is a component of the blood
j. eating prescribed foods in specified amounts
k. a basic nutrient which is essential for building and repairing body tissue

C.   Read each function and name the nutrients which perform each function.   Consider all six nutrients; some nutrients will be listed more than once.

FUNCTION	NUTRIENTS
Furnish heat and energy	
Build and repair tissues	
Regulate body processes	

Chapter 2
The Body's Use of Food

OBJECTIVES

After studying this chapter, the student should be able to:

- Explain the process of digestion, absorption and metabolism.
- Label the organs and glands in the digestive system.
- List enzymes and/or digestive juices secreted by each organ and gland in the digestive system.
- State one function of the thyroid gland.
- Define calorie.
- Calculate individual minimum caloric requirements.

Although the body is infinitely more complex than the automobile engine, it may be compared to the engine because both require fuel in order to run. The body's fuel is, of course, food. In order for the body to use its fuel the food must first be prepared by the body. This is done through the processes of digestion and absorption. The actual use of the food as fuel, resulting in energy, is called *metabolism*.

DIGESTION

The first step in the body's preparation of its food is digestion. *Digestion* is the process whereby food is broken down into smaller parts, chemically changed, and moved through the gastrointestinal system. The *gastrointestinal* or *digestive system* consists of the body structures which participate in digestion. As the process of digestion is discussed, refer to figure 2-1, and note the locations of the structures which perform the functions of digestion.

Digestion occurs through two types of action: mechanical and chemical. With mechanical action, food is broken up by the teeth. It is then moved along the gastrointestinal tract through the esophagus, stomach, and intestines. This movement is caused

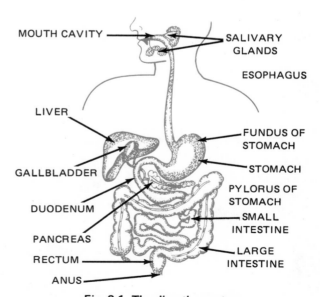

Fig. 2-1 The digestive system

by a rhythmic contraction of the muscular walls of the tract called *peristalsis.*

During chemical digestion, the composition of food is changed. Chemical changes occur through the addition of water and the splitting, or breaking down, of the food molecules. This process is called *hydrolysis.* Food is broken down into nutrients that the tissues can absorb and use. Hydrolysis is brought about essentially by enzymes, table 2-1. An *enzyme* is an organic substance that causes chemical changes in other substances. Enzymes are usually named for the substance on which they act, for example, the enzyme *sucrase* acts on sucrose, and the enzyme *maltase* acts on maltose.

Digestion in the Mouth

Digestion begins in the mouth where the food is broken up by the teeth and mixed with saliva. *Saliva* is a secretion of the salivary glands which contains a digestive enzyme called *ptyalin* (also called salivary amylase) that acts on starch. However, because food is normally held in the mouth for such a short time, very little starch is chemically changed here. The final chemical digestion of starch occurs in the small intestine.

Digestion in the Stomach

Peristalsis and gravity transfer food from the mouth to the stomach via the esophagus. The *esophagus* is the tube connecting the mouth and the stomach. The stomach has three main functions in digestion. It serves to:

- temporarily store food
- mix food with gastric juices
- provide a slow, controlled emptying of food into the small intestine

The stomach consists of the upper portion known as the *fundus;* the middle area known as the *body;* and the end nearest the intestine called the *pylorus.*

TABLE 2-1 Enzymes and Foods Acted Upon

	Enzyme	Food Acted Upon
Mouth	Ptyalin	Starch
Stomach	Pepsin	Proteins
	Rennin	Proteins in milk
	Gastric lipase	Emulsified fat
Small Intestine	Pancreatic amylase	Starch
	Pancreatic proteases (trypsin) (chymotrypsin) (carboxypeptidases)	Proteins
	Pancreatic lipase (steapsin)	Fats
	Lactase	Lactose
	Maltase	Maltose
	Sucrase	Sucrose
	Peptidases	Proteins

Food accumulates in the fundus and moves to the body where it mixes with the gastric juices. *Gastric juices* are digestive secretions of the stomach. The gastric juices contain hydrochloric acid and the enzymes, *pepsin, rennin* and *gastric lipase. Hydrochloric acid* breaks the food down, so the enzymes can work on the food, helps to dissolve some minerals, and destroys much of the bacteria present on food. *Pepsin* changes proteins into smaller forms. *Rennin* acts on the protein in milk, causing it to curdle. *Gastric lipase* acts on emulsified fats such as are found in cream and egg yolk. An emulsified fat is a fat finely divided and held in suspension by another liquid.

Disgestion in the Small Intestine

After the food has been thoroughly mixed with gastric juices, it becomes a semi-liquid mass called *chyme* (pronounced kime). In this form it moves through the pylorus by peristalsis into the *duodenum,* the first section of the small intestine.

When food reaches the small intestine, the gallbladder is triggered into releasing a

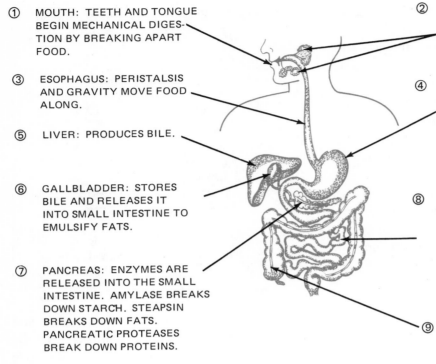

① MOUTH: TEETH AND TONGUE BEGIN MECHANICAL DIGESTION BY BREAKING APART FOOD.

② SALIVARY GLANDS: BEGIN CHEMICAL DIGESTION AS PTYALIN BEGINS TO CHANGE STARCH TO MALTOSE.

③ ESOPHAGUS: PERISTALSIS AND GRAVITY MOVE FOOD ALONG.

④ STOMACH: HYDROCHLORIC ACID PREPARES THE GASTRIC AREA FOR ENZYME ACTION. PEPSIN BREAKS DOWN PROTEINS. RENNIN BREAKS DOWN MILK PROTEINS. LIPASE ACTS ON EMULSIFIED FATS.

⑤ LIVER: PRODUCES BILE.

⑥ GALLBLADDER: STORES BILE AND RELEASES IT INTO SMALL INTESTINE TO EMULSIFY FATS.

⑧ SMALL INTESTINE: PRODUCES ENZYMES, PREPARES FOODS FOR ABSORPTION. LACTASE CONVERTS LACTOSE, MALTASE CONVERTS MALTOSE, SUCRASE CONVERTS SUCROSE, TO FORM SIMPLE SUGARS. PEPTIDASES REDUCE PROTEINS TO AMINO ACIDS.

⑦ PANCREAS: ENZYMES ARE RELEASED INTO THE SMALL INTESTINE. AMYLASE BREAKS DOWN STARCH. STEAPSIN BREAKS DOWN FATS. PANCREATIC PROTEASES BREAK DOWN PROTEINS.

⑨ LARGE INTESTINE: ABSORBS WATER; COLLECTS FOOD RESIDUE FOR EXCRETION.

Fig. 2-2 Basic functions of the digestive organs

substance called bile. Bile is produced in the liver but stored in the gallbladder. *Bile* emulsifies fats after it is secreted into the small intestine. This action enables the enzymes to digest the fats more easily.

Chyme also triggers the pancreas to secrete its juice into the small intestine. Juice secreted from the pancreas contains the following enzymes:

- *Trypsin, chymotrypsin,* and *carboxypeptidases,* which split proteins into smaller substances. These are called pancreatic proteases because they are protein-splitting enzymes produced by the pancreas.
- *Pancreatic amylase,* which converts starches (polysaccharides) to simple sugars.
- *Steapsin,* a lipase which reduces fats to fatty acids and glycerol.

The small intestine itself produces an intestinal juice which contains the enzymes *lactase, maltase* and *sucrase.* These enzymes split lactose, maltose and sucrose, respectively, into simple sugars. The small intestine also produces enzymes called *peptidases* which break down proteins into amino acids.

ABSORPTION

After digestion, the next major step in the body's preparation of its food is absorption. *Absorption* is the passage of nutrients into the body fluids and tissues. In order to be absorbed, nutrients must be in their simplest forms: carbohydrates have been broken down to the simple sugars (glucose, fructose and galactose); proteins to amino acids; and fats to fatty acids and glycerol. Most absorption of nutrients occurs in the small intestine although there is some occurring in the large intestine. Water is absorbed in the mouth, stomach, small intestine and large intestine.

Absorption in the Small Intestine

The small intestine is approximately twenty-two feet long. Its inner surface contains many fingerlike projections called *villi*. Each villus contains numerous blood *capillaries* (tiny blood vessels) and *lacteals* (lymphatic vessels). The villi absorb nutrients from the chyme by way of these blood capillaries and lacteals; these nutrients are eventually transferred to the bloodstream. Glucose, fructose and galactose; amino acids; minerals; and water-soluble vitamins are absorbed by the capillaries. Fructose and galactose are subsequently carried to the liver where they are converted to glucose. Lacteals absorb glycerol and *fatty acids* (end products of fat digestion), in addition to the fat-soluble vitamins.

Absorption in the Large Intestine

By the time the chyme reaches the large intestine most digestion and absorption is complete. However, some digestive juices are carried into the large intestine in the chyme and continue their work for a time. A major task of the large intestine is to absorb water. The large intestine also collects food residue. *Food residue* is that part of food which is not digested and consequently, not absorbed. Undigested food is subsequently excreted as feces by way of the rectum. In healthy people, 99 percent of carbohydrate, 95 percent of fat, and 92 percent of protein is absorbed. It is important that the diet contain some bulk (also called fiber or indigestible residue). *Bulk* is that part of the food eaten which body enzyme action cannot digest. Examples of bulk are the outer hull on corn kernels or wheat grain; celery strings; and apple skins. Including bulk in the diet promotes the health of the large intestine. *Fiber*, or bulk, in the diet helps to produce softer stools and more frequent bowel movements.

METABOLISM

After digestion and absorption, nutrients are carried by the blood to the cells of the body. Within the cells, nutrients are changed into energy through a complex process called metabolism. During metabolism, nutrients are combined with oxygen within each cell. This is known as *oxidation.* Oxidation reduces carbohydrates and fats ultimately to carbon dioxide and water; proteins are reduced to carbon dioxide, water and nitrogen.

As nutrients are oxidized, energy and its by-product, heat, are released. When this released energy is used to build new substances from simpler substances, the process is called *anabolism.* An example of anabolism is the formation of new body tissues. When released energy is used to break down substances into simpler substances, the process is called *catabolism.* Catabolism occurs in the breakdown of tissue as with surgery, burns, and during periods of high fever. This building up and breaking down of substances (metabolism) is a continuous process within the body and requires a continuous supply of nutrients. Whenever the body performs work, it uses energy. It does not matter whether the work is *voluntary*, such as walking and swimming, or *involuntary*, such as breathing and digesting food. More energy is needed to perform work which is difficult than to perform work which is easy. The body usually stores an excess of nutrients and is able to use these stores during times of need.

Metabolism and the Thyroid Gland

Metabolism is governed primarily by the secretions of the thyroid gland. These secretions are *thyroxine* and *triiodothyronine* (T_3). When the thyroid gland secretes too much of these hormones, a condition known as *hyperthyroidism* may result. In such a case, the body metabolizes its food too quickly, and weight is lost. When too little thyroxine and T$_3$ are secreted, the condition called *hypothyroidism* may occur. In this case, the body metabolizes food too slowly and the patient tends to become sluggish and accumulate fat.

BASAL METABOLISM RATE

Energy is needed for maintenance of body tissue and temperature, for growth and for physical and mental activity. The rate at which energy is needed just for body maintenance is called the *basal metabolism rate* (BMR). Medical tests can determine a person's BMR. When a BMR test is given, the body is at rest and performing only necessary involuntary functions. Respiration, circulation, cell activity and maintenance of body temperature are examples of these functions. Voluntary activity is not measured in a BMR test.

DETERMINING ENERGY NEEDS

The unit used to measure the fuel value of food is the *calorie* (sometimes called the kilocalorie or Kcal), or in the metric system, the *joule*. One calorie is equal to 4.184 joules, but this may be rounded off to 4.2 joules. A *calorie* is the amount of heat needed to raise the temperature of one kilogram of water one degree Celsius (°C).

The number of calories in a food is its *caloric value*. Caloric values of foods vary greatly. Values vary because foods contain varying amounts of nutrients. In addition, nutrients differ in the number of calories they contain. One gram of carbohydrate yields 4 calories or 17 joules; one gram of protein yields 4 calories or 17 joules; and one gram of fat yields 9 calories or 38 joules. The caloric or energy values of foods are scientifically determined by a device known as the *bomb calorimeter*. As a reference, the number of calories in average servings of common foods are listed in Table A-6 of the Appendix.

Calculating Caloric Requirements

A person's average daily *caloric requirement* is the number of calories needed by an individual in a twenty-four hour period. Caloric requirements are determined by one's age, size, sex and activity.

Children, in proportion to their weight, require more calories than adults because they are growing and are usually more active than adults. As people age, their basal metabolism rates decline and their physical activities are usually reduced. These reductions cause their caloric requirements to be lowered as well.

Tall people with large body frames require more calories than short people with small body frames. Larger people have more body mass to maintain and to move around than do smaller people. Men usually require more food than women. Activity, however, is the greatest single factor determining energy needs as can be seen in table 2-2.

The Food and Nutrition Board of the National Research Council has estimated average minimum caloric requirements of certain population groups as shown in table 2-3. Many people have caloric needs which are higher than the minimum requirements shown.

At times, it is necessary or desirable to obtain a more specific estimate of one's minimum caloric requirement than an average provides. The specific caloric requirement is obtained by first determining a person's basal metabolic rate (BMR). The BMR equals one calorie per kilogram of body weight, per hour. The BMR, plus 50 percent of that total, equals the person's minimum caloric requirement. To obtain the minimum caloric requirement:

(1) Change body weight from pounds to kilograms by dividing the body weight by 2.2 (2.2 pounds = 1 kilogram)

(2) Multiply the number of kilograms of body weight times 24 (hours per day).

(3) Multiple the answer in step 2 by .50 (50 percent).

(4) Add the answers in steps 2 and 3. The sum is the daily minimum caloric requirement.

TABLE 2-2

ENERGY EXPENDITURE IN DAILY ACTIVITIES

Activity Category*	Man, 70 kg			Woman, 58 kg	
	Time (hr)	Rate (kcal/ min)	Total [kcal (k J)]	Rate (kcal/min)	Total [kcal (k J)]
Sleeping, reclining	8	1.0-1.2	540(2270)	0.9-1.1	440(1850)
Very light	12	up to 2.5	1300(5460)	up to 2.0	900(3750)
Seated and standing activities, painting trades, auto and truck driving, laboratory work, typing, playing musical instruments, sewing, ironing					
Light	3	2.5-4.9	600(2520)	2.0-3.9	450(1890)
Walking on level 2.5-3 mph, tailoring, pressing, garage work, electrical trades, carpentry, restaurant trades, cannery workers, washing clothes, shopping with light load, golf, sailing, table tennis, volleyball					
Moderate	1	5.0-7.4	300(1260)	4.0-5.9	240(1010)
Walking 3.5-4 mph, plastering, weeding and hoeing, loading and stacking bales, scrubbing floors, shopping with heavy load, cycling, skiing, tennis, dancing					
Heavy	0	7.5-12.0		6.0-10.0	
Walking with load uphill, tree felling, work with pick and shovel, basketball, swimming, climbing, football					
Total	24		2740(11,500)		2030(8,530)

Source: Food and Nutrition Board, National Academy of Sciences, National Research Council.

* Data from Durnin and Passmore, 1967.

TABLE 2-3. Average Minimum Caloric Requirements Per Day

	Age (years)	Weight (kg)	Weight (lbs)	Height (cm)	Height (in)	Energy (kcal)*
Infants	0.0-0.5	6	14	60	24	kg x 117
	0.5-1.0	9	20	71	28	kg x 108
Children	1-3	13	28	86	34	1,300
	4-6	20	44	110	44	1,800
	7-10	30	66	135	54	2,400
Males	11-14	44	97	158	63	2,800
	15-18	61	134	172	69	3,000
	19-22	67	147	172	69	3,000
	23-50	70	154	172	69	2,700
	51+	70	154	172	69	2,400
Females	11-14	44	97	155	62	2,400
	15-18	54	119	162	65	2,100
	19-22	58	128	162	65	2,100
	23-50	58	128	162	65	2,000
	51+	58	128	162	65	1,800
Pregnant						+300
Lactating						+500

Source: Food and Nutrition Board, National Academy of Sciences, National Research Council.

*Kilojoules (kJ) = 4.2 x kcal.

For example, assume a woman weighs 110 pounds.

1) One kilogram equals 2.2 pounds. Therefore, 110 pounds must be divided by 2.2. The woman weighs 50 kilograms.

2) Multiply the 50 kilograms by 24 hours. This gives a total of 1200 calories, the estimated basal metabolism rate.

3) Multiply the 1200 calories by .50 (50 percent). The total is 600 calories.

4) Add 1200 calories plus 600 calories for a minimum daily caloric requirement of 1800 calories.

A person who takes in fewer calories than he or she burns usually becomes thinner. If a person takes in more calories than he or she burns, the body stores them as *adipose tissue* (fat). Some adipose tissue is necessary to protect the body and support its organs. Adipose tissue also helps to regulate body temperature, just as insulation helps regulate the temperature of a building. An excess of adipose tissue, however, leads to obesity which can endanger health.

SUMMARY

The body is comparable to an automobile engine because each requires fuel. Food acts as fuel and must be prepared by the body itself through a series of processes: digestion, absorption, and metabolism. Digestion is the process whereby food is broken down into smaller parts, chemically changed, and moved along the gastrointestinal tract. Mechanical digestion refers to that part of the process performed by the teeth and muscles of the digestive system. Chemical digestion refers to that part of the process wherein food is broken down to nutrients which the blood can absorb. Chemical changes are performed mainly by enzymes. Following digestion, food is absorbed by the blood, primarily in the small intestine and then carried to all body tissues. After absorption, food is metabolized. During metabolism, food is combined with oxygen in a process called oxidation. Energy released during oxidation is measured by the calorie or joule. Caloric values of foods vary as well as people's caloric (energy) requirements. Requirements vary according to a person's age, size, sex, and activity.

DISCUSSION TOPICS

1. Describe the process of digestion.

2. Of what value are enzymes to digestion? Name 5 enzymes and the nutrients on which they act.

3. Describe absorption of nutrients.

4. Of what value is indigestible residue in the diet? What are some examples of foods that provide it?

5. Describe metabolism.

6. What is the BMR? If anyone in the class has undergone a BMR test, ask her or him to describe it.

7. Explain why the body requires food even during sleep.

8. Why is it incorrect to say: "He ate 2000 calories today"? What did he eat? What are calories? What are joules? How are they comparable?

9. Explain the differences between the terms, *caloric value* and *caloric requirement*.

10. What does it mean to be overweight? What is the most common cause of overweight? What reasons do people give for being overweight? How can one prevent excessive weight gain? How can overweight people reduce? How may overweight endanger health?

SUGGESTED ACTIVITIES

a. Trace figure 2-1. On the traced figure, insert the names of the body structures without referring back to the original illustration.

b. Using the method of calculating a person's minimum caloric requirement as given in this chapter, calculate your minimum caloric requirement. Convert it to joules.

c. Using table 2-3, and table A-6 (in the Appendix) plan a menu for one day which would satisfy the caloric requirement of a 40-year-old woman who weighs 128 pounds.

d. Adapt the preceding menu to the needs of a 22-year-old man who weighs 147 pounds.

e. Using table 2-3, and A-6 (in the Appendix), compile a list of foods, especially vegetables, fruits, milk, eggs and meat, which would satisfy the caloric requirement of a woman who is nursing her baby. She is 30 years old and weighs 128 pounds. Compute the grams of protein included.

f. Adapt the preceding menu to the needs of the woman after weaning her baby.

WORD STUDY

absorption	caloric	chemical
adipose tissue	requirement	digestion
amylase	caloric value	chyme
anabolism	calorie	digestion
basal metabolism	calorimeter	duodenum
rate (BMR)	capillary	emulsified fats
bile	catabolism	endocrine glands

enzyme	joule	peptidases
esophagus	lactase	peristalsis
feces	lacteals	protease
food residue	maltase	ptyalin
fundus (of stomach)	mechanical digestion	pylorus
gastric juices	metabolism	rennin
gastric lipase	obesity	saliva
gastrointestinal system	oxidation	salivary amylase
hormone	pancreas	sucrase
hydrochloric acid	pancreatic amylase	thyroid gland
hydrolysis	pancreatic lipase	thyroxine
hyperthyroidism	pancreatic protease	triiodothyronine (T_3)
hypothyroidism	pepsin	villi

REVIEW

A.   Complete the following statements.

1. Food is broken down for body use during the process known as _____ _____ .

2. Food is combined with oxygen during the process called _____ _____ .

3. The tube connecting the mouth and stomach is the _____ _____ .

4. The two kinds of digestive action are _____ and _____ .

5. The rhythmic contraction of the muscular walls of the digestive tract is called _____ .

6. Proteases, lipases, and amylases are examples of _____ _____ .

7. Saliva contains the digestive enzyme called _____ .

8. Hydrochloric acid, pepsin, and rennin are all secretions of the _____ _____ .

9. The semiliquid mass of food which has been mixed with gastric juices is called _____ .

10. The passage of nutrients into the body fluids and tissues is called _____ .

11. Metabolism is primarily governed by the secretions of the_____ _____ .

12. The unit used to measure the fuel value of food is the _____ _____ or the _____ .

13. The average daily total of calories needed by an individual is called the _____ .

14. A condition of extreme overweight is called _____ .

15. The rate at which energy is needed just for body maintenance is called the _____ .

B.   Label the structures on the following diagram.

C.   In the space opposite each enzyme or secretion, name the structure which *secretes* it.

1. ptyalin   _____ .

2. hydrochloric acid _____ .

3. pepsin   _____ .

4. rennin   _____ .

5. trypsin   _____ .

6. steapsin   _____ .

7. lactase   _____ .

8. maltase   _____ .

9. peptidases   _____ .

10. bile   _____ .

D.   Briefly answer the following questions.

1. Name the four steps in computing an individual's minimum caloric requirements.

2. Where does the major absorption of nutrients take place?

3. How does an enzyme get its name?

Chapter 3
Carbohydrates and Fats

OBJECTIVES

After studying this chapter, the student should be able to:

- Name six sources of carbohydrates and six sources of fat.
- Identify the way carbohydrates and fats are classified.
- Identify the number of calories provided per gram of carbohydrate or fat.
- Identify the steps in digestion, absorption and metabolism of carbohydrates and fats.

Energy foods are those which can be rapidly oxidized by the body to release heat and energy. In this chapter, the two major sources of energy (carbohydrates and fats) will be discussed.

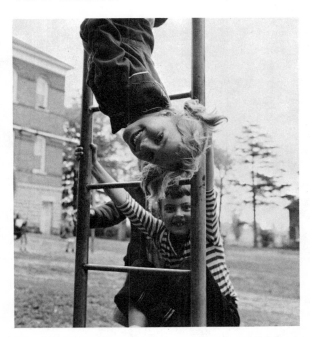

Fig. 3-1 Vigorous play is important for children to develop strong muscles and good coordination. They must be supplied with sufficient carbohydrates and fats in their diets to provide adequate energy. *(Courtesy of the National Education Association)*

CARBOHYDRATES

Carbohydrates are the least expensive and most abundant of the energy nutrients. Foods rich in carbohydrates grow easily in most climates. They keep well and are generally easy to digest. Carbohydrates provide the major source of calories for people all over the world. They provide approximately half the calories for people living in the United States. Carbohydrates are named for the chemical elements of which they are composed: carbon, hydrogen and oxygen.

Functions

Providing energy and heat is the major function of carbohydrates. Each gram of carbohydrate provides 4 calories (17 joules). This is the same number of calories provided by proteins. However, protein metabolism is not as complete as carbohydrate metabolism; this makes carbohydrate a more efficient energy nutrient. When carbohydrates provide energy, they spare proteins for another essential use: building and repairing body tissues. This function is known as the *protein sparing action* of carbohydrates. Carbohydrates are also essential for the metabolism of fats.

Food Sources

The principal sources of carbohydrates are plants. Examples of foods rich in carbohydrates are bread, cereals, crackers, macaroni products, rice, potatoes, corn, peas, beans, bananas, apples, pears, sweet desserts, sugars, syrups, honey, and candy.

Classification

Carbohydrates may be divided into three groups: monosaccharides, disaccharides, and polysaccharides. *Monosaccharides* (also known as simple or single sugars) are the simplest form of carbohydrates. They are sweet, require no digestion and can be absorbed directly into the bloodstream from the

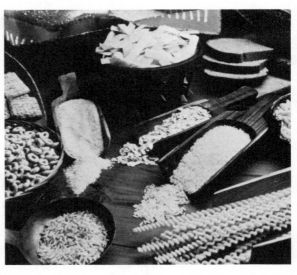

Fig. 3-2 Good sources of carbohydrates. *(Courtesy Tupperware)*

TABLE 3-1   Carbohydrates

BEST SOURCES	FUNCTIONS	DEFICIENCY SYMPTOMS

Sugars (monosaccharides and disaccharides)
  sugars
  candy, syrups
  jams and jellies
  honey
  molasses
  cakes and cookies
	Furnish heat and energy
	Aid in metabolism of fats
		Loss of weight

Starch (polysaccharides)
  flour
  macaroni products
  bread
  crackers
  cereals
  potatoes
  corn
  lima beans
  green peas
  bananas, pears, apples
	Furnish heat and energy
	Aid in metabolism of fats
	
	The fruits and vegetables also provide bulk and some vitamins and minerals
		Loss of weight

Cellulose (polysaccharide)
  bran, whole grain cereals
  green and leafy vegetables
  fruits, especially
    apples, pears, oranges
    grapefruit
	Provides bulk necessary for peristalsis	Possible constipation

small intestine. The simple sugars, *glucose, fructose,* and *galactose* are monosaccharides. *Glucose,* also called dextrose, is the form of carbohydrate to which all other forms are converted for eventual metabolism. *Fructose,* also called levulose and fruit sugar, is found with glucose in many fruits and vegetables and in honey. It tastes especially sweet. *Galactose* is a product of the digestion of milk. It is not found naturally.

Disaccharides are sometimes called double sugars. They are sweet and must be changed to simple sugars before they can be absorbed. Disaccharides include the sugars, *sucrose, maltose,* and *lactose. Sucrose* is the form of carbohydrate present in granulated, powdered, and brown sugar and in molasses. It is one of the sweetest and least expensive sugars. Its sources are sugar cane, sugar beets, and the sap from maple trees. *Maltose* is an intermediate product in the digestion of starch within the body. It is manufactured from starch by enzyme action and is not found naturally. *Lactose* is the sugar found in milk. It is distinct from most other sugars because it is not found in plants. Lactose is less sweet than the other single or double sugars. For this reason, it is sometimes added to beverages in order to increase their caloric value while not greatly changing the flavor.

Polysaccharides are complex compounds that are not sweet. Their solubility and digestibility vary.

Starch is a polysaccharide found in grains and vegetables. Vegetables contain less starch than grains because vegetables have a higher moisture content. The starch in grain is found mainly in the *endosperm* (center part of the grain). This is the part from which white flour is made. The tough outer covering of grain kernels is called the *bran*, figure 3-3. The bran is used in coarse cereals and whole wheat flour. Although the *germ* is the smallest part of the cereal grain, it is the life center.

Wheat germ is included in products made of whole wheat. It may also be purchased and used in baked products or as an addition to breakfast cereals. Wheat germ is a rich source of vitamin B complex, vitamin E, minerals, and protein.

Before the starch in grain can be used for food, the bran must be broken down. The heat and moisture of cooking break this outer covering, making the food more flavorful and more digestible. Although bran itself is indigestible, it is important that some be included in the diet because of the fiber it provides.

Glycogen is sometimes called animal starch because animals store carbohydrates in the form of glycogen. Glucose is converted

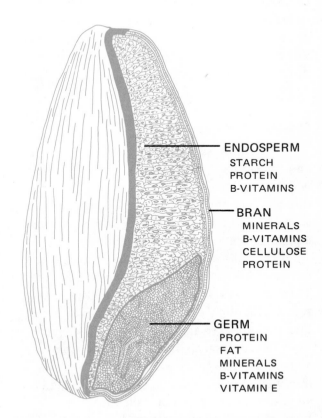

ENDOSPERM
STARCH
PROTEIN
B-VITAMINS

BRAN
MINERALS
B-VITAMINS
CELLULOSE
PROTEIN

GERM
PROTEIN
FAT
MINERALS
B-VITAMINS
VITAMIN E

Fig. 3-3 A grain of wheat has three parts. All parts are used in whole wheat flour; only the endosperm is used in white flour.

to glycogen for storage. Glycogen is converted back to glucose when the body requires fuel for heat and energy.

Cellulose, also called roughage, is a fibrous form of carbohydrate which makes up the framework of plants. Cellulose has no energy value and is insoluble and indigestible. Its function is to provide bulk for the intestines. Cellulose aids in carrying food along the digestive tract by providing the fiber necessary for normal peristalsis. This action helps to prevent constipation. Studies have indicated that the average person needs approximately four to seven grams of cellulose each day.

The major sources of cellulose are bran, whole grain cereals and fibrous fruits and vegetables. These foods leave a high residue of cellulose after digestion. Highly processed or refined foods such as white bread, macaroni products and pastries leave little or no residue because cellulose has been removed during processing.

Digestion and Absorption

The monosaccharides, *glucose, fructose,* and *galactose,* are single or simple sugars which may be absorbed from the intestine directly into the bloodstream. They are subsequently carried to the liver where fructose and galactose are changed to glucose.

The disaccharides, *sucrose, maltose* and *lactose* require an additional step of digestion. They must first be converted to the simple sugar, glucose, before they can be absorbed into the bloodstream.

The polysaccharides are more complex and their digestibility varies. After the cellulose wall is broken down, starch is changed to an intermediate product called *dextrin;* it is then changed to maltose and finally to glucose. Cooking can change starch to dextrin. For example, when bread is toasted, it turns golden brown and tastes sweeter because the starch has been changed to dextrin.

The digestion of starch begins in the mouth where the enzyme ptyalin begins to change starch to dextrin. The second step occurs in the stomach where the food is mixed with gastric juices. The final step occurs in the small intestine where the digestible carbohydrates are changed to simple sugars and subsequently absorbed by the blood.

Metabolism and Elimination

All carbohydrates are changed to the simple sugar glucose before metabolism can take place. After the blood has carried the glucose to the cells, it can be oxidized. Frequently, the volume of glucose which reaches the cells exceeds the amount the cells can use. In these cases, glucose is converted to glycogen to be stored in the liver and muscles. Glycogen is broken down and released as glucose is needed for energy or heat. This process is controlled mainly by the insulin secreted by the islets of Langerhans in the pancreas. When the secretion of insulin is impaired or absent, as in diabetes, insulin must be supplied to the patient. In such a case, the diabetic patient's intake of carbohydrates must be carefully controlled to balance the prescribed dosage of insulin.

Oxidation of glucose results in energy and its by-product, heat. With the exception of cellulose, the only waste products of carbohydate metabolism are carbon dioxide and water. It is a very efficient nutrient.

Dietary Requirements

While there is no specific daily dietary requirement for carbohydrate, the Food and Nutrition Board of the National Research Council recommends that people have 50 to 100 grams of digestible carbohydrate each day. Because overweight is a major health problem in the United States, it should be noted that eating an excess of carbohydrates is one of the most common causes of obesity. Although some of the surplus carbohydrate is changed to glycogen, the major part of any surplus becomes adipose tissue. Also, an excess of carbohydrate in the form of sugar can spoil an appetite for other nutrients which are more important. Too many carbohydrates may cause tooth decay, and may irritate the lining of the stomach causing flatus. A deficiency of carbohydrate usually results in loss of weight and possible metabolic problems.

FATS

Fats furnish the most concentrated form of energy. Each gram of fat provides 9 calories or 38 joules. Most foods high in fat are more expensive than those high in carbohydrates. Fats provide approximately 40 percent of the calories for people in the United States. Like carbohydrates, fats are composed of carbon, hydrogen, and oxygen, but in different proportions. Fats are sometimes called *lipids*, a term which is used for oily substances which are not soluble in water.

Functions

In addition to providing energy and heat, fats are important in the function and structure of body tissues. Some fats act as carriers of essential fatty acids and vitamins. Fats give a feeling of *satiety* (satisfaction) after meals. The satisfaction that fats provide is due partly to the flavor they give other foods and partly to their slow rate of digestion which prevents hunger.

Food Sources

Fats are present in both plants and animals. Examples of foods rich in fat are butter, margarine, cooking oils, mayonnaise, cream, rich pastries, fatty meats and egg yolk.

TABLE 3-2 Fats

BEST SOURCES	FUNCTIONS	DEFICIENCY SYMPTOMS
Butter	Furnish heat and energy	Loss of weight
Lard or lard substitutes	Carry fat-soluble vitamins	Retarded growth
Margarine	Supply essential	Abnormal skin
Meat fats	fatty acids	
Bacon	Give satiety to meals	
Oils		
Nuts		
Cheese		
Cream		
Egg yolk		

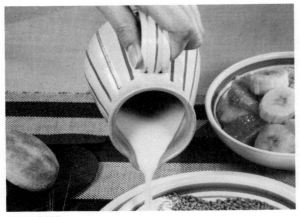

A. CREAM

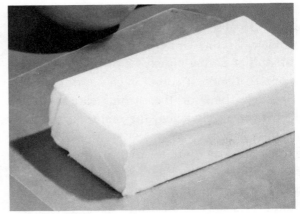

B. MARGARINE

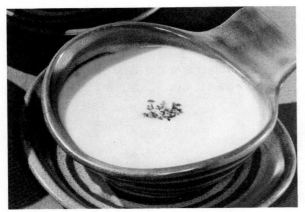

C. CREAMED SOUP

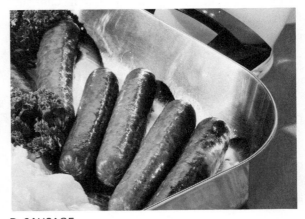

D. SAUSAGE

Fig. 3-4 A fat may be hidden in other foods or used as a food itself.

Classification

Fats may be classified as visible fats and invisible fats. The *visible fats* are the foods which are purchased and used as fats such as butter, margarine, and cooking oils. *Invisible fats* (hidden fats) are those found in meats, milk, cheese, eggs, and pastries. Fats are further classified as saturated, monounsaturated, or polyunsaturated, according to their chemical composition. Fats are composed of fatty acids which can be divided into these three groups.

When a fat is *saturated*, each carbon atom in the fatty acid carries all the hydrogen atoms possible. Examples of saturated fats are the fats in meat, eggs, whole milk and whole milk cheeses, cream, ice cream, butter, hydrogenated fats, and chocolate.

If a fat is *monounsaturated,* there is one place among its carbon atoms where there are fewer hydrogen atoms attached than in saturated fats. Examples of monounsaturated fats are olive oil, avocados, and cashew nuts.

If a fat is *polyunsaturated*, there are two or more places among its carbon atoms where there are fewer hydrogen atoms attached than in saturated fats. Examples of polyunsaturated fats include vegetable oils, margarines containing liquid vegetable oils, mayonnaise, fish, and peanuts.

Saturated fats are usually solid at room temperature.   Polyunsaturated   fats   are

TABLE 3-3 Types of Fat in Common Foods

High in Saturated Fats	High in Polyunsaturated Fats	High in Monounsaturated Fats
Meat—beef, veal*, lamb, pork, and their products, such as cold cuts, sausages	Liquid vegetable oils corn, cottonseed, safflower, soybean	Olive oil
Eggs	Margarines containing	Olives
Whole milk	substantial amounts of the above oils	Avocados
Whole milk cheese	in liquid form	Cashew nuts
Cream, sweet and sour	Fish	
Ice cream	Mayonnaise, salad dressing	
Butter and some margarines	Nuts—walnuts, filberts, pecans, almonds,	
Lard	peanuts	
Hydrogenated shortenings	Peanut butter	
Chocolate	Products made from or with the above	
Coconut and coconut oil		
Products made from or with the above		

Source: Bureau of Nutrition, Dept. of Health, City of New York
*Lean veal is low in total fat

usually soft or oily. Manufacturers add hydrogen to the oily vegetable fats to make them solid. This process, called *hydrogenation*, turns vegetable oils into saturated fats. Margarine is made from the inexpensive vegetable oils in this way. The margarine is churned with milk to enhance its flavor. Vitamin A, and sometimes vitamin D, is added to make it nutritionally equal to butter. When it has been enriched with these vitamins, it is called *fortified* margarine.

A fatty substance called *cholesterol* exists in saturated fats and in body cells. A certain amount of cholesterol is essential for health, and the body manufactures (synthesizes) it from food. There is some evidence, however, that an excess of saturated fats in the diet raises the blood cholesterol level which, in turn, increases the probability of heart disease. For this reason, it may be advisable to use foods containing the polyunsaturated fats as much as possible, rather than those containing saturated fats.

Digestion and Absorption

The chemical digestion of fats occurs mainly in the small intestine. Fats are not digested in the mouth. They are digested only slightly in the stomach where gastric lipase acts on emulsified fats such as those found in cream and egg yolk. Fats must be mixed well with the gastric juices before entering the small intestine. In the small intestine, bile emulsifies the fats and the enzyme steapsin (pancreatic lipase) reduces them to fatty acids and glycerol, which the body subsequently absorbs. Ninety-five percent of the fats eaten are digested. However, the digestion of fats is very complex. Usually soft fats, or fats that melt at low temperatures, are easier to digest than the hard fats in meats.

Fats are insoluble in water, which is the main component of blood. Because of this, special carriers must be provided in order for the fats to be absorbed and transported by the blood to body cells. In the initial stages of absorption, bile joins with the products of fat digestion to carry fat. Later, protein combines with the final products of fat digestion to form special carriers called *lipoproteins*. The lipoproteins subsequently carry the fats to the body cells by way of the blood.

Metabolism and Elimination

Fats are carried by way of lipoproteins to body cells where metabolism occurs. Fatty acids are broken down to carbon dioxide and water, releasing energy. The portion of fat which is not needed for immediate use is stored as adipose tissue. Carbon dioxide and water are waste products which are removed from the body by the circulatory, respiratory and excretory systems.

Dietary Requirements

Although there is no specific daily dietary requirement for fats, the American Heart Association suggests that people limit their fat intake. They suggest that no more than 35 percent of the total calories should come from fats.

Certainly an excess of fat should be avoided in the diet. Each gram of fat yields more than twice the energy of one gram of carbohydrate or protein, and therefore, an excess can easily cause overweight.

SUMMARY

Energy foods are those which can be rapidly oxidized to release energy and heat. The two major sources of energy are carbohydrates and fats. They are both composed of carbon, hydrogen, and oxygen, but in different amounts. One gram of carbohydrate provides 4 calories (17 joules) and one gram of fat provides 9 calories (38 joules). Carbohydrates are less expensive and more abundant than fats.

The principal sources of carbohydrates are plant products such as sugars, breads, cereals, pasta, rice, potatoes and bananas. In addition to providing energy, carbohydrates are essential for fat metabolism. Digestion of carbohydrates begins in the mouth, continues in the stomach and is completed in the small intestine.

Fats are found in both plants and animals. Specific sources include butter, margarine, cooking oils, mayonnaise, cream and fatty meats. Besides providing energy, fats are important in the function and structure of body tissues. Some fats are carriers of fatty acids and vitamins; they also give satiety to meals. Digestion of fats occurs mainly in the small intestine, where they are reduced to fatty acids and glycerol. Eating an excess of either fats or carbohydrates can result in obesity.

DISCUSSION TOPICS

1. What are the three basic groups of carbohydrates?
   Name several foods for each group.

2. Discuss the effects of regularly eating an excess of carbohydrates.

3. Which polysaccharides (starches) might be considered a dietary staple for the following nationalities?

   - Italian
   - Mexican
   - Chinese
   - American Indian
   - French

4. Why should people eat roughage? Name three food sources of roughage.

5. Describe the digestion and metabolism of carbohydrates.

6. Of what value are fats to the body? What are some good food sources of fats.

7. Classify each of the following fats, indicating if they are saturated, monounsaturated, or polyunsaturated. Are they visible or invisible?

   - lard
   - vegetable shortening
   - vegetable oil
   - butter
   - margarine
   - chocolate

8. Describe the digestion and metabolism of fats.

9. Compare the energy yields of carbohydrates and fats. Why does a fat provide a more concentrated form of energy?

10. Which of the two energy nutrients studied in this chapter is generally more expensive to supply through food items? Give reasons why you believe this is true.

SUGGESTED ACTIVITIES

a. Hold a soda cracker in your mouth until you notice the change in flavor as the starch changes to dextrin.

b. Toast a slice of bread and describe the change in appearance and flavor that occurred in the carbohydrate.

c. Make a chart of the six sugars and their sources discussed in this chapter. Indicate whether they are single or double sugars.

d. Using hospital sources, find out how glucose may be given to patients too weak to take food. Under what circumstances may glucose or sugar foods be given? In what emergencies must the diabetic patient be given sugar?

e. Visit a grocery store. Compare the costs of six foods that are good sources of carbohydrates with six foods that are good sources of fats.

f. Make a list of the foods you have eaten in the past 24 hours. Circle the carbohydrate-rich foods and underline the fats. Approximately what percentage of your calories were in the form of carbohydrate? In the form of fats? Could your diet be improved? If so, how?

g. Trace figure 2-1 in chapter 2. Use it to explain the digestion of carbohydrates, using words and arrows.

h. Trace figure 2-1 in chapter 2. Use it to explain the digestion of fats, using both words and arrows.

i. Role play a situation between a diet counselor and a teenage girl who has placed herself on an extreme low calorie diet. She refuses to eat anything that she believes contains fat and will take very little carbohydrate. Explain to her the functions of carbohydrates and fat in the human body.

j. Make a list of foods which contain large amounts of saturated fats. Beside each food listed, write the name of another food which could be used as a substitute, but which contains largely polyunsaturated fats.

WORD STUDY

bran	germ	monounsaturated fats
carbohydrate	glucose	pancreas
cellulose	glycogen	polysaccharide
cholesterol	hydrogenation	polyunsaturated fats
dextrin	insulin	refined foods
diabetes	invisible fats	residue
disaccharide	islets of Langerhans	roughage
endosperm	lactose	satiety
fats	lipid	saturated fats
fortified margarine	lipoproteins	sucrose
fructose	maltose	synthesis
galactose	monosaccharide	visible fats

REVIEW

A.   Multiple choice. Select the *letter* which precedes the best answer.

1. The three main groups of carbohydrates are
    a. fats, proteins, and minerals
    b. glucose, fructose, and galactose
    c. monosaccharides, disaccharides, and polysaccharides
    d. sucrose, cellulose, and glycogen

2. Galactose is a product of the digestion of
    a. milk
    b. meat
    c. breads
    d. vegetables

3. A simple sugar to which all forms of carbohydrates are ultimately converted is
    a. sucrose
    b. glucose
    c. galactose
    d. maltose

4. Wheat germ is a source of vitamins
    a. B complex and D
    b. B complex and C
    c. B complex and E
    d. none of these

5. A fibrous form of carbohydrate which cannot be digested is
    a. glucose
    b. glycogen
    c. cellulose
    d. fat

6. Glycogen is stored in the
    a. heart and lungs
    b. liver and muscles
    c. pancreas and gallbladder
    d. small and large intestines

7. Fats may be classified as
    a. visible and invisible
    b. saturated, monounsaturated, and polyunsaturated
    c. neither of the above
    d. both a and b

8. Fats are sometimes called
    a. lipids   c. lactose
    b. lipoproteins   d. lacteals

9. Two foods which contain large amounts of saturated fats are
    a. lamb and ice cream   c. mayonnaise and peanut butter
    b. margarine and jam   d. chocolate and fish

10. The digestion of fats occurs mainly in the
    a. small intestine   c. stomach
    b. large intestine   d. mouth

B. Match the term listed in column II with its definition in column I.

Column I

_____ 1. least expensive energy nutrient
_____ 2. adipose tissue
_____ 3. carbohydrate as stored in the liver
_____ 4. disaccharide
_____ 5. center part of grain
_____ 6. outer covering of grain
_____ 7. number of calories per gram of
            carbohydrate
_____ 8. number of calories per gram of fat
_____ 9. fats that are solid at room temperature
_____ 10. fats that are liquid or soft at room
            temperature

Column II

a. body fat
b. endosperm
c. carbohydrate
d. four
e. six
f. nine
g. glucose
h. saturated
i. bran
j. glycogen
k. polyunsaturated
l. sucrose

Chapter 4
Proteins

OBJECTIVES
After studying this chapter, the student should be able to:
- State the function of protein in the body.
- Identify the elements of which proteins are composed.
- Describe the effects of protein deficiency.
- State the energy yield of proteins.
- Identify at least six food sources of complete proteins and six food sources of incomplete proteins.

Body cells are constantly wearing out; as a result, they are continuously in need of replacement. Protein is the basic material of every body cell. It is the only nutrient that can make new cells and rebuild tissue. Therefore, an adequate amount of protein in the diet is essential for normal growth and development and for the maintenance of health. Protein is appropriately named: it is a word of Greek derivation, and means "of first importance."

PROTEINS
Like carbohydrates and fats, proteins contain carbon, hydrogen, and oxygen, but in different proportions. In addition, proteins contain nitrogen; and some contain sulfur, phosphorus, iron, and iodine as well. Each gram of protein provides 4 calories (17 joules).

Proteins coagulate (thicken) when heated or when acid is added to them. For example, when an egg is cooked, it becomes thick and firm. Meat which is cooked at too high a temperature becomes tough. When lemon juice is added to milk, the protein in the milk coagulates, and the milk appears curdled.

Functions
The primary function of protein is to build and repair body tissues. Proteins are important components of hormones and enzymes and as such they play major roles in the regulation of the body processes of digestion and metabolism. They can provide energy if and when the supply of carbohydrates and fats is insufficient.

TABLE 4-1. Amino Acids

Essential	Nonessential
Histidine*	Alanine
Isoleucine	Arginine
Leucine	Asparagine
Lysine	Aspartic acid
Methionine	Cysteine
Phenylalanine	Cystine
Threonine	Glutamic acid
Tryptophan	Glutamine
Valine	Glycine
	Hydroxyproline
	Proline
	Serine
	Tyrosine

*Histidine is only known to be essential for infants.

Classification

Proteins are composed of chemical compounds containing nitrogen which are known as *amino acids*. These amino acids are sometimes called the building blocks of proteins. Scientists have identified 22 amino acids but found only nine of them to be essential to humans, table 4-1. An essential amino acid is one which is absolutely necessary for normal growth and development. A nonessential amino acid can be produced by the body if an adequate supply of nitrogen is provided.

The quality of a protein depends on the number and types of amino acids it contains. Proteins containing all essential amino acids are *complete proteins*. A complete protein can build and repair tissue. The best sources of complete proteins are animal foods.

Incomplete proteins are those which lack one or more of the essential amino acids. Consequently, incomplete proteins cannot build tissue without the help of other proteins. The value of each is increased when it is eaten in combination with another incomplete protein at the same meal. This way one incomplete protein may provide the essential amino acids missing in the other. The combination may thereby provide all nine essential amino acids. Incomplete proteins are found in plant foods.

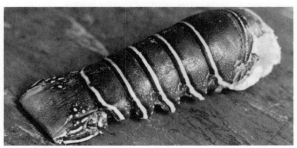

A. SHELLFISH

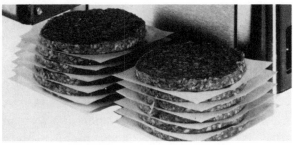

B. GROUND BEEF

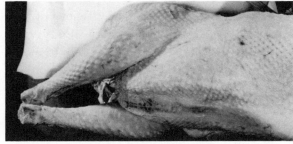

C. CHICKEN

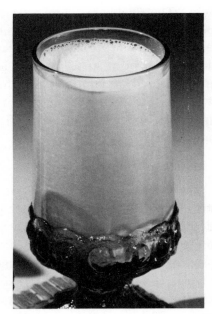

D. MILK

Fig. 4-1 Complete proteins are supplied by animal food sources.

Food Sources of Proteins

Proteins are found in both animal and plant foods. The animal food sources provide the highest quality, or complete proteins. They include meats, fish, poultry, eggs, milk and cheese.

Proteins found in plant foods are of a lower quality than those found in animal foods. Even so, plant foods are important sources of protein. Examples of plant foods containing protein are corn, grains, nuts, sunflower seeds, sesame seeds and legumes such as soybeans, navy beans, pinto beans, split peas, chick peas, and peanuts.

Plant proteins can be used to produce *textured protein* products, also called analogs. These products are made by extracting the protein from plants, (usually soybeans) and spinning it into fibers of nearly pure protein. The fibers are colored, flavored, and shaped into a product that resembles and tastes like meat. Textured protein can also be used as a filler in other foods, such as ground meat. Textured protein increases the protein content of the food to which it is added. It may be used as an economical meat replacement.

Digestion and Absorption

The mechanical digestion of protein begins in the mouth where the teeth grind the food into small pieces. Chemical digestion begins in the stomach. Hydrochloric acid prepares the stomach so the enzyme *pepsin* can begin its task of reducing proteins to polypeptides. In young children, the enzyme *rennin* coagulates milk in the stomach which prevents the milk from passing through the stomach too quickly. It is believed that adults do not produce rennin.

After the partially digested proteins (polypeptides) reach the small intestine, three pancreatic enzymes (trypsin, chymotrypsin and carboxypeptidase) continue chemical digestion. Two intestinal peptidases finally reduce the proteins to amino acids.

After digestion, the amino acids in the small intestine are absorbed by the blood and carried to all body tissues.

Metabolism and Elimination

The body needs varying compositions of the amino acids to build and repair the different tissues of the body. All essential amino acids must be present to build and repair the cells as needed. Surplus amino acids are sent back to the liver where they are dismantled by splitting off the nitrogen. The remaining parts are used for energy or stored as glycogen or adipose tissue. The end products of the metabolism of amino acids are carbon dioxide, water, and nitrogen. Some of the nitrogen is sent to the kidneys and excreted as urea; some nitrogen may be kept and used again to make simple amino acids as the body requires.

Dietary Requirements

A person's daily protein requirement depends on his size, age, and physical condition. A large person has more body cells to maintain than a small person. A growing child, a pregnant woman or a woman who is breastfeeding needs more protein per pound of body weight than an average adult. When digestion is inefficient, fewer amino acids are absorbed by the body, consequently raising the protein requirement. In addition extra protein is usually required after surgery and for patients with severe burns. The Food and Nutrition Board of the National Academy of Sciences has compiled a chart of recommended daily protein allowances for average groups of people, table 4-2.

TABLE 4-2. Daily Protein Requirement

	Age (years)	Weight (kg)	Weight (lbs)	Height (cm)	Height (in)	Protein (g)
Infants	0.0-0.5	6	14	60	24	kg x 2.2
	0.5-1.0	9	20	71	28	kg x 2.0
Children	1-3	13	28	86	34	23
	4-6	20	44	110	44	30
	7-10	30	66	135	54	36
Males	11-14	44	97	158	63	44
	15-18	61	134	172	69	54
	19-22	67	147	172	69	54
	23-50	70	154	172	69	56
	51+	70	154	172	69	56
Females	11-14	44	97	155	62	44
	15-18	54	119	162	65	48
	19-22	58	128	162	65	46
	23-50	58	128	162	65	46
	51+	58	128	162	65	46
Pregnant						+30
Lactating						+20

Source: Food and Nutrition Board, National Academy of Sciences. Washington D.C., 1974

Nutritional edema may occur when people are unable to obtain an adequate supply of protein. They may lose appetite, strength, and weight and wounds may heal very slowly. Patients suffering from nutritional edema become lethargic and depressed. *Edema* is the retention of fluids in body tissues, resulting in an extremely swollen appearance. Edema occurs because the body draws water into its cells as if to compensate for the lack of protein. This water is excreted when sufficient protein is eaten.

Children who lack sufficient protein do not grow to their potential size. Babies born to mothers eating insufficient protein during pregnancy may have permanently impaired mental capacities. There are two deficiency diseases caused by a grossly inadequate supply of protein which affect children. *Marasmus* afflicts very young children who lack protein and energy foods. The infant with marasmus appears emaciated, but does not have edema. His hair is dull and dry, and his skin is thin and

TABLE 4-3 Protein in an Average Diet for One Day

Food Group	Amt. in g.	Household Measure	Energy (kcal.)	Protein (g.)
Milk or equivalent	488	2 c. (1 pint)	320	17
Meat, fish, poultry, or egg	120	4 oz., cooked	376	30
Vegetables:				
Potato, cooked	100	1 medium	65	2
Deep green or				
yellow, cooked	75	1/2 c.	27	2
Other, raw or cooked	75	1/2 c.	45	2
Fruits:				
Citrus	100	1 serving	43	1
Other	100	1 serving	85	..
Bread, white enriched	100	4 slices	270	9
Cereal, whole grain	130	2/3 c. cooked or		
or enriched	30	1 oz. dry	89	3
Butter or margarine	14	1 Tbsp.	100	..
Totals			1420	66
Compare with recommended allowances				
Males (70 kg., 23-50 yrs. old)			2700	56
Females (58 kg., 23-50 yrs. old)			2000	46

Source: Mitchell, et al. *Nutrition in Health and Disease.* J. B. Lippincott Co., 1976

wrinkled, figure 4-2. The other protein deficiency disease which affects children is *kwashiorkor*. Kwashiorkor results in edema, painful skin lesions, and hair changes, figure 4-3.

SUMMARY

Protein is the only nutrient containing nitrogen, an element which is necessary for growth and the maintenance of health. In addition to building and repairing body tissues, proteins regulate body processes and can supply energy. Each gram of protein provides 4 calories (17 joules). Proteins are composed of amino acids, nine of which are essential for growth and repair of body tissues. Complete proteins contain all of the essential amino acids and can build tissues. The best sources of complete protein are animal foods such as

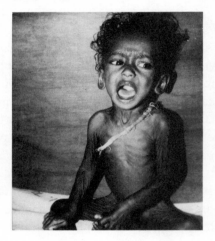

A. Visible signs of marasmus include extreme wasting, wrinkled skin and irritability.

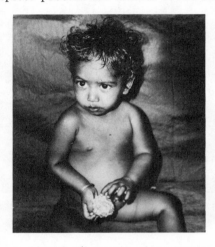

B. After 4 1/2 months of nutritional therapy, the same child shows great improvement.

Fig. 4-2 A child with marasmus may not recover completely, but is greatly helped by nutritional therapy. *(World Health Organization)*

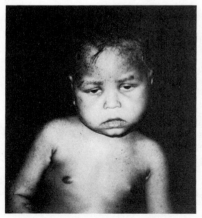

A. Edema, skin lesions and hair changes are common signs of kwashiorkor.

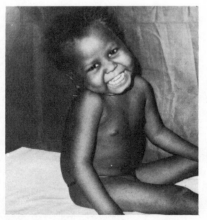

B. Only one month after receiving a proper diet, hunger, discomfort and visible signs of disease are greatly reduced.

Fig. 4-3 Effects of kwashiorkor can be partly eliminated by putting protein back into the diet. *(World Health Organization)*

meat, fish, poultry, eggs, milk, and cheese. Incomplete proteins do not contain all of the essential amino acids and cannot build tissues. The best sources of incomplete proteins are legumes, corn, grains, and nuts. The nutritional value of incomplete protein foods may be increased by eating two or more incomplete protein foods at the same meal. Chemical digestion of proteins occurs in the stomach and small intestine. Proteins are reduced to amino acids and ultimately absorbed into the blood through the small intestine.

A severe deficiency of protein in the diet may cause marasmus or kwashiorkor in children, and may result in impaired physical and mental development.

DISCUSSION TOPICS

1. Why are proteins especially important to children, pregnant women, and people who are ill?
2. What is the composition of proteins?
3. What functions do proteins perform in the body?
4. After having read chapters 3 and 4, discuss why it may be unwise to use protein foods as energy foods.
5. Discuss protein deficiency and the effects it may have on children and pregnant women.
6. Describe the digestion of proteins.
7. Describe the metabolism of proteins.
8. Tell what amino acids are and explain their importance. Tell where they are found.
9. Describe textured protein products. If anyone in class has eaten textured protein, ask her/him to describe the taste, color, appearance, and cost of the food.
10. Discuss why foods rich in complete proteins are usually more expensive than foods containing incomplete proteins.

SUGGESTED ACTIVITIES

a. Cook an egg at a low temperature and another at a high temperature. Observe, taste, and discuss the differences. Do the same with two portions of ground meat, being careful not to burn them. What characteristics of protein foods do these demonstrations indicate?
b. Keep a record of the foods you eat in a 24-hour period. Using table A-6 in the Appendix, compute the grams of protein consumed. Did your diet provide the recommended amount of protein as indicated in table 4-2 of this chapter?
c. Make a chart for display in the classroom showing complete and incomplete protein foods.
d. Add 1 teaspoon of lemon juice to 1/2 cup of milk. Observe, taste and discuss the result.

e. Plan a day's menu for yourself; include foods especially rich in complete proteins.
   1. Alter your planned menu; replace some of the complete protein foods with those containing incomplete proteins.
   2. Visit a local supermarket and compute the cost of the menu that contains complete proteins. Compute the cost of the menu that contains the incomplete proteins. Which is less expensive? Why?
   3. Adapt the planned menu to suit a 30-year-old pregnant woman, weighing 128 pounds.

WORK STUDY

amino acids	marasmus
coagulate	nitrogen
complete protein	nutritional edema
incomplete protein	proteins
kwashiorkor	textured protein

REVIEW

A.   Multiple Choice. Select the *letter* which precedes the best answer.

1. The building blocks of proteins are
    a. ascorbic acids
    b. amino acids
    c. nitrogen and sulphur only
    d. meat and fish

2. Proteins can
    a. provide energy and heat
    b. build body tissue
    c. repair body tissue
    d. perform all of these functions

3. Corn, peas, and beans
    a. are complete protein foods
    b. are incomplete protein foods
    c. contain no protein
    d. lose proteins during cooking

4. A person's daily protein requirement depends on
    a. age
    b. size
    c. physical condition
    d. all of these factors

5. Protein deficiency may result in
    a. beriberi   c. nutritional edema
    b. goiter   d. leukemia

6. Good sources of complete protein foods are
   a. eggs and ground beef
   b. breads and cereals
   c. butter and margarine
   d. legumes and nuts

7. One gram of protein provides
   a. 4 calories
   b. 9 calories
   c. 19 joules
   d. 37.8 joules

8. The chemical digestion of protein occurs in
   a. the mouth and stomach
   b. the mouth and small intestine
   c. the stomach and small intestine
   d. all of these

9. Complete proteins contain all the essential
   a. nutrients
   b. ascorbic acid
   c. amino acids
   d. calories and joules

10. The *primary* function of protein is to
    a. build and repair body cells
    b. provide heat and energy
    c. digest minerals and vitamins
    d. none of these

B. Arrange the following foods into two lists, one containing those that are the best sources of complete proteins and one containing those that are the best sources of incomplete proteins.

scrambled eggs
lima beans
corn on the cob
hot chocolate milk
chick peas and rice
skim milk
beefburgers
baked navy beans
filet of sole
fried chicken
peanuts
Swiss cheese

C. Match the term in column I with its definition in column II.

Column I	Column II
_____ 1. rennin	a. chemical element in an amino acid
_____ 2. amino acids	b. disease of severe protein deficiency
_____ 3. corn	c. reduces proteins to smaller substances in the stomach
_____ 4. pepsin	d. coagulates milk
_____ 5. roast beef	e. retention of body fluids
_____ 6. legumes	f. carbohydrate
_____ 7. kwashiorkor	g. 22 building blocks of protein
_____ 8. edema	h. lima beans
_____ 9. nitrogen	i. example of incomplete protein
_____ 10. textured protein	j. example of complete protein
	k. meat substitute

Chapter 5
Minerals

OBJECTIVES

After studying this chapter, the student should be able to:

- List at least two food sources of given mineral elements.
- List one or more functions of given mineral elements.
- Describe the recommended method of avoiding mineral deficiencies.

Chemical analysis would show that the human body is made up of specific chemical elements. Four of these elements, oxygen, carbon, hydrogen and nitrogen, make up 96 percent of body weight, table 5-1. All the remaining elements, called *mineral elements* or just *minerals,* represent only four percent of body weight. Nevertheless, each of these minerals is essential in a specific amount for good health. A *mineral* is an *inorganic* (non-living) element which may help to build tissues, regulate body fluids or assist in various body functions. Minerals are found in all body tissues. They cannot provide energy by themselves, but in their role as body regulators, they contribute toward the production of energy within the body.

Minerals are found in water and in *natural* (unprocessed) foods, together with proteins, carbohydrates, fats, and vitamins. Minerals in the soil are absorbed by growing plants. Humans obtain minerals by eating plants grown in mineral-rich soil, or by eating animals which in turn have eaten plants. The specific mineral content of food is determined by burning the food and then chemically analyzing the remaining ash. Highly processed or refined foods such as sugar and white flour contain almost no minerals. Iron is added to some flour and baked

TABLE 5-1. Chemical Elements in the Human Body

Element	Percent	Element	Percent
Oxygen	65%	Sodium	.15%
Carbon	18%	Magnesium	.05%
Hydrogen	10%	Iron	.004%
Nitrogen	3%	Manganese	.0003%
Calcium	1.5-2.2%	Copper	.00015%
Phosphorus	.8-1.2%	Iodine	.00004%
Potassium	.35%	Cobalt	
Sulfur	.25%	Fluorine	minute traces
Chloride	.15%	Zinc	

products which are then labelled *enriched*. A balanced diet supplies all the minerals in amounts necessary to maintain health.

Minerals may be divided into two groups. One group contains the major or *macrominerals* which are required in large amounts, at least 100 milligrams per day. The second group contains the *microminerals* or trace elements. This group is so named because the minerals within it are required in very small amounts, no more than a few milligrams a day. Table 5-2 names the macrominerals and microminerals (trace elements).

Scientists lack exact information on some of the trace elements although they do know that trace elements are essential to good health. The study of these elements continues in order to learn their precise relationships to human nutrition.

The Food and Nutrition Board of the National Academy of Sciences–National Research Council has recommended daily dietary allowances for six minerals. According to the standards of this agency, there is sufficient information to set allowances for only six minerals, table 5-3.

TABLE 5-2. Macrominerals and Microminerals (Trace Elements)

Macrominerals	Microminerals (Trace Elements)
Calcium	Iron
Phosphorus	Copper
Magnesium	Iodine
Sodium	Manganese
Potassium	Zinc
Chloride	Fluorine
Sulfur	Cobalt
	Chromium
	Molybdenum
	Selenium

TABLE 5-3. Recommended Daily Mineral Needs

	Age (years)	Weight (kg)	Weight (lbs)	Height (cm)	Height (in)	Calcium (mg)	Phosphorus (mg)	Iodine (μg)	Iron (mg)	Magnesium (mg)	Zinc (mg)
Infants	0.0-0.5	6	14	60	24	360	240	35	10	60	3
	0.5-1.0	9	20	71	28	540	400	45	15	70	5
Children	1-3	13	28	86	34	800	800	60	15	150	10
	4-6	20	44	110	44	800	800	80	10	200	10
	7-10	30	66	135	54	800	800	110	10	250	10
Males	11-14	44	97	158	63	1,200	1,200	130	18	350	15
	15-18	61	134	172	69	1,200	1,200	150	18	400	15
	19-22	67	147	172	69	800	800	140	10	350	15
	23-50	70	154	172	69	800	800	130	10	350	15
	51+	70	154	172	69	800	800	110	10	350	15
Females	11-14	44	97	155	62	1,200	1,200	115	18	300	15
	15-18	54	119	162	65	1,200	1,200	115	18	300	15
	19-22	58	128	162	65	800	800	100	18	300	15
	23-50	58	128	162	65	800	800	100	18	300	15
	51+	58	128	162	65	800	800	80	10	300	15
Pregnant						1,200	1,200	125	18+	450	20
Lactating						1,200	1,200	150	18	450	25

Source: Food and Nutrition Board, National Academy of Sciences–National Research Council, 1974.

TABLE 5-4 Minerals

MINERALS	BEST SOURCES	FUNCTIONS	DEFICIENCY SYMPTOMS

Calcium	Milk
	Cheese
	Some dark green,
	    leafy vegetables
		Normal development and
		maintenance of bones and
		    teeth
		Clotting of the blood
		Nerve irritability
		Normal heart action
		Normal muscle activity
		Activates enzymes
			Retarded growth
			Poor tooth and bone
			    formation
			Rickets
			Slow clotting
			    time of blood
			Tetany

Phosphorus	Milk and cheese
	Egg yolk
	Meat
	Poultry
	Fish
	Whole grain cereals
	Legumes
	Nuts
		Normal development and
		    maintenance of bones
		    and teeth
		Cell activity
		Maintenance of normal
		    acid-base balance of
		    the blood
		Normal muscle activity
		Metabolism of carbohy-
		    drates and fats
			Retarded growth
			Poor tooth and bone
			    formation
			Rickets
			Weakness
			Anorexia
			Pain in bones
			(Symptoms are rare)

Sodium	Salt Meat Poultry Fish Eggs Milk	Fluid balance Acid-base balance Osmosis Regulates muscle and nerve irritability Glucose absorption	Nausea Exhaustion Muscle cramps
Potassium	Meat Poultry Whole grains Leafy vegetables Legumes Oranges Bananas Prunes	Osmosis Fluid balance Acid-base balance Regular heart rhythm Regulation of nerve impulse conduction Cell metabolism	Muscle weakness Apathy Abnormal heartbeat

Chloride	Salt
	Meat
	Milk
	Eggs
		Osmosis
		Fluid balance
		Acid-base balance
		Formation of hydrochloric
		    acid
			Very rare, but may occur
			    after prolonged vomiting
			Nausea
			Exhaustion

Magnesium	Meat
	Nuts
	Milk
	Seafood
	Cereal grains
	Fresh green vegetables
		Constituent of bones
		Necessary for healthy
		    muscles and nerves
		Metabolism
			Unusual heart action
			Mental, emotional and
			    muscle disorders

Sulfur	Protein Foods	For building hair, nails, and all body tissues	Unknown

(TABLE 5-4. Cont'd.)

MINERALS	BEST SOURCES	FUNCTIONS	DEFICIENCY SYMPTOMS
Iodine (trace)	Salt water fish Foods grown in soil bordering salt water Iodized salt	Formation of hormones in thyroid gland	Goiter
Iron (trace)	Liver and other organ meats Muscle meats Legumes Dried fruits Egg yolk Whole grain or enriched breads and cereals Dark green and leafy vegetables Potatoes	Essential for formation of hemoglobin of the red blood cells	Anemia characterized by weakness, dizziness, loss of weight and pallor
Copper (trace)	Liver Nuts Kidney Raisins Brains Cocoa Legumes	Essential for formation of hemoglobin of the red blood cells Component of enzymes	Anemia (see iron)
Manganese (trace)	Whole grains Legumes Nuts Tea	Component of enzymes Glucose utilization	Unknown
Zinc (trace)	Seafood Oysters Liver Meat Eggs Milk	Component of insulin and enzymes Wound healing	Thought to be dwarfism, hypogonadism, anemia
Cobalt (trace)	Supplied in Vitamin B_{12}	A component of vitamin B_{12}, necessary for formation of the red blood cells	Unknown
Fluorine (trace)	Fluoridated water	Increases resistance to tooth decay	Tooth decay

CALCIUM AND PHOSPHORUS

Calcium and phosphorus together are necessary for the formation of healthy bones and teeth. Calcium also helps to maintain normal clotting of the blood and the action of the heart, muscles, and nerves. Phosphorus is important in the metabolism of carbohydrates and fats. It is important in cell activities and for a proper acid-base balance of the blood.

The best sources of calcium are milk and milk products. Calcium is also found in some dark green leafy vegetables. Phosphorus is obtained from eating milk, cheese, egg yolk, meat, poultry, and fish.

Calcium and phosphorus deficiencies may result in rickets. *Rickets* is a disease which occurs in early childhood and results in poorly formed bone structure. It causes

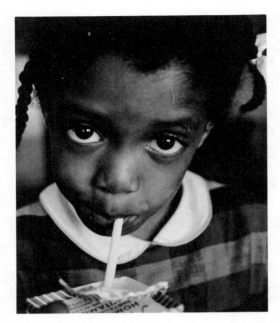

Fig. 5-1 Milk is an important source of calcium and phosphorus. These minerals are essential for the normal growth and development of bones and teeth. *(Courtesy of the National Education Association)*

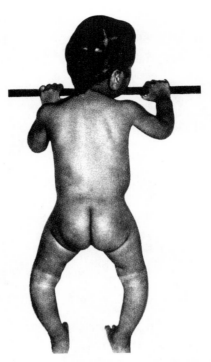

Fig. 5-2 One of the symptoms of rickets is bowed legs, a symptom appearing after the child has learned to walk. *(Courtesy of the Upjohn Co., and Dr. R. L. Nemir.)*

bowed legs and enlarged wrists or ankles. Severe cases can result in stunted growth. Insufficient calcium in the blood may cause a condition characterized by involuntary muscle movement, *tetany.*

Except during adolescence, pregnancy, and lactation, the recommended allowance for calcium and phosphorus for both sexes from the age of one year is 800 milligrams. During adolescence, pregnancy or lactation, calcium and phosphorus requirements are higher. Milk and cheese provide large quantities of calcium in small servings. For example, one cup of milk provides 300 milligrams of calcium; one ounce of cheddar cheese provides 250 milligrams of calcium. Phosphorus is widely distributed in foods and therefore a deficiency is rare.

SODIUM, POTASSIUM AND CHLORIDE

Sodium, potassium, and chloride are essential for normal *osmosis* (the entering and

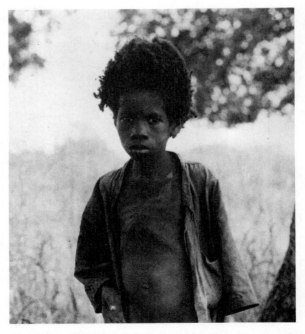

Fig. 5-3 Calcium deficiency can cause bone malformation as seen in this child's chest. *(World Health Organization)*

leaving of materials through the body cell walls). These minerals also help maintain the acid-base balance and the fluid balance of the body. Upsets in this balance may result in *dehydration* (loss of body fluid) or edema (abnormal accumulation of body fluids). Edema is frequently associated with *cardiovascular* (heart) and *nephritic* (kidney) conditions. In such cases sodium may be restricted in the diet because it contributes to edema.

The metabolism maintains a constant acid-base balance in the body. Cells function best in a neutral or slightly *alkaline* (base) medium. Sodium, potassium, and chloride are essential for maintaining this balance and deficiencies of these minerals can upset it. If too much acid is lost (which may happen during severe nausea), tetany due to *alkalosis* (too little acid) may develop. If the alkaline reserve is deficient due to starvation or faulty metabolism as in the case of diabetes, *acidosis* (too much acid) may develop.

MAGNESIUM

Magnesium is vital to both hard and soft body tissues and is essential for metabolism. Its deficiency can result in mental, emotional, and muscular disorders. An inadequate diet, an unusual loss of body fluids, or faulty metabolism may cause a magnesium deficiency.

Eating a balanced diet is the best method of avoiding magnesium deficiency. See table 5-3 for the recommended daily dietary allowances. The best sources of magnesium are meats, milk, cereals, green vegetables, and nuts.

SULFUR

Sulfur is necessary to all body tissues. It is a component of one of the amino acids and consequently is found in most protein foods. An adequate amount of protein in the diet insures an adequate supply of sulfur.

IRON AND COPPER

Iron and copper are both absolutely essential for healthy blood. Iron is a necessary part of *hemoglobin*, the coloring matter of red blood cells. Hemoglobin allows the red blood cells to combine with oxygen in the lungs and carry it to the body tissues. When red blood cells are worn out, the body collects the used iron and sends it to the *bone marrow* (the soft vascular tissue in the bone center) to be used in the manufacture of new red blood cells. Without copper, the body could not produce these cells.

Red meats (especially liver), egg yolks, dried fruits, whole grain cereals, and legumes are good sources of these minerals. Iron is also present to some extent in dark green leafy vegetables, enriched cereals, and potatoes.

Deficiencies in iron and copper can result in *nutritional anemia*. Anemia is the lack of an adequate number of red blood cells and/or hemoglobin. Because the bloodstream cannot carry enough oxygen to the cells, the anemic person suffers from dizziness and weakness, which are two symptoms of a lack of oxygen. The person loses weight and has a lowered resistance to disease.

The recommended daily requirements for iron is increased for adolescent girls and women of childbearing age in order to prevent deficiencies resulting from the effects of menstruation and pregnancy. Women should make a special effort to include iron-rich foods in their diets. Depending upon the individual, an iron supplement may be ordered by the physician.

IODINE

Iodine is necessary for the normal functioning of the thyroid gland. The thyroid gland determines the rate of metabolism. The best sources of iodine are seafood, plants grown in soil near the sea, and iodized salt. *Iodized salt* is common table salt which has

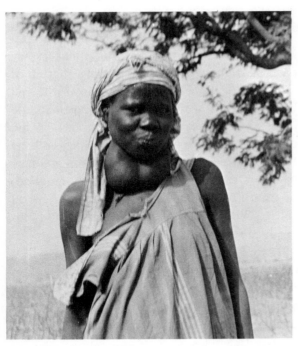

Fig. 5-4   In goiter, which results primarily from iodine deficiency, the thyroid gland enlarges. *(Courtesy of the Food and Agriculture Organization of the United Nations)*

had iodine added to it in an amount that, if used in normal cooking, provides sufficient iodine.

When the thyroid gland lacks sufficient iodine, it cannot function normally. This gland then grows larger than it should, forming a lump on the neck called a *goiter*, figure 5-4. If the lack of iodine is severe, it may retard the manufacture of thyroxine and T_3, the hormones secreted by the thyroid gland. This will lower the basal metabolism rate.

MANGANESE

Manganese is a constituent of several enzymes and is necessary for glucose utilization. It is found in nuts, whole grains, tea, and legumes. Effects of manganese deficiency are unknown.

ZINC

Zinc is a component of insulin and of several enzymes. It is found in seafood, liver, meat, eggs, and milk. Deficiency symptoms are thought to include dwarfism, hypogonadism and anemia.

COBALT

Cobalt is a component of vitamin B_{12}, which is necessary for the formation of red blood cells. A balanced diet usually provides an adequate amount of this mineral. Effects of its deficiency are unknown.

FLUORINE

Fluorine is a normal constituent of the bones and teeth. Its main function is to reduce tooth decay. Its principal source is water that contains fluorine. A deficiency of fluorine may result in tooth decay.

COOKING FOODS CONTAINING MINERALS

Most of the minerals in food occur as salts which are soluble in water. Therefore, the minerals leave the food and remain in the cooking water. Foods should be cooked in as little water as possible and the cooking liquid saved to be used in soups, gravies, and white sauces. Using this liquid improves the flavor of foods to which it is added. If there is a considerable amount of fat in the liquid, chill the liquid until the fat accumulates on the top. The fat can then be easily removed.

SUMMARY

Minerals are necessary to promote growth and regulate body processes. They are found in soil and water and come to people via their food and drink. Deficiencies can result in conditions such as rickets, anemia, and goiter. A well-balanced diet can prevent these deficiencies. Because minerals are soluble in water, the water used in cooking mineral-rich foods should be saved and used in preparing other foods.

DISCUSSION TOPICS

1. Discuss the special importance of calcium and phosphorus to children.

2. In class discussions, list ways of supplying an adequate amount of calcium for an adult who dislikes milk. Plan a day's menu for this adult.

3. Ask if any member of the class has suffered from anemia. If so, ask the class member to describe the symptoms and treatment. What measures are being taken to prevent a recurrence of the condition?

4. What is a goiter? Has anyone observed a goiter? If so, describe it. What causes goiter?

SUGGESTED ACTIVITIES

a. Ask a biology teacher to demonstrate the process of osmosis. Discuss its function in the body.

b. Ask a chemistry teacher to explain the properties of acids, alkalies, and salts to the class. Have the teacher relate these properties to the use of minerals by the body.

c. Using outside sources, prepare a report on how sodium and potassium regulate the body's fluid balance.

d. Plan a day's menu. List the minerals found in the foods included.

e. List the foods you have eaten in the past 24 hours. List the minerals in these foods. Note whether there appear to be mineral deficiencies. Make a list of foods which could be added to your diet in order to make up for the mineral deficiencies.

f. Name four foods rich in at least three minerals.

WORD STUDY

acidosis	goiter	nephritic
alkalosis	hemoglobin	nutritional anemia
bone marrow	hypogonadism	osmosis
cardiovascular	iodized salt	rickets
dehydrated	macrominerals	tetany
dwarfism	microminerals	trace element

REVIEW

A. Multiple Choice. Select the *letter* which precedes the best answer.

1. Minerals are inorganic elements that
   a. help to build tissues
   b. are found in all body tissues
   c. regulate various body functions
   d. all of the above

2. The trace elements in the human body are defined as
    a. those minerals that cannot be detected in laboratory tests
    b. those essential minerals found in very small amounts
    c. those minerals which are not essential to health
    d. only those minerals which are found in the blood

3. Calcium is necessary for
    a. healthy bones and teeth
    b. normal clotting of the blood
    c. action of the heart and muscles
    d. all of the above

4. Phosphorus is found in
    a. poultry and fish
    b. common table salt
    c. vegetable oils
    d. leafy vegetables

5. The coloring matter of the blood is
    a. hemoglobin
    b. lymph
    c. marrow
    d. plasma

6. Some of the common symptoms of nutritional anemia are
    a. muscle spasms and pain in the liver
    b. bowed legs and an enlarged thyroid gland
    c. edema and loss of vision
    d. dizziness and weakness

7. Iodine is essential to health because it
    a. is necessary for red blood cells
    b. strengthens bones and teeth
    c. helps the blood to carry oxygen to the cells
    d. affects the rate of metabolism

8. Sodium is often restricted in cardiovascular and nephritic conditions because it
    a. causes the heart to beat slowly
    b. encourages the growth of the heart
    c. contributes to edema
    d. raises the blood sugar

9. Iron is known to be a necessary component of
    a. thyroxine
    b. adipose tissue
    c. hemoglobin
    d. amino acids

10. Liquid from cooking vegetables should be used in preparing other dishes because
    a. mineral salts are soluble in water
    b. the hydrogen and oxygen in water aid the digestion of minerals
    c. the amino acids are soluble in water
    d. none of the above

B.   Complete the following statements.

1.   This mineral is essential for healthy bones and teeth. Its best sources are milk and cheese. It works closely with phosphorus. It is _____ .

2.   This mineral is essential for the formation of hemoglobin. Some of its best sources are meats, legumes, and whole grain cereals. It works closely with copper. It is _____ .

3.   This mineral is essential for a healthy thyroid gland. Its best natural sources are seafood and foods grown in soil bordering the sea. It is _____ .

4.   This mineral is essential for osmosis, maintenance of body neutrality and water balance. It is sometimes restricted in cardiovascular conditions. It works closely with chloride. It is _____ .

5.   This trace mineral increases resistance to tooth decay. It is _____ .

6.   This mineral is essential for healthy muscles and nerves. It is found in meat, milk, cereal grains and fresh green vegetables. Its deficiency may result in mental, emotional, and muscular disorders. It is _____ .

7.   This mineral is essential for regular heart rhythm. It is found in meats, oranges, bananas, and prunes. Its deficiency may result in an abnormal heartbeat. It is _____ .

8.   This mineral is essential in the production of red blood cells. It works closely with iron. It is found in organ meats. Its deficiency may result in anemia. It is _____ .

9.   This mineral is essential for healthy bones and teeth. It is found in milk and meats. It works closely with calcium. It is _____ .

10. This mineral, along with sodium and potassium, is essential for normal osmosis. It is found in table salt, meat, milk, and eggs. It is _____ .

C.   Match the item in column I with its description in column II.

Column I	Column II
_____ 1. nutritional anemia	a. red coloring matter in blood
_____ 2. bone marrow	b. the passing of materials through cell walls
_____ 3. hemoglobin	c. involuntary muscle movement
_____ 4. goiter	d. disease resulting in poorly formed bones
_____ 5. iodized salt	e. lack of iron
_____ 6. osmosis	f. dry from loss of water
_____ 7. tetany	g. essential mineral needed in very small amounts
_____ 8. rickets	h. soft tissue filling bone cavity
_____ 9. trace element	i. salt with iodine removed
_____10. dehydrated	j. salt with iodine added
	k. enlarged thyroid gland

Chapter 6
Vitamins

OBJECTIVES

After studying this chapter, the student should be able to:

- Identify at least two food sources of each vitamin.
- State one or more functions of each vitamin.
- Identify the diseases or symptoms caused by vitamin deficiencies.
- Explain the terms, fat-soluble vitamins and water-soluble vitamins.

Vitamins are organic compounds which are essential for body processes. Vitamins themselves do not provide energy; they enable the body to use the energy provided by fats, carbohydrates, and proteins. The name *vitamin* implies their importance. *Vita* in Latin, means life. The existence of vitamins has been known since early in the twentieth century. It was discovered that animals fed diets of pure proteins, carbohydrates, fats, and minerals did not thrive as did those fed normal diets (which included vitamins).

Vitamins were originally named by letter. However, some are currently named according to their chemical composition. After its initial discovery, vitamin B proved to be more than one compound, so it was divided into specific groups (B_1, B_6 and B_{12} etc). As a whole the group is called "B complex."

Vitamins are found in minute amounts in natural foods. The specific amounts and kinds of vitamins in foods vary. Sometimes a *precursor*, or *a provitamin* is found in foods. This is a substance from which the body can manufacture a specific vitamin.

Vitamin deficiencies can occur and can result in disease. However, a person who eats a well-balanced diet usually avoids vitamin deficiencies. The term *avitaminosis* means "without vitamins." This word followed by the name of a specific vitamin is used to indicate a serious lack of that particular vitamin. *Hypervitaminosis* is the excess of one or more vitamins. Either a lack or excess of vitamins can be detrimental to a person's health.

Extra amounts of vitamins taken beyond those received in the diet are called *vitamin supplements*. These are available in concentrated forms such as tablets or capsules. Vitamin concentrates are sometimes termed natural or *synthetic* (man made). Some people believe a meaningful difference exists between the two types and that the natural are far superior in quality to the synthetic. However, according to the United States Federal Drug Administration (FDA), the body cannot in any way distinguish between a vitamin of plant or animal origin and one manufactured in a laboratory.

Synthetic vitamins are frequently added to foods during processing. When this is done, the foods are described as *enriched* or *fortified*. Examples of these foods are enriched breads and cereals to which thiamine, niacin, riboflavin and iron have been added.

Vitamins A and D are added to fortified margarine and milk. Occasionally vitamins are lost during food processing. In most cases, food producers can replace these vitamins with synthetic vitamins, making the processed food nutritionally equal to the natural, unprocessed food. Foods in which vitamins are replaced are called *restored* foods.

Because some vitamins are easily destroyed by light, air, heat, and water, it is important to know how to preserve the vitamin content of food during its preparation and cooking. It may be helpful to study the following list.

- Buy the freshest, unbruised vegetables and fruits. Use them raw when possible.
- Prepare fresh vegetables and fruits just before serving.
- Heat canned vegetables quickly and in their own liquid.
- Follow package directions when using frozen vegetables or fruit.
- Use as little water as possible and have it boiling when adding vegetables.

- Cover the pan (except for the first few minutes when cooking strongly flavored vegetables) and cook as short a time as possible.
- Save the cooking liquid for later use in soups, stews, and gravies.
- Store fresh vegetables and most fruits in a cool, dark place.

FAT-SOLUBLE VITAMINS

Vitamins are classified as fat soluble or water soluble. The fat-soluble vitamins, A, D, E, and K, are chemically similar, and all of them are soluble in fat. They are not lost easily in cooking and they can be stored in the body. Deficiencies are slower to appear than those caused by lack of the water-soluble vitamins (B complex and C). The vitamin values of A, D, and E are given in *International Units* (IU); Vitamin A is also given in *retinol equivalents* (RE). All other vitamin values are given in milligrams (mg) or micrograms, (μg), table 6-1.

TABLE 6-1 Recommended Daily Vitamin Allowances

	Age (years)	Weight (kg)	(lbs)	Height (cm)	(in)	Fat-Soluble Vitamins				Water-Soluble Vitamins						
						Vitamin A Activity (RE)	(IU)	Vitamin D (IU)	Vitamin E Activity (IU)	Ascorbic Acid (mg)	Folacin (μg)	Niacin (mg)	Riboflavin (mg)	Thiamine (mg)	Vitamin B$_6$ (mg)	Vitamin B$_{12}$ (μg)
Infants	0.0-0.5	6	14	60	24	420	1,400	400	4	35	50	5	0.4	0.3	0.3	0.3
	0.5-1.0	9	20	71	28	400	2,000	400	5	35	50	8	0.6	0.5	0.4	0.3
	1-3	13	28	86	34	400	2,000	400	7	40	100	9	0.8	0.7	0.6	1.0
	4-6	20	44	110	44	500	2,500	400	9	40	200	12	1.1	0.9	0.9	1.5
	7-10	30	66	135	54	700	3,300	400	10	40	300	16	1.2	1.2	1.2	2.0
Males	11-14	44	97	158	63	1,000	5,000	400	12	45	400	18	1.5	1.4	1.6	3.0
	15-18	61	134	172	69	1,000	5,000	400	15	45	400	20	1.8	1.5	2.0	3.0
	19-22	67	147	172	69	1,000	5,000	400	15	45	400	20	1.8	1.5	2.0	3.0
	23-50	70	154	172	69	1,000	5,000		15	45	400	18	1.6	1.4	2.0	3.0
	51+	70	154	172	69	1,000	5,000		15	45	400	16	1.5	1.2	2.0	3.0
Females	11-14	44	97	155	62	800	4,000	400	12	45	400	16	1.3	1.2	1.6	3.0
	15-18	54	119	162	65	800	4,000	400	12	45	400	14	1.4	1.1	2.0	3.0
	19-22	58	128	162	65	800	4,000	400	12	45	400	14	1.4	1.1	2.0	3.0
	23-50	58	128	162	65	800	4,000		12	45	400	13	1.2	1.0	2.0	3.0
	51+	58	128	162	65	800	4,000		12	45	400	12	1.1	1.0	2.0	3.0
Pregnant						1,000	5,000	400	15	60	800	+2	+0.3	+0.3	2.5	4.0
Lactating						1,200	6,000	400	15	80	600	+4	+0.5	+0.3	2.5	4.0

Source: Food and Nutrition Board, National Academy of Sciences, National Research Council, 1974

Vitamin A

Vitamin A (retinol) promotes growth and is essential in maintaining healthy eyes and skin. In addition, it aids in the prevention of infections by helping to maintain healthy *mucous membranes* (the lining of the nose, throat, other air passages, the gastrointestinal tract and genitourinary tract). Its deficiency symptoms include night blindness; dry, rough skin; skin lesions; loss of balance; decreased sensitivity to taste and smell; and increased susceptibility to infections. Avitaminosis A can result in blindness or *xerophthalmia,* a condition characterized by dry, lusterless mucous membranes of the eye.

Food sources of vitamin A include animal foods such as liver, butter, cream, whole milk, whole milk cheese, egg yolk, fish liver oils, and fortified margarine. *Carotene* is a precursor of vitamin A and is found in dark green and yellow vegetables and fruits. The presence of carotene makes these foods good sources of vitamin A.

A well-balanced diet is the preferred way to obtain the required amounts of vitamin A. The use of vitamin supplements should be discouraged. An excess of vitamin A can have serious consequences. Hypervitaminosis A can result in loss of appetite and hair, dry skin, unusual *pigmentation* (coloring of the skin) and bone pain. See table 6-1 for the recommended daily dietary allowances as prescribed by the Food and Nutrition Board of the National Research Council-National Academy of Sciences.

Vitamin D

Vitamin D (calciferol) helps regulate the metabolism of calcium and phosphorus in the body. The action with these minerals makes vitamin D essential for strong, healthy bones and teeth. A deficiency of vitamin D may result in rickets in children. In adults a deficiency may result in *osteomalacia*, a softening of the bones because of a loss of calcium.

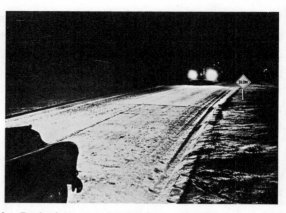

A. Both the normal individual and the person suffering from a deficiency of vitamin A see the headlights of an approaching car.

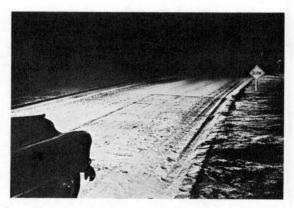

B. After the car has passed the normal individual sees a wide stretch of road.

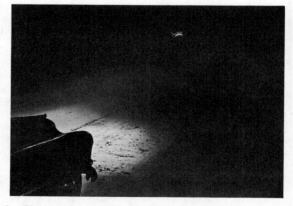

C. The person deficient in vitamin A can barely see a few feet ahead and cannot see the road sign at all.

Fig. 6-1 Comparison to normal vision demonstrates reduced visibility caused by night blindness. (*Courtesy of Upjohn Company*)

The best source of vitamin D is the sun. Humans have an ingredient in the skin which forms vitamin D when exposed to sunlight. The amount of vitamin D that is formed depends on the individual's pigmentation and the amount of sunlight available. The best food sources of vitamin D are fatty fish, liver, eggs, and butter. Because of the rather limited number of food sources of vitamin D and the unpredictability of sunshine, health authorities decided that vitamin D should be added to a common food source such as milk. Consequently, most milk available in the United States today has been *irradiated* (fortified) with 400 IU of vitamin D per quart. Drinking one quart of irradiated milk each day fulfills the recommended daily dietary allowances for people six months to twenty-two years of age, and for pregnant and lactating women. While the vitamin D requirement for adults over the age of twenty-two has not been established, it is believed that their needs can be met by an average exposure to sunlight. People who are seldom outdoors should use dietary sources also.

Hypervitaminosis D must be avoided because it can cause calcium and phosphorus deposits in soft tissues of the body. Symptoms of hypervitaminosis D include nausea, weakness, *anorexia* (loss of appetite) and constipation.

Vitamin E

The precise function of vitamin E in humans has not been well defined. Studies indicate that vitamin E is essential for normal reproduction in some animals, but there is no evidence that vitamin E is essential for human reproduction. Vitamin E appears to be important to the health of red blood cells in humans. Some claim that vitamin E concentrates help prevent or cure heart disease, cancer, muscular dystrophy, sterility, ulcers, burns, and other skin problems. None of these claims has been substantiated by clinical evidence.

Vitamin E is found in many common foods, although animal foods are the poorest sources. Wheat germ and wheat germ oils are two of the best sources.

Because of its wide availability in foods, a deficiency of vitamin E is very rare. It has occurred in some premature infants. A symptom of vitamin E deficiency is an increase in the rate of *hemolysis* (the destruction of red blood cells). See table 6-1 for the recommended daily dietary allowances.

Vitamin K

Vitamin K is necessary for proper clotting of the blood. Approximately half of the vitamin K in the body comes from food eaten. The other half is synthesized by bacteria in the intestines. Vitamin K deficiency is rare; it may be caused by the body's failure to absorb or metabolize the vitamin. The use of mineral oil interferes with the absorption of fat-soluble vitamins and is to be discouraged. A deficiency may also be caused by *antibiotic therapy* (the ingestion of antibiotic drugs to combat infection) which interferes with the bacterial synthesis of vitamin K. Vitamin K deficiency causes increased clotting time of blood and a greater tendency to *hemorrhage* (bleed). The best sources of vitamin K are spinach, cabbage, kale, cauliflower, peas, and cereals. Animal foods are generally poor sources.

Hypervitaminosis K can be *toxic*. The indiscriminate use of vitamin K concentrates should be avoided. Precise dietary requirements have not been determined.

WATER-SOLUBLE VITAMINS

Water-soluble vitamins dissolve in water and are easily destroyed by air and in cooking. They cannot be stored in the body. The water-soluble vitamins include vitamin B complex and vitamin C.

Vitamin B Complex

Toward the end of the nineteenth century, a doctor in Indonesia discovered that chickens which were fed table scraps of polished rice developed symptoms much like those of his patients suffering from beriberi. When these same chickens were later fed brown (unpolished) rice, they recovered.

Some years later, this mysterious component of unpolished rice was recognized as an essential food substance and was named vitamin B. Subsequently, it was named vitamin *B complex* because the vitamin was found to be composed of several compounds. The B complex vitamins include thiamine (B_1), riboflavin, niacin, B_6, cobalamin (B_{12}), folacin, pantothenic acid and biotin.

Thiamine. *Thiamine* is essential for proper carbohydrate metabolism. A deficiency of thiamine can result in impaired carbohydrate metabolism. Symptoms of thiamine deficiency include the loss of appetite, fatigue, nervous irritability, indigestion and constipation. An extreme deficiency of this vitamin causes beriberi.

Thiamine is found in many foods but generally in very small quantities. (See table A-6 in the Appendix). Most breads and cereals are enriched with thiamine so that most people can easily fulfill their recommended daily dietary requirement. The best natural food sources of thiamine are dry yeast, wheat germ, pork and organ meats.

Riboflavin. *Riboflavin* is essential for carbohydrate, fat, and protein metabolism. It is also necessary for healthy skin around the mouth and for healthy functioning of the eyes. A deficiency of riboflavin can result in

cheilosis, (a condition characterized by sores on the lips and cracks at the corners of the mouth) and eye sensitivity, characterized by itching, burning, and eye fatigue.

Riboflavin is found in many plant and animal foods, but in small quantities. The best sources are milk, organ meats, green leafy vegetables, and enriched cereals. Because of the small quantities of riboflavin in foods, deficiencies of riboflavin may develop. The generous use of milk in the diet is a good way of preventing a deficiency of this vitamin. See table 6-1 for the recommended daily dietary allowances.

Niacin. This vitamin is also called *nicotinic acid*. Niacin is essential for carbohydrate, fat, and protein metabolism and for the prevention of pellagra. *Pellagra* is a disease characterized by sores on the skin, diarrhea, and general irritability. Pellagra is rare in the United States.

The best sources of niacin are meats, poultry, and fish. Whole grain and enriched cereals also contain some niacin. Milk and eggs do not provide niacin but they do provide its precursor, *tryptophan*. Consequently milk is considered a good source of niacin.

Hypervitaminosis of niacin has been shown to adversely affect the heart and liver. Self-prescribed doses of the vitamin concentrate should be discouraged. See table 6-1 for the recommended daily dietary allowances.

Vitamin B_6. Although the vitamin B_6 is known to be essential to man, its specific function is still being studied. It is associated with the metabolism of proteins. Its deficiency symptoms may include *anemia* and abnormalities of the nervous system. Its best food sources are pork, organ meats, and legumes. See table 6-1 for the recommended daily dietary allowances.

Vitamin B₁₂ (Cobalamin). Vitamin B_{12} is essential for healthy red blood cells and nerve tissue and is involved in metabolism. It is given *parenterally* (by intravenous or intramuscular injections) as treatment for pernicious anemia. *Pernicious anemia* is a severe blood disease characterized by a decrease in the number of red blood cells. The anemia is caused by a body defect which inhibits red blood cell formation. The number of cells decreases but the size of the cells increases. The best food sources of vitamin B_{12} are organ meats (especially liver), milk, and eggs. See table 6-1 for the recommended allowances.

Folacin. Folacin, like vitamin B_{12}, is essential for the formation of red blood cells and for normal metabolism. Its deficiency results in anemia, *glossitis* (inflammation of the tongue) and gastrointestinal problems. The best sources of folacin are dark green leafy vegetables, liver, yeast, and fruit. See table 6-1 for the recommended daily dietary allowances.

Pantothenic Acid. Pantothenic acid is involved in the metabolism of carbohydrates, fats, and proteins. Its deficiency has not been recognized in humans. The word *pantothenic* is of Greek derivation and means "from many places". This is appropriate as this vitamin is found extensively in foods, especially animal foods. Its best sources are organ meats, salmon, eggs, yeast, whole grain cereals, and legumes. Its recommended daily dietary allowances have not been established.

Biotin. Biotin participates in metabolism. Its deficiency symptoms include nausea, anemia, anorexia, depression, and glossitis. The best food sources of biotin include organ meats, peanuts and mushrooms. Dietary allowances have not been established.

VITAMIN C

Vitamin C is also known as *ascorbic acid.* This vitamin appears to have several functions in the human body, but they are not yet well understood. It has an important role in the formation of *collagen,* a protein substance that holds body cells together. This makes it essential for wound healing. It is also important in metabolism. There are many who believe that this vitamin plays an important role in fighting infections. However, the position of the Food and Nutrition Board of the National Research Council-National Academy of Sciences is that this claim has not been sufficiently established.

The deficiency of vitamin C results in delayed wound healing, bleeding, sore gums, and mouth, and in severe cases, scurvy. *Scurvy* is a disease characterized by bleeding gums, loose teeth, sore joints and muscles, and loss of weight. In extreme cases it can result in death.

The best sources of vitamin C are citrus fruits (oranges, lemons, limes, grapefruit and tangerines) cantaloupe, strawberries, tomatoes, cabbage, and potatoes. See table 6-1 for the recommended daily dietary allowances.

SUMMARY

Vitamins are organic compounds that regulate body functions and promote growth. Each vitamin has a specific function or functions within the body. Food sources of vitamins vary, but generally a well-balanced diet provides sufficient vitamins to fulfill body requirements. Vitamin deficiencies can result from inadequate diets or from the body's inability to utilize vitamins. Vitamins are available in concentrated forms, but their use should be carefully monitored as overdoses can be detrimental to health. Vitamins A, D, E and K are fat-soluble. Vitamin B complex and Vitamin C are water-soluble. Water-soluble vitamins can be destroyed during food preparation. It is important that care is taken during the preparation of food so as to preserve the vitamin content.

TABLE 6-2 Vitamins

VITAMINS	BEST SOURCES	FUNCTIONS	DEFICIENCY SYMPTOMS
Fat-Soluble Vitamins			

Vitamin A	Fish liver oils
	Liver
	Butter, margarine (fortified)
	Whole milk, cream, cheese
	Egg yolk
	Vegetables (green and yellow)
	Fruits (yellow)
		Growth
		Health of eyes
		Structure and functioning
		  of the cells of the skin
		  and mucous membranes
			Functional disorders of
			  the eye (night blindness)
			Increased susceptibility
			  to infections
			Changes in skin and
			  membranes

Vitamin D	Sunshine
	Fatty fish
	Milk (irradiated)
	Egg yolk
	Liver
		Growth
		Regulating calcium and
		  phosphorus
		  metabolism
		Building and maintain-
		  ing normal bones
		  and teeth
			Rickets
			Soft bones
			Poor tooth development
			Osteomalacia

Vitamin E	Wheat germ and wheat
	  germ oils
	Vegetable oils
	Margarine
	Legumes
	Peanuts
	Dark green, leafy
	  vegetables
		Not conclusively defined
		  in humans; may affect
		  the red blood cells
			Increased rate of hemo-
			  lysis of the red blood
			  cells

Vitamin K	Spinach
	Kale
	Cabbage
	Cauliflower
	Cereals
		Normal clotting of
		  blood
			Slow clotting of blood
			Hemorrhagic disease in
			  newborn

**Water-Soluble
  Vitamins**
 	
Thiamine (B_1)
	Wheat germ
	Lean pork
	Yeast
	Legumes
	Whole grain and enriched
	  cereal products
	Liver
	Heart
	Kidney
		Carbohydrate
		  metabolism
		Healthy appetite
		Functioning of nerves
			Loss of appetite
			Irritability
			Less resistance to fatigue
			Constipation

Riboflavin	Milk, cheese
	Enriched bread and cereals
	Green, leafy vegetables
	Eggs
	Liver, kidney, heart
		Carbohydrate, fat, and
		  protein metabolism
		Health of the mouth
		  tissue
		Healthy eyes
			Cheilosis
			Blurring of vision
			Intolerance to light

TABLE 6-2 (continued)

VITAMINS	BEST SOURCES	FUNCTIONS	DEFICIENCY SYMPTOMS
Niacin (Nicotinic Acid)	Meats (especially organ meats) Poultry and fish Milk Enriched breads and cereals Milk	Prevention of pellagra Carbohydrate, fat, and protein metabolism	Glossitis Skin eruptions Nausea Diarrhea Nervous disorders Anorexia Pellagra
Vitamin B$_6$	Pork Organ meats Legumes Whole grain cereals	Metabolism of proteins	Anemia Dermatitis Kidney stones Depression Anorexia Nausea
Vitamin B$_{12}$ (Cobalamin)	Liver, kidney Muscle meats Milk, cheese Eggs	Metabolism Healthy red blood cells Treatment of pernicious anemia	Anemia
Folacin	Dark green, leafy vegetables Liver Yeast Fruit	The blood-forming system Metabolism	Anemia Glossitis Diarrhea
Pantothenic Acid	Heart, liver, kidney Eggs Peanuts Whole grain cereals	Various steps in metabolism	Unknown
Biotin	Organ Meats Mushrooms Peanuts	Various steps in metabolism	Skin disorders Nervous disorders Anorexia Anemia
Vitamin C (Ascorbic Acid)	Citrus fruits, pineapple Melons Berries Tomatoes Cabbage Broccoli Green Peppers	Maintaining collagen Healthy gums Aids in wound healing	Sore gums Tendency to bruise easily Scurvy

DISCUSSION TOPICS

1. How do vitamins help to provide energy to the body?
2. Discuss possible times when avitaminosis of one or more vitamins may occur.

3. Discuss any vitamin deficiencies which class members have observed. What treatments were prescribed?

4. Discuss why it may be unwise for anyone but a physician to prescribe vitamin supplements.

5. Discuss the terms enriched, fortified, and restored. What do they mean in relation to food products?

6. Discuss the proper storage and cooking of foods in order to retain their vitamin content.

7. If any member of the class has experienced night blindness ask him or her to describe it. Discuss how this condition occurs, how it may be alleviated and how it can be prevented.

8. Ask if any class member has observed a child with rickets. Discuss the appearance of a child with rickets. Discuss how this disease can be prevented.

SUGGESTED ACTIVITIES

a. Prepare two packages of a frozen vegetable. Cook one package according to the directions on the package and the other in 2 cups of water for 30 minutes. Compare them for palatability. Discuss their probable vitamin and mineral content.

b. Many foods are described as enriched, fortified, and restored. Visit a supermarket and make lists of foods described by each term.

c. Write a menu for one day which is especially rich in the B-complex vitamins. Underline the foods that are the best sources of these vitamins.

d. Organize a "spelldown", asking the functions and sources of vitamins.

e. List the foods you have eaten in the past 24 hours. Write the name of a vitamin beside the food for which it is a rich source. What percentage of your day's food did *not* contain vitamins? Could this diet be nutritionally improved? How?

f. Plan a day's menu for a person who has been instructed to eat an abundance of foods rich in vitamin A.

WORD STUDY

anorexia	cheilosis	glossitis
antibiotic therapy	citrus fruit	hemolysis
ascorbic acid	cobalamin	hemorrhage
avitaminosis	collagen	hypervitaminosis
beriberi	enriched foods	irradiate
biotin	fat soluble	mucous membrane
calciferol	folic acid	niacin
carotene	fortified foods	osteomalacia

pantothenic acid	restored foods	tryptophan
pellagra	riboflavin	vitamin
parenteral	scurvy	vitamin supplements
pernicious anemia	thiamine	water soluble
pigmentation		xerophthalmia

REVIEW

A. Multiple Choice. Select the *letter* preceding the best answer.

1. The daily vitamin requirement is best supplied by
   a. eating a well-balanced diet
   b. eating one serving of citrus fruit for breakfast
   c. taking one of the many forms of vitamin supplements
   d. eating at least one serving of meat each day

2. All of the following measures preserve the vitamin content of food except
   a. using vegetables and fruits raw as often as possible
   b. preparing fresh vegetables and fruits just before serving
   c. adding raw, fresh vegetables to a small amount of cold water and heating to boiling
   d. storing fresh vegetables in a cool place

3. Fat-soluble vitamins
   a. cannot be stored in the body
   b. are lost easily during cooking
   c. are dissolved by water
   d. are slower than water-soluble vitamins to exhibit deficiencies

4. Night blindness is caused by a deficiency of
   a. vitamin A   c. niacin
   b. thiamine   d. vitamin C

5. Good sources of thiamine include
   a. citrus fruits and tomatoes   c. carotene and fish-liver oils
   b. wheat germ and liver   d. nuts and milk

6. Water-soluble vitamins include
   a. A, D, E, and K
   b. A, B_6, and C
   c. thiamine, niacin, and calciferol
   d. thiamine, riboflavin, niacin, B_6, B_{12}

7. Injections of vitamin B_{12} are given in the treatment of
   a. scurvy   c. pellagra
   b. pernicious anemia   d. beriberi

8. Blindness can result from a severe lack of
   a. vitamin K   c. thiamine
   b. vitamin A   d. vitamin E

9. Organ meats are good sources of the following vitamins:
    a. thiamine, riboflavin, B_{12} c. vitamins D and E
    b. biotin, vitamin C   d. all of these
10. Irradiated milk is a good source of
    a. vitamin E   c. vitamin K
    b. vitamin D   d. vitamin C
11. Good sources of Vitamin C are
    a. meats   c. breads and cereals
    b. milk and milk products   d. citrus fruits
12. The vitamin that aids in the prevention of rickets is
    a. vitamin A   c. vitamin C
    b. thiamine   d. vitamin D
13. The vitamin that is necessary for the proper clotting of the blood is
    a. vitamin A   c. vitamin D
    b. vitamin K   d. niacin
14. The three vitamins with which breads and cereals are commonly enriched are
    a. vitamins A, D, and K
    b. thiamine, riboflavin, and niacin
    c. vitamins E, B_6, and B_{12}
    d. ascorbic acid, pantothenic acid, and folacin
15. The vitamin that is known to prevent scurvy is
    a. vitamin A   c. vitamin C
    b. vitamin B complex   d. vitamin D
B. Match the vitamins listed in column I with their characteristics listed in column II.

Column I	Column II
_____ 1. vitamin A	a. also called vitamin C
_____ 2. thiamine	b. also called amino acids
_____ 3. riboflavin	c. essential for reproduction in some animals
_____ 4. niacin	d. substance the body converts to vitamin A
_____ 5. vitamin E	e. primarily found in polished rice
_____ 6. vitamin D	f. deficiency causes night blindness
_____ 7. vitamin B_{12}	g. best-known treatment for pernicious anemia
_____ 8. ascorbic acid	h. extreme deficiency may cause beriberi
_____ 9. vitamin K	i. severe deficiency may result in rickets
_____ 10. carotene	j. deficiency may cause pellagra
	k. essential for proper clotting of the blood
	l. deficiency may cause cheilosis

C. Briefly answer the following questions.
  1. What vitamins are fat soluble? Name three characteristics of fat-soluble vitamins.
  2. What vitamins are water soluble? Name three characteristics of water-soluble vitamins.

SECTION EVALUATION 1 BASIC NUTRITION

A. Complete the following statements by filling in the blanks.

1. Many Americans are _____ because of insufficient exercise and overindulgence in high-calorie foods.

2. Chemical substances essential to life which are provided only by proteins are called _____ .

3. The primary function of carbohydrates and fats is to supply _____ and _____ .

4. The primary function of proteins is to _____ .

5. The amount of water each person should consume daily is _____ .

6. The type of carbohydrate that is indigestible but necessary for proper elimination is _____ .

7. The products of digestion are changed into heat and energy through a metabolic process called _____ .

8. Energy needs are determined by age, size, sex, and _____ .

9. The gland controlling the rate of metabolism is the _____ .

10. The unit used in measuring the fuel value of food is the _____ .

11. Fatty tissue is also known as _____ .

12. Two examples of foods rich in fats are _____ and _____ .

13. Calcium and phosphorus together are necessary for _____ .

14. Iron is necessary for healthy _____ .

15. Liver is an excellent source of the mineral _____ .

16. Seafood and iodized salt are excellent sources of the mineral_____ .

17. The vitamins which are easily destroyed by heat, air, light, or water are _____ .

18. The four vitamins that are fat soluble are _____ .

19. Night blindness is a symptom of _____ deficiency.

20. An extreme deficiency of thiamine can result in a disease called _____ .

21. Another name for vitamin C is _____ .

22. Pellagra may be prevented by eating a diet containing _____ .

23. Citrus fruits are excellent sources of vitamin_____ .

24. A severe deficiency of vitamin D during early childhood can result in _____ .

25. The vitamin essential for proper clotting of the blood is _____ .

B.   Match the term in column I with its definition in column II.

Column I   Column II

_____ 1. glucose   a. common table sugar

_____ 2. sucrose   b. indigestible carbohydrate

_____ 3. fat   c. organic substance that changes other substances

_____ 4. cellulose   d. enlarged thyroid gland

_____ 5. glycogen   e. protein deficiency

_____ 6. amino acids   f. simple sugar

_____ 7. enzyme   g. carbohydrate as stored in the liver

_____ 8. kwashiorkor   h. insufficient red blood cells

_____ 9. goiter   i. provides 9 calories per gram

_____ 10. anemia   j. building blocks of protein

                             k. vitamin K

C.   Multiple Choice. Select the *letter* which precedes the best answer.

1. Food is moved along the digestive tract by
    a. ciliated epithelium along the length of the alimentary canal
    b. a muscular action known as peristalsis
    c. the currents formed by digestive juices
    d. all of the above

2. Digestion in the mouth includes
    a. only chemical digestion
    b. only mechanical digestion
    c. both chemical and mechanical digestion
    d. none of the above

3. Gastric juice contains
    a. hydrochloric acid   c. ptyalin
    b. salivary amylase   d. bile

4. Before it can be absorbed into the bloodstream, starch must be broken
    down to
    a. glucose   c. glycogen
    b. hydrochloric acid   d. amino acids

5. If fat is not used immediately following metabolism, it is stored as
    a. alkalosis   c. glycerol
    b. adipose tissue   d. amino acids

6. During hydrogenation
    a. the end products of digestion are changed into heat and energy
    b. hydrogen is added to oily fats to solidify them
    c. margarine has calories added to make it as nourishing as butter
    d. proteins are changed into amino acids

7. When there is little or no protein in the diet
   a. an accumulation of excess fluid may develop in body tissues
   b. hemorrhage may occur if the skin is broken
   c. the number of white blood cells becomes excessive
   d. an excess of adipose tissue develops

8. Sodium and potassium are important in a well-balanced diet because they
   a. help maintain the fluid balance of the body
   b. prevent circulatory infections from spreading
   c. prevent anemia and hemoglobin deficiency
   d. prevent goiter and other thyroid disorders

9. Injections of vitamin B_{12} are ordered for the treatment of
   a. pernicious anemia   c. scurvy
   b. pellagra   d. wounds

10. Vitamin C is used in the treatment of
    a. pernicious anemia and goiter   c. beriberi and night blindness
    b. pellagra and heart disease   d. wounds and scurvy

D.   Briefly answer the following questions.

1. What are the factors which determine energy needs? How is each of these factors important?

2. Describe digestion. Include mechanical and chemical digestion, peristalsis, gastric juices, pancreatic juices, bile, fundus of stomach, alimentary canal, esophagus, ptyalin, hydrochloric acid and enzymes.

3. Name the six essential nutrients. List their functions and at least three food sources of each.

4. Of what chemical elements are proteins composed? Why are proteins essential to life?

5. Name five ways in which the vitamin content of foods can be preserved?

6. a. What are the caloric values of the following nutrients?
   10 grams of protein:
   20 grams of carbohydrate:
   5 grams of fat:

   b. Which nutrient is the cheapest source of energy?

Section 2

MEAL PLANNING

Chapter 7

The Basic Four Food Groups

OBJECTIVES

After studying this chapter, the student should be able to:

- Define a balanced diet.
- Identify the Basic Four food groups.
- Identify the chief nutrients provided by each of the four food groups.
- Identify at least two foods contained in each of the four food groups.
- Determine the recommended number of servings per day for each food group.

The statement, "eat a balanced diet" may have been repeated so many times that its importance is being overlooked. Its value is so great, however, that it deserves serious consideration by people of all ages. A *balanced diet* is one that includes the six essential nutrients in adequate amounts to preserve and promote good health.

The question arises as to how one might attain a balanced diet. The Food and Nutrition Board of the National Academy of Sciences-National Research Council has established recommended daily dietary allowances of the essential nutrients whose human requirements have been established. Table A-6 in the Appendix gives the nutritive values of the edible foods. It is important to

remember that the edible portion is only that part of the food that can be eaten. Daily review of these lists would certainly provide enough information to plan a balanced diet. However, ordinary meal planning would be quite time-consuming if the table had to be consulted each time a meal was planned. Fortunately, nutritionists have devised an elementary method that simplifies planning a balanced diet. This method is based on the Basic Four food groups. A thorough knowledge of these food groups makes planning nutritious meals fast and easy. In using this simple guide, it is essential that the diet be selected primarily from these four broad food groups: the meat group; vegetable and fruit group; milk and milk products group; and the bread and cereal group.

TABLE 7-1 Recommended Daily Dietary Allowances

	Age (years)	Weight (kg)	Weight (lbs)	Height (cm)	Height (in)	Energy (kcal)	Protein (g)	Fat-Soluble Vitamins			Water-Soluble Vitamins							Minerals					
								Vitamin A Activity (RF)c (IU)	Vitamin D (IU)	Vitamin E Activity (IU)	Ascorbic Acid (mg)	Folacinf (µg)	Niacing (mg)	Riboflavin (mg)	Thiamine (mg)	Vitamin B6 (mg)	Vitamin B12 (µg)	Calcium (mg)	Phosphorus (mg)	Iodine (µg)	Iron (mg)	Magnesium (mg)	Zinc (mg)
Infants	0.0-0.5	6	14	60	24	kgx117	kgx2.2	420 1,400	400	4	35	50	5	0.4	0.3	0.3	0.3	360	240	35	10	60	3
	0.5-1.0	9	20	71	28	kgx108	kgx2.0	400 2,000	400	5	35	50	8	0.6	0.5	0.4	0.3	540	400	45	15	70	5
Children	1-3	13	28	86	34	1,300	23	400 2,000	400	7	40	100	9	0.8	0.7	0.6	1.0	800	800	60	15	150	10
	4-6	20	44	110	44	1,800	30	500 2,500	400	9	40	200	12	1.1	0.9	0.9	1.5	800	800	80	10	200	10
	7-10	30	66	135	54	2,400	36	700 3,300	400	10	40	300	16	1.2	1.2	1.2	2.0	800	800	110	10	250	10
Males	11-14	44	97	158	63	2,800	44	1,000 5,000	400	12	45	400	18	1.5	1.4	1.6	3.0	1,200	1,200	130	18	350	15
	15-18	61	134	172	69	3,000	54	1,000 5,000	400	15	45	400	20	1.8	1.5	2.0	3.0	1,200	1,200	150	18	400	15
	19-22	67	147	172	69	3,000	54	1,000 5,000	400	15	45	400	20	1.8	1.5	2.0	3.0	800	800	140	10	350	15
	23-50	70	154	172	69	2,700	56	1,000 5,000		15	45	400	18	1.6	1.4	2.0	3.0	800	800	130	10	350	15
	51+	70	154	172	69	2,400	56	1,000 5,000		15	45	400	16	1.5	1.2	2.0	3.0	800	800	110	10	350	15
Females	11-14	44	97	155	62	2,400	44	800 4,000	400	12	45	400	16	1.3	1.2	1.6	3.0	1,200	1,200	115	18	300	15
	15-18	54	119	162	65	2,100	48	800 4,000	400	12	45	400	14	1.4	1.1	2.0	3.0	1,200	1,200	115	18	300	15
	19-22	58	128	162	65	2,100	46	800 4,000	400	12	45	400	14	1.4	1.1	2.0	3.0	800	800	100	18	300	15
	23-50	58	128	162	65	2,000	46	800 4,000		12	45	400	13	1.2	1.0	2.0	3.0	800	800	100	18	300	15
	51+	58	128	162	65	1,800	46	800 4,000		12	45	400	12	1.1	1.0	2.0	3.0	800	800	80	10	300	15
Pregnant						+300	+30	1,000 5,000	400	15	60	800	+2	+0.3	+0.3	2.5	4.0	1,200	1,200	125	18+	450	20
Lactating						+500	+20	1,200 6,000	400	15	80	600	+4	+0.5	+0.3	2.5	4.0	1,200	1,200	150	18	450	25

Source: Food and Nutrition Board, National Academy of Sciences-National Research Council, 1974

At least a minimum number of servings is taken from each of the four food groups. Serving sizes vary according to the type of food and the individual eating the food. Small servings are allowed for young children and extra large for very active adults and teenagers. Pregnant women or mothers who are breast feeding require additional milk.

It is advisable to have some meat, poultry, fish, eggs, milk or a milk product at each meal. The protein which is generously provided in these foods gives satiety (satisfaction) to meals.

Meals can be planned using foods in the four groups and additional foods not listed in these groups. The foods must provide enough calories to satisfy energy requirements for the day. Children need enough food energy to support normal growth and provide the energy which they expend each day. Adults need enough food energy to maintain body weight at a level most favorable to health and well-being.

Table 7-2 gives an analysis of the nutrients supplied by a menu based on the Basic Four food groups. The menu provides a balanced diet for a female between the ages of twenty-three and fifty years of age. Note that the nutrient values exceed the allowances but that the caloric value closely follows the amount recommended. The total caloric value is very important. Both caloric and nutrient content of the menu must be considered when planning meals.

THE VEGETABLE AND FRUIT GROUP

All vegetables and fruits are included in this group. Those vegetables and fruits that are especially rich sources of vitamins A and C are emphasized. **Four or more** servings of different fruits and vegetables should be eaten each day. Foods in this group provide sugar and cellulose in addition to vitamins A, E, K, B complex, and C, and the minerals iron, calcium, phosphorus, potassium, and magnesium. Usually one-half cup of each is considered a serving.

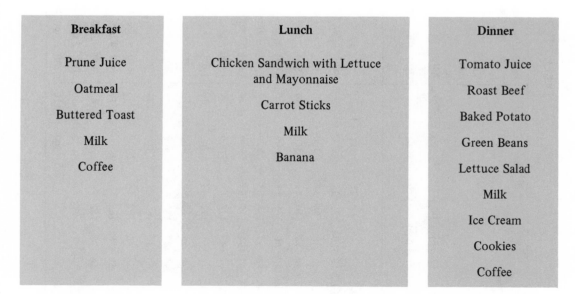

Breakfast	Lunch	Dinner
Prune Juice	Chicken Sandwich with Lettuce and Mayonnaise	Tomato Juice
Oatmeal	Carrot Sticks	Roast Beef
Buttered Toast	Milk	Baked Potato
Milk	Banana	Green Beans
Coffee		Lettuce Salad
		Milk
		Ice Cream
		Cookies
		Coffee

Fig. 7-1 Three meals a day can provide a well-balanced diet of the Basic Four food groups. (See table 7-2 for an analysis of this menu.)

TABLE 7-2 Nutrients Provided by the Sample Menu*†

	1/2 cup prune juice	1 cup oatmeal	3 slices enriched bread	1 tablespoon butter	3 cups whole milk	3 ounces chicken	4 large lettuce leaves	1 tablespoon mayonnaise	1/2 carrot	1 medium banana	1/2 cup tomato juice	5.4 ounces lean roast beef	1 baked potato	1/2 cup green beans	3 fluid ounces ice cream	1 tablespoon "French" dressing	2 chocolate chip cookies	Total	Recommended Daily Allowances
Protein (g)	.5	5	6	Tr	27	20	2	Tr	.5	1	1	48	3	1	2	Tr	2	119	46
Calcium (mg)	18	22	63	3	864	8	68	3	9	10	9	20	9	31	73	2	8	122	800
Iron (mg)	5.2	1.4	1.8	0	.3	1.4	1.4	.1	.2	.8	1.1	6	.7	.4	Tr	.1	.4	21.3	18
Vitamin A (IU)	-	0	Tr	470	1050	80	1900	40	2750	230	970	Tr	Tr	340	220	-	20	8070	4000
Thiamine (mg)	.015	.19	.18	-	.21	.05	.06	Tr	.015	.06	.06	.12	.1	.045	.02	-	.02	1.14	1.0
Riboflavin (mg)	.015	.05	.15	-	1.23	.16	.08	.01	.015	.07	.03	.36	.04	.055	.11	-	.02	2.39	1.2
Niacin (mg)	.5	.2	1.8	-	.6	7.4	.4	Tr	.15	.8	.95	8.6	1.7	.3	.1	-	.2	23.7	13
Vitamin C (mg)	2.5	0	Tr	0	6	-	18	-	2	12	20	-	20	7.5	1	-	Tr	89	45
Calories	100	130	210	100	480	115	20	100	10	100	23	250	90	15	95	65	100	2003	2000

* Menu selected from the Basic Four food groups.

† Daily allowance established for a female between the ages of 23 and 50 years, weighing 128 lbs.

TABLE 7-3. Fruit and Vegetable Group

FRUITS AND VEGETABLES RICH IN VITAMIN C		
oranges	cantaloupe	collard greens
grapefruit	guavas	turnip greens
limes	tomatoes	watercress
lemons	cabbage	kale
tangerines	broccoli	parsley
strawberries	Brussels sprouts	green and red peppers

FRUITS AND VEGETABLES RICH IN VITAMIN A		
collard and beet greens	watercress	apricots
Swiss chard	winter squash	cantaloupe
chicory	carrots	mangoes
escarole	pumpkin	papayas
kale	sweet potatoes	
spinach	yams	

The best sources of vitamin C are the juicy fruits and the dark green vegetables. Fruits and vegetables which are dark green or yellow are good sources of vitamin A. Sometimes the same fruit or vegetable is an excellent source of both vitamins A and C. At least one serving from the fruit and vegetable group should be selected from those high in vitamin A and one from those high in vitamin C. The remaining two or more servings can be selected according to taste from other available vegetables and fruits. It is important that care be taken during the preparation of these foods so as to minimize any nutrient loss.

MILK AND MILK PRODUCTS GROUP

All types of milk and milk products are included in this group. Butter is excluded because of its very high fat content, and proportionately low protein and calcium content. This group provides proteins, fats, carbohydrates, calcium, phosphorus, vitamin A,

TABLE 7-4 Milk and Milk Products Group

TYPES OF MILK	TYPES OF MILK PRODUCTS
whole milk	yogurt
skim milk	cheese
evaporated milk	ice cream
condensed milk	ice milk
dry milk	
buttermilk	

riboflavin, and niacin. Fortified milk or fortified milk products also contain vitamin D.

The number of servings varies according to age and condition. The serving size is 8 fluid ounces of milk or its equivalent according to calcium content. The following dairy foods contain calcium equal to that found in one cup of milk:

- two 1-inch cubes of cheddar cheese

- 1-1/2 cups of cottage cheese
- 1-1/2 cups of ice cream or ice milk

It must be noted that milk used in making cream sauces, gravies, or baked products should be counted as part of the requirement. A cheese sandwich would fulfill one of the serving requirements and a serving of ice cream or ice milk could fulfill half of one of the serving requirements. These examples show that drinking milk is not the only way to fulfill the milk requirement.

THE BREAD AND CEREAL GROUP

All whole grain, enriched, or restored breads and cereals are included in the bread and cereal group. This group provides carbohydrate, thiamine, niacin, B_6, iron, phosphorus, and magnesium.

The average person should have **4 or more servings** daily from the bread and cereal group. Each of the following constitutes one serving: 1 slice of bread, 1 roll, 1 biscuit, about 2/3 cup cooked cereal, and 1 cup dry cereal.

THE MEAT GROUP

All meats, fish, poultry, eggs, and meat *alternates* (substitutes) are included in this group. Foods from the meat group provide protein, some fat, iron, copper, sodium, potassium, chloride, magnesium, phosphorus, zinc, vitamins A, B complex, and D.

One should have **2 or more servings** from this group each day. Approximately three ounces of boneless meat, poultry, fish, or meat alternate constitute one serving. Meat alternates such as beans and nuts can be good sources of protein and are usually less expensive than meats, fish and poultry.

SUMMARY

The simplest and most efficient method of maintaining a balanced diet is to plan meals

TABLE 7-5 Recommended Servings of Milk Per Day

Children under 9 years	2 to 3 servings
Children 9 to 12	3 or more servings
Teenagers	4 or more servings
Adults	2 or more servings
Pregnant women	4 or more servings
Mothers who are breast feeding	4 or more servings

TABLE 7-6 Bread and Cereal Group

breads
  whole wheat
  dark rye
  enriched
cornmeal, whole grain or enriched
rolls or biscuits made with whole wheat or enriched flour
flour, enriched
  whole wheat, other whole grain
oatmeal bread
grits, enriched

cereals
  whole wheat
  rolled oats
  brown rice
  converted rice
  other cereals, if whole grain or restored
noodles, spaghetti, macaroni

TABLE 7-7 Meat Group

MEATS	MEAT ALTERNATES
beef	dried beans
lamb	dried peas
veal	lentils
pork, except bacon	nuts
organ meats, such as heart, liver, kidney brain, tongue, sweetbread	peanuts
	peanut butter
	soybean flour
	soybeans
poultry, such as chicken, duck, goose, turkey	
fish, shellfish	
lunch meats such as bologna liverwurst	

using the Basic Four food groups as a guide. These four groups are: vegetables and fruits; milk and milk products; meats; and breads and cereals. Each group has a specified number of servings required. Other foods may be added as desired if the requirements of the Basic Four are not eliminated and if the other foods do not raise the total caloric value of the diet above that recommended.

DISCUSSION TOPICS

1. Name the Basic Four food groups. Of what value are they when planning meals?

2. What groups of nutrients are provided in the vegetable and fruit group? The milk group? The meat group? The bread and cereal group?

3. How does the careful use of the Basic Four food groups eliminate the need to check menus with a chart of the recommended daily dietary allowances?

4. Discuss the sale of hollow calorie foods in school cafeterias. Is it a good policy? If so, why? If not, why not? What would your position be on this subject if you were principal of an elementary school? Of a junior or senior high school?

SUGGESTED ACTIVITIES

a. Visit a meat market and identify the various meat group sources (sweetbreads, muscle meats, shellfish, etc.). What essential nutrients does each of these foods provide? Price these foods at the store. Look up a recipe for each and explain its preparation to the class. If possible, prepare it for the class.

b. Organize a campaign to educate your fellow students in regard to the Basic Four food groups. Consider using classroom and lunchroom bulletin boards, flyers, assembly programs with speakers or a short play and lunchroom demonstrations of foods and their preparation.

c. Buy some fruits and vegetables that are new to you. Bring these to class, prepare and sample them. Perhaps these might be added to your home menus from time to time.

d. Using a restaurant menu, choose a breakfast, lunch, and dinner. Check the selection of foods used with the Basic Four food groups. Are they balanced meals? Discuss the problems which people who eat all their meals in restaurants might have in maintaining a well-balanced diet.

e. Using the following table, fill in the "Menus" column with the foods eaten in the past two days. In the "Food Groups Used" column list the groups to which each food belongs. To evaluate personal dietary habits, fill in the "Food Groups Not Used" column. Compare the table with those of the rest of the class and discuss how eating habits may be improved.

	MENUS	FOOD GROUPS USED	FOOD GROUPS NOT USED
Breakfast			
Lunch			
Dinner			
Snacks			

WORD STUDY

balanced diet	edible portion	serving size
Basic Four food groups	meat alternate	sweetbreads

REVIEW

Multiple Choice. Select the *letter* which precedes the best answer.

1. A balanced diet is one that includes
    a. equal amounts of carbohydrates and fats
    b. no animal products
    c. all six essential nutrients
    d. more vegetables than fruits

2. The Basic Four food groups include
    a. vegetables and fruits   c. breads and cereals
    b. milk and meats   d. all of these

3. The size of a serving from the meat group should be approximately
    a. 1/4 pound   c. 3 ounces
    b. 1 ounce   d. 1/2 pound

4. Foods included in the normal diet should
    a. provide enough calories to satisfy energy requirements
    b. contain an adequate amount of the essential nutrients
    c. be based on the Basic Four food groups
    d. all of the above

5. When a food lends satiety to meals, it
    a. is always fattening
    b. provides enormous amounts of bulk
    c. gives satisfaction
    d. is very chewy

6. When planning meals
    a. the nutrient content of meals is the main consideration
    b. both nutrient content and caloric value must be considered
    c. only the caloric value need be considered
    d. none of the above is true

7. Fruits and vegetables should be eaten
    a. no more than twice a day
    b. no more than three times a week
    c. at least four times a day
    d. at least six times a day

8. Fruits and vegetables are rich sources of
    a. vitamins   c. proteins
    b. fats   d. all of these

9. Teenagers should have a serving of milk (or its substitute)
    a. not more than twice a day
    b. at least four times a day
    c. not more than four times a week
    d. not at all if they are overweight

10. Milk products are made from milk and include
    a. butter and margarine
    b. yogurt and cottage cheese
    c. bean curd and coconut milk
    d. all of the above

11. Milk and its products provide rich sources of
    a. proteins and fats
    b. carbohydrates
    c. minerals and vitamins
    d. all of the above

12. Breads and cereals should be eaten at least
    a. once a day   c. three times a day
    b. twice a day   d. four times a day

13. Breads and cereals are rich sources of
    a. vitamin D   c. carbohydrates
    b. fats   d. all of these

14. Foods from the meat group should be served at least
    a. once a day   c. three times a day
    b. twice a day   d. four times a day

15. Foods from the meat group are rich sources of
    a. proteins   c. vitamin C
    b. carbohydrates   d. all of these

Chapter 8
Planning Appetizing Meals

OBJECTIVES

After studying this chapter, the student should be able to:

- State and define criteria for planning appetizing meals.
- Identify the purpose of a menu pattern.
- Adapt a menu pattern to suit individual requirements or preferences.

To build and maintain healthy bodies, the knowledge of basic nutrition must be combined with imagination when planning meals. Appetite appeal is as important as nutritive value in meal planning because the best food is nutritious only when it is eaten. Although the Basic Four food groups serve as the elementary guide in meal planning, the following criteria must also be considered: variety, appearance, flavor and aroma, texture, satiety, and individual likes and dislikes.

Variety

Even favorite foods become less interesting when they are prepared day after day without variation. The finest cut of steak is no longer appetizing if it is served seven days a week. It is important to consider variety within each of the Basic Four food groups each day.

Appearance

Because the initial reaction to food is based on its appearance, it is essential to consider the colors and shapes of food when planning meals. Colors and shapes should vary and blend in a harmonious way. Although a meal of tomato soup, corned beef, red cabbage, beets, and raspberry sherbet is nutritious, it lacks variety in color. Melon balls, fish balls, small boiled potatoes, brussels sprouts, and cherries lack variety in shape.

Flavor and Aroma

Flavor and aroma are so closely related that they are best considered together. Imagine eating a meal of onion soup, spiced sausage, mustard, sauerkraut, and hot peppers. Compare it, in terms of flavor and aroma, with a meal of chicken consomme, unspiced veal, mashed potatoes, and custard. Both

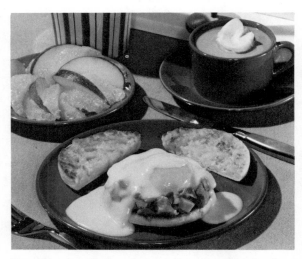

Fig. 8-1 Breakfast can stimulate the appetite by a pleasing variety of shape and color of food. *(Courtesy of National Dairy Council)*

menus are unappetizing. The first has too many foods with strong flavor and aroma, and the second has an excess of bland foods. *Bland* foods have mild flavors.

Texture

The *texture* (consistency or feel) of foods must also vary. Wouldn't cream soup, baked fish, mashed potatoes, squash, and rice pudding make a dull meal? On the other hand, jaws would tire while eating a meal in which all of the foods required considerable chewing.

Satiety

A feeling of satiety, or satisfying fullness in the stomach, should linger after a meal, but the individual should not feel as if he or she has overeaten. One reason meals should include some protein and fat is that these nutrients stay in the stomach longer than carbohydrates, thus giving satiety value to the meal. Carbohydrate is necessary, however, to satisfy taste and provide quick energy.

Individual Likes and Dislikes

It is especially important to consider the individual likes and dislikes of various family members. If a particular food is disliked by everyone, it may be possible to substitute its nutritional equal. When a particular food is disliked by only one member of the family, it is advisable to serve it during that person's absence. Naturally, family and religious customs are respected when planning meals.

THE MENU PATTERN

A pattern must be used in planning a meal just as in sewing a garment. Figure 8-2 shows basic menu patterns for a day, based on the Basic Four food groups. Evaluate them in terms of nutritional adequacy. Most people add to the basic patterns.

The menus in figure 8-3 are based on the menu patterns in figure 8-2. Evaluate them in terms of nutritional adequacy, attractiveness, economy, and efficiency of preparation.

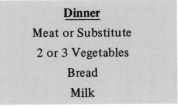

Breakfast	Lunch	Dinner
Fruit	Meat or Substitute	Meat or Substitute
Cereal	Fruit or Vegetable	2 or 3 Vegetables
Bread	Bread	Bread
Milk	Milk	Milk

Fig. 8-2 A day's menu pattern is formed from the Basic Four food groups.

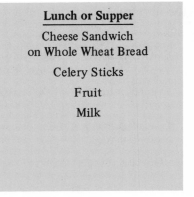

Breakfast	Dinner	Lunch or Supper
Orange Juice	Meat Loaf	Cheese Sandwich on Whole Wheat Bread
Cereal	Baked Potato	Celery Sticks
Milk-Sugar	Corn Pudding	Fruit
Toast	Coleslaw	Milk
Butter-Jelly	Bread-Butter	
Milk	Ice Cream	
(Coffee for adults)	Milk	
	(Coffee, Tea for adults)	

Fig. 8-3 These three meals demonstrate how foods are selected from menu patterns.

Adapting the Menu Pattern

Sometimes there are family members such as young children, elderly people, or the ill, who are unable to conform to the family meal plan. In such circumstances the menu should be adapted to suit the person with the particular needs. This means minor changes are made in the basic plan.

Individual variations in the menu should require little or no extra preparation. Suppose the sample menu were planned for a family which included a young couple, a 3-year-old boy, and an 80-year-old grandmother. The foods served should appeal to everyone and be easy for the elderly woman and the child to chew and digest.

In figure 8-3, breakfast is especially adaptable because a variety of ready-to-eat cereals can be served. The remaining foods on the menu should be suitable for everyone. The coleslaw on the sample dinner menu might present a problem, but a substitution of a cooked vegetable for the grandmother and the little boy could solve it. For lunch or supper, the cheese sandwiches might be made with enriched white bread instead of whole wheat, and a cooked vegetable could be substituted for the celery sticks. If a fresh fruit is served for dessert, it should be something easily chewed and digested, such as a banana.

If a member of the family is ill, that person may require a special diet prescribed by the doctor. Even in such cases, the family menu should be adapted whenever possible to save time and expense in preparation and to make the patient feel that he or she is not causing extra work.

Weekly Planning

Efficiency in planning is increased by planning meals for several days or a week at one time. It is also economical to plan several meals at one time to allow for adequate use of leftovers, figure 8-4. The nurse as well as the homemaker soon learns that practical shortcuts are invaluable. Modern convenience foods may be used as often as the budget and family desires will allow. *Convenience foods* are partially prepared foods such as frozen foods, baking mixes, TV dinners, etc. Meals that can be prepared in the oven are efficient and economical.

SUMMARY

The Basic Four food groups serve as a guide for planning nutritionally sound menus. To stimulate appetites, meals should provide satiety value and variety in color, flavor, aroma, texture, and shape. Menus should be flexible so they can be easily adapted to the special needs of individual family members. This flexibility helps save time and money. Planning several meals at one time is efficient and economical. The use of leftovers, convenience foods, and oven meals should be considered in weekly planning.

VEGETABLES AND FRUITS

COOKED SNAP BEANS, LIMA BEANS, CORN, PEAS and CARROTS: casseroles, croquettes, meat and vegetable pie, salads, sauces, souffles, soup, stew, stuffed peppers, stuffed tomatoes, vegetables in cheese sauce

COOKED LEAFY VEGETABLES (CHOPPED): creamed vegetables, soup, meat loaf, meat patties, omelet, souffle

COOKED POTATOES: croquettes, fried or creamed potatoes, meat-pie topping, potatoes in cheese sauce, stew or chowder

COOKED or CANNED FRUITS: fruit cup, fruit sauces, jellied fruit, quick breads, salads, shortcake, upsidedown cake, yeast breads

Fig. 8-4 Using leftovers from the Basic Four food groups (continued)

━━━━━━━━━ MILK & MILK PRODUCTS ━━━━━━━━━

SOUR MILK: cakes, cookies, quick breads

SOUR CREAM: cakes, cookies, dessert sauces, meat stews, pie or cake fillings, salad dressing, sauce for vegetables

━━━━━━━━━ BREADS & CEREALS ━━━━━━━━━

COOKED WHEAT, OAT and CORN CEREALS: fried cereal, meat loaf or patties, souffles, sweet puddings

COOKED RICE, NOODLES, MACARONI and SPAGHETTI: casseroles, meat or cheese loaf, timbales

STALE BREAD: slices for French toast, dry crumbs for apple betty, croquettes, fondues, coating for fried chops, soft crumbs for bread pudding, meat loaf, stuffings

CAKE and COOKIES: apple betty, cake balls with fruit or chocolate sauce, cottage pudding, crumb crust pies, refrigerator cake, trifle (cake strips with custard sauce)

━━━━━━━━━ MEAT ━━━━━━━━━

EGG YOLKS: cakes, cookies, cornstarch pudding, custard and custard sauce, eggnog, pie and cake fillings, salad dressing, sauce for vegetables

EGG WHITES: cakes, frostings, fruit whip, meringue, souffles

HARD-COOKED EGG or YOLK: casserole dishes, garnish, salads, sandwiches

COOKED MEATS, POULTRY and FISH: casserole dishes, hash, meat patties, meat pies, salads, sandwiches, stuffed vegetables

Fig. 8-4 Using leftovers from the Basic Four food groups

DISCUSSION TOPICS

1. What criteria, in addition to the Basic Four food groups, should be considered when planning family meals? Why?

2. Evaluate the menu in figure 8-3 in terms of its appetite appeal.

3. How may leftover meats be used?

4. How may leftover vegetables be used?

5. Why is it advisable to adapt the family meal to suit the special needs of the patient rather than prepare a separate meal for the patient?

6. Discuss the advantages and disadvantages of convenience foods.

SUGGESTED ACTIVITIES

a. Visit a local supermarket and make a list of the various convenience foods available. Compare their prices to the same foods that have not been partially prepared.

b. Look up recipes which use leftover roast beef. Present them to the class.

c. Plan a week's menu for a family of four who have no special dietary needs. Use the sample menus as a guide for listing the foods in proper order. Consider each of the following criteria in planning the menu:

nutritive quality   attractiveness
economy   efficiency of preparation

d. Select a menu for one day from the planned menu in activity c. Adapt it for a visiting grandmother who has difficulty chewing.

WORD STUDY

aroma	convenience foods	flavor
bland	custom	texture
consistency		

REVIEW

A.   Multiple Choice. Select the *letter* which precedes the best answer.

1. An example of a meal plan that lacks variety is preparing
   a. two vegetables for dinner every day
   b. various dishes using meat each day
   c. a fried egg with cinnamon toast each morning
   d. fruit for lunch and dinner on the same day

2. Food products that are partially prepared commercially are called
   a. hollow calorie foods   c. bland foods
   b. convenience foods   d. brand name foods

3. The appearance of food refers to the way it
   a. tastes   c. looks
   b. smells   d. all of these

4. The flavor of food refers to its
   a. taste   c. satiety value
   b. smell   d. cost

5. The aroma of food refers to its
   a. appearance   c. taste
   b. smell   d. satiety value

6. The texture of consistency of food refers to its
   a. appearance   c. aroma
   b. feel   d. satiety value

7. Menus should be evaluated in terms of
   a. nutritional adequacy
   b. attractiveness and economy
   c. efficiency of preparation
   d. all of the above

8. Changing a menu to meet the special needs of a family member is called
   a. planning the menu
   b. adapting the menu
   c. the pattern of the menu
   d. varying the menu

9. Two examples of bland foods are
   a. grapefruit and oranges
   b. mashed potatoes and custard
   c. Italian sausage and salami
   d. all of the above

10. Foods which provide satiety value
    a. also provide large amounts of vitamin C
    b. give a lasting feeling of satisfying fullness in the stomach
    c. are those which all family members like
    d. are sugars and starches

B. Plan two dinners, selecting menus from the foods listed below. Consider variety in color, texture, and flavor. Adapt the steak menu to suit an 80-year-old woman who finds it difficult to chew.

Baked halibut, broiled steak, creamed corn, stewed tomatoes, jellied vegetable salad, tossed green salad, mashed potatoes, baked potatoes, cherry upside-down cake, rice pudding with pineapple.

C. Briefly answer the following questions.

1. In addition to the Basic Four food groups, name seven other criteria which should be considered when planning meals.

2. Why should several meals be planned at one time?

3. Why is it important for a meal to be attractive?

Chapter 9
Developing Good Eating Habits

OBJECTIVES

After studying this chapter, the student should be able to:

- Identify at least three bad eating habits.
- Describe the development of food customs.
- List some food habits of various age groups and cultural groups.
- Adapt a menu for a cultural group with strict dietary laws.

The rules of good nutrition are more easily recited than practiced. It is important not only to study these rules, but to follow them daily. It is much easier to help other people correct their eating habits after evaluating and correcting one's own eating habits.

Some of the most common bad eating habits include eating an excess of foods containing fats and carbohydrates, attempting to control weight gain by crash reducing diets, and skipping meals. Obesity and/or malnutrition may be caused by an excess of carbohydrates or fats in the diet. This is especially true if foods containing these two nutrients are substituted for foods containing the other essential nutrients. *Crash reducing diets* typically consist of only a narrow selection of foods, thus limiting the types of nutrients obtained. Skipping meals also limits the intake of nutrients. Ironically, this may also cause an increase in the total daily caloric intake since one is apt to overeat after being without food for a long period of time. Habits are not easily changed. However, the key to change rests on understanding the reasons eating patterns develop.

FOOD CUSTOMS

People from each country have favorite foods. Frequently, there are distinctive food customs originating in just a small section or area of a particular country. Some religions demand particular food customs. Because most people prefer the foods they were accustomed to while growing up, food habits are often based on nationality and religion.

When people move from one country to another, or from one area to another, their economic circumstances sometimes change. They may be introduced to new foods and new food customs. Although their original food customs may have been nutritionally adequate, their new environment may cause them to change their eating habits. For example, if milk was a staple in their diet before moving and is unusually expensive in the new environment, milk may be replaced by a nutritionally inferior beverage such as soda, coffee, or tea. Candy, a luxury in their former environment, may be inexpensive and popular in their new environment. As a result, a family might increase consumption of candy and reduce purchases of a more nutritious food. Someone who is not familiar

TABLE 9-1 Cultural Food Habits

Group	Foods Most Used	Possible Deficiencies

Greek
 	
Turkish
 	
Armenian
	Goat's milk, cheese, yogurt
	Vegetables cooked in olive oil —
	    peas, beans, lentils
	Salads in oil, vinegar
	Fruits — nuts — pastry
	Meat — lamb in combination with rice
	    and vegetables
	Cracked wheat
		Butter
		Potatoes
		Fresh fruits
		Raw vegetables
		Meat

Italian	Pastas (macaroni products)
	Sausages, veal, pressed meat, bread,
	    spaghetti
	Tomato, cheese sauces, olive oil
	Green vegetables, fresh fruits, goat's
	    milk, cheese (if cost does not
	    prohibit)
	Highly seasoned food
		Milk
		Fresh meats
		Without a garden
		    they will lack
		    fresh vegetables
		    and fruits of
		    prohibitive
		    cost
		Lack of iron and
		    other minerals
		Lack of whole
		    grain cereals

U.S. South	Hot breads, corn bread, rice, sweet
	    potatoes, hominy grits, greens, beans,
	    black-eyed peas cooked with fresh or
	    salt pork
	Game meat
	Fish, chicken, watermelon, molasses
		Milk, butter,
		    cheese, eggs,
		    meat, raw
		    vegetables

U.S
Mid-West
	Meat (beef, pork) potatoes,
	    gravies
	Canned and frozen vegetables
	Bread and cakes
	Dairy products
		Salads
		Green and raw
		    vegetables
		Minerals

Chinese	Vegetables, dried and fresh
	    meats, small amounts of fish
	    and poultry, pork
	Rice or wheat cereals
		Low in fat, milk,
		    cream or butter
		    and raw vegetables
		Insufficient meat
		    and green and
		    yellow vegetables
		Vitamins A, B, C

Mexican	Dried beans, chili peppers, corn, rice,
	    tortillas, tomatoes,
	    fruits
		Whole grain cereals
		    (other than corn)
		Milk

Puerto- Rican	Rice, beans Plantains Beef, chicken, and pork	Eggs Milk Fresh vegetables

TABLE 9-1   Cultural Food Habits (cont'd.)

Group	Foods Most Used	Possible Deficiencies
Jewish	Fish (fresh and salt) and smoked meat (beef, veal organs) Chicken (always on Sabbath) Meat and vegetable soup Rich pastries Whole grain breads and cereals Noodles, matzos (at Passover) Milk, cheese dishes Dried fruit and nuts Highly seasoned foods Horseradish	Low in fresh fruit and vegetables

with the nutritive values of foods can easily make such mistakes in their food selection. Food customs are largely influenced by the foods that are easily available and least expensive.

The meal patterns of nationalities and religious groups different from one's own may seem strange. However, the foods used often fall into the Basic Four food groups making the diet nutritionally adequate. When a patient's eating habits need to be corrected, such corrections are easier if the food customs of the patient are known. To gain this knowledge, it is advisable to talk with the patient and learn about his background. This knowledge can be used to plan nourishing menus consisting of foods that are appetizing to the patient. The necessary adjustments in the diet can then be made gradually and effectively.

Specific Cultural Diet Patterns

Specific cultural diet patterns are given in table 9-1. Certain religious restrictions may also influence dietary habits.

- Seventh Day Adventists do not eat meat, fish, or poultry.

- Mormons do not drink coffee or tea.

- Orthodox Jewish people follow the restrictions given in figure 9-1.

- Roman Catholics may refrain from eating meat on certain fast days.

In addition to religious restrictions, one can see the effect of culture on diet by comparing food habits of selected groups in Table 9-1.

NUTRITIONAL NEEDS OF VARIOUS AGE GROUPS

Good nutrition is essential for people of all ages. However, each age group has its own special nutritional needs and problems.

Childhood

Although specific nutritional requirements change as children grow, nutrition always affects physical, mental, and emotional growth and development. Studies indicate that the size and mental ability of an individual are directly influenced by the diet during the early years. Children who have an inadequate supply of proteins and calories during their early years may be shorter and less intellectually able than children who receive an adequate diet.

When people develop poor eating habits as children, they are apt to continue them throughout their lives. Poor dietary habits can aggravate emotional and physical problems such as irritability, anxiety, fatigue, and even illness. Because children learn partly by imitation, learning good eating habits is easier if the parents have good eating habits. Nutritious foods should be available at snack time as well as at mealtime.

Forbidden Foods

Flesh of animals without cloven (split) hoof or which do not chew their cud.
Hindquarters of any animals. Shellfish.
Fish without scales or fins. Fowl that are birds of prey. All creeping things and insects.

Rules in Food Preparation or Consumption

Slaughtering must be done by a qualified person and in a prescribed manner. The meat or poultry must be drained of blood, first by severing the jugular vein and carotid artery, then by soaking in brine before cooking.
Meat or meat products may not be prepared or eaten with milk or milk products.
The dishes used in the preparation and serving of one must be kept separate from the other.
A specified time, 6 hours, must elapse between consumption of meat and milk.
The mouth must be rinsed after eating fish and before eating meat.
There are prescribed fast days — Passover Week, Yom Kippur and Feast of Purim.
No cooking is done on the Sabbath — from sundown Friday to sundown Saturday.
Food may not be used from a Kosher market that remains open on the Sabbath.

Fig. 9-1   The Orthodox Jewish group follows strict dietary laws.

It is important to remember that because the rate of growth is not constant, children's appetites vary. Their likes and dislikes also may change. It may be helpful to introduce new foods gradually. Allowing the child to assist in marketing and in the preparation of a new food is often a good way of arousing interest in the food and a desire to eat it. Children very often prefer foods that are simply prepared and are fearful of foods covered by sauce or gravy.

Adolescence

Adolescence is typically a period of rapid growth which is accompanied by an enormous appetite. When good eating habits have been established during childhood and there is nutritious food available, the teenager's food habits should present no problem.

Adolescents are imitators, like children, but instead of imitating adults, adolescents prefer to imitate their peers and do what is popular. Unfortunately, the foods that are popular are often hollow calorie foods such as potato chips, sodas, and candy. Hollow calorie foods provide mainly carbohydrates and some fat, and almost no proteins, minerals, or vitamins.

When the adolescent's food habits need improvement, it is wise for the adult to tactfully inform him of his nutritional needs and of the inferiority of the hollow calorie foods. The adolescent has a natural desire for independence and may resent being told what to do.

Before attempting to change an adolescent's food habits, his or her food choices should be carefully checked for nutrient content. It is too easily assumed that because the adolescent chooses the food, the food is automatically a poor choice in regard to nutrient content. This is not always the case. Some favorite foods of teenagers such as pizza, franks, hamburgers, milk shakes, and hot chocolate (if made with milk) contain many of the essential nutrients. These same foods also have relatively high caloric values. If the adolescent has a problem maintaining a minimum weight, he or she may need some advice in regard to diet.

Middle Age

Middle age is a period when the physical activities of young adulthood typically begin to decrease, resulting in a lowered caloric requirement for most individuals. At this age women seldom have young children to supervise, and the strenuous physical labor of some male occupations is delegated to younger men. Middle-aged people may tire more easily than they did when they were younger. Therefore, they may not get as much exercise during their leisure hours as they did in earlier years. Because appetite and food intake may not decrease, there is a common tendency toward overweight during this period. It is wise to compare the Recommended Daily Dietary Requirements with the actual nutrients and calories consumed by the middle-aged individual in a typical day. This would indicate to the individual that an adjustment may need to be made.

Although the nutritional needs for growth have disappeared by middle age, the nutritional needs for a constant state of good health remain. The healthy body continues replacing worn out cells and producing heat and energy until death.

Old Age

If the established food habits of the older person are poor, such habits will undoubtedly have been a long time in the making. These habits will not be easy to change. Poor food habits which begin during old age have more complex causes. Decreased income during retirement, physical disability, and inadequate cooking facilities may cause difficulties in food selection and preparation. Anorexia caused by grief, loneliness, boredom, or difficulty in chewing may decrease food consumption. The adjustment of food habits depends upon a consideration of the individual's total situation.

A person's typical daily food intake should be compared with the Recommended Daily Dietary Requirements. However, older people's needs vary considerably. Consequently the older person should be examined by a doctor to determine specific requirements. Generally, caloric requirements are reduced, largely because physical activity is reduced.

TABLE 9-2   Energy Needs for Various Ages

	Age (years)	Weight (kg)	Weight (lbs)	Height (cm)	Height (in)	Energy (kcal)[b]
Infants	0.0-0.5	6	14	60	24	kgx117
	0.5-1.0	9	20	71	28	kgx108
Children	1-3	13	28	86	34	1,300
	4-6	20	44	110	44	1,800
	7-10	30	66	135	54	2,400
Males	11-14	44	97	158	63	2,800
	15-18	61	134	172	69	3,000
	19-22	67	147	172	69	3,000
	23-50	70	154	172	69	2,700
	51+	70	154	172	69	2,400
Females	11-14	44	97	155	62	2,400
	15-18	54	119	162	65	2,100
	19-22	58	128	162	65	2,100
	23-50	58	128	162	65	2,000
	51+	58	128	162	65	1,800
Pregnant						+300
Lactating						+500

Source: Food and Nutrition Board, National Academy of Sciences — National Research Council, 1974

SUMMARY

Food habits usually originate from national or religious customs. When such customs result in inadequate diets, corrections should be made gradually. Corrections are easier and more effectively made when the reasons for the food habits are understood.

DISCUSSION TOPICS

1. Discuss the reasons why nurses and homemakers should practice the rules of good nutrition themselves.

2. How do food habits originate?

3. From personal experience, explain why certain foods are enjoyed more than others that are commonly available in the local area.

4. What effects does environment have on particular food habits? When do the effects of a new environment improve diets and when do they impair them?

5. Discuss the dangers of skipping meals.

SUGGESTED ACTIVITIES

a. Give a series of short reports on food customs. Each student should select a different country or area within a country for study. After the reports have been presented, hold a class discussion on whether climate, availability of food, and economic factors determine the food customs of the country studied. Include the following points in the reports.

What is the climate of the country? What crops are grown? Are modern methods of agriculture used? Does the country have to depend on imports for a large part of its food supply? If so, what foods are imported? Is a large part of the population poor? What foods are most popular? Are they produced in the country itself? Are they expensive or cheap?

b. Plan a menu for a Roman Catholic fast day.

c. Investigate the lunch program of a local school. Have a panel discussion on its purpose, limitations, favorable characteristics, and suggested improvements.

d. Make attractive posters for the school lunchroom or cafeteria in which the improvement of eating habits is stressed.

WORD STUDY

adolescence	cultural	fast day
beverage	environment	peer
crash reducing diet	family custom	religious custom

REVIEW

A. Multiple Choice. Select the *letter* preceding the best answer.

1. Food customs means one's
   a. food nutrients
   b. food habits
   c. food requirements
   d. all of the above

2. Some bad eating habits which are common include
   a. skipping meals
   b. eating an excess of carbohydrates and fats
   c. using crash reducing diets
   d. all of the above

3. The basis for food customs may be
    a. religion
    b. nationality
    c. foods available locally
    d. all of these

4. Moving to a new environment or experiencing a change in salary
    a. rarely changes established food habits
    b. usually influences established food habits
    c. always reduces the amount of food eaten
    d. never reduces the quality of food eaten

5. Crash reducing diets
    a. may limit the types of nutrients obtained
    b. are an acceptable way to control weight gain
    c. contain a wide selection of foods
    d. all of the above

6. Diet during childhood directly influences the individual's
    a. size
    b. mental ability
    c. physical development
    d. all of these

7. As a rule, adolescents
    a. avoid hollow calorie foods
    b. present no problems in regard to food habits
    c. eat very small quantities
    d. imitate the food habits of their peers

8. During middle age,
    a. appetites automatically decrease
    b. caloric requirements are often reduced
    c. the body stops replacing worn cells and tissues
    d. all of the above

9. When food habits change during old age, the reason may be
    a. decreased income
    b. physical disabilities
    c. anorexia
    d. all of these

10. A diet of dried beans, corn and chili peppers would most likely be used by a (an)
    a. Mexican family
    b. Italian family
    c. Armenian family
    d. Orthodox Jewish family

B. Adapt the following menu for a person of the Orthodox Jewish faith, using figure 9-1.

    Baked Ham

    Scalloped Potatoes

    Buttered Peas

    Bread and Butter

    Fresh Fruit

    Milk or Coffee

Chapter 10
Evaluating and Preserving Food Quality

OBJECTIVES

After studying this chapter, the student should be able to:

- State the criteria for evaluating the quality of meat, poultry, fish, eggs, vegetables, and fruit.
- Describe methods of storing and cooking various kinds of food in order to preserve nutrient content.
- Identify the different types of milk and explain how milk is pasteurized.
- State why food additives are used.

Today's supermarkets provide such a variety of foods that it is essential for the *consumer* (one who buys and uses marketed items) to be able to determine the *nutritional value* (nutrient content) of foods. In addition, the consumer should have a basic knowledge of quality, appropriate uses, preparation, and storage of foods in order to buy wisely. There is no use in purchasing a food just because it is rich in a specified nutrient if the food cannot be properly stored or prepared.

Today's consumer may also be interested in food additives. *Food additives* are chemical substances added to food during the processing, storage, or packaging. There are two types of additives: the intentional additives which are added to perform specific functions in food, and the incidental additives which were not intentionally added, but which may be there as a result of some stage of production or packaging. All additives are chemicals. However, some additives are produced in nature and some are produced in laboratories. Additives are added to various foods to enrich nutrient content, retard spoilage, enhance flavor, or to maintain appearance,

consistency and texture, tables 10-1 and 10-2. Salt is one of the earliest known additives.

There is controversy regarding the addition of additives to foods. The food industry maintains that without some additives, foods would not grow or keep as well as they now do. Without additives, an increase in food spoilage could increase food costs. Some people want additives eliminated altogether on grounds that additives may cause disease. The Federal Food and Drug Administration (FDA) requires proof of the safety of food additives. However, scientific measures of safety change with ongoing research.

BEVERAGES

Beverages are fluids which relieve thirst, aid in regulating body processes, and provide nourishment. Water is the base of all beverages. It is usually served in addition to another beverage at meals. Water is necessary to regulate body processes.

Milk is an important beverage because of its high nutritive value. Chocolate flavored syrup or eggs may be added to increase its nutritive and caloric value or change its flavor.

TABLE 10-1. Reasons for Using Additives

To impart and maintain desired consistency—emulsifiers distribute tiny particles of one liquid in another to improve texture homogeneity and quality. Stabilizers and thickeners give smooth uniform texture and flavor and desired consistency.

To improve nutritive value—medical and public health authorities endorse this use to eliminate and prevent certain diseases involving malnutrition. Iodized salt has eliminated simple goiter. Vitamin D in dairy products and infant foods has virtually eliminated rickets. Niacin in bread, cornmeal and cereals has eliminated pellagra in the southern states.

To enhance flavor—many spices and natural and synthetic flavors give us a desired variety of flavorful foods such as spice cake, gingerbread and sausage.

To control acidity or alkalinity—leavening agents are used in the baking industry in cakes, biscuits, waffles, muffins and other foods. Similar additives make fruits and potatoes easier to peel for canning; others neutralize sour cream in making butter.

To maintain appearance, palatability and wholesomeness—by delaying deterioration of food due to microbial growth or oxidation. Food spoilage caused by mold, bacteria and yeast is prevented or slowed by certain additives. Antioxidants keep fats from turning rancid and certain fresh fruits from darkening during processing when cut and exposed to air.

To give desired and characteristic color—to increase acceptability and attractiveness by correcting objectionable natural variations.

To mature and bleach—and to modify gluten to improve baking, to improve appearance of certain cheeses and to meet the desire for white wheat flour by changing the natural yellow pigments.

Other functions—such as humectants to retain moisture in some foods and to keep others, including salts and powders, free-flowing.

Source: Manufacturing Chemists Association

TABLE 10-2. Additives and the Foods in which they are Used

ADDITIVE	FOODS
lecithin, mono- and diglycerides, gum arabic, agar-agar, methyl cellulose	baked goods, cake mixes, salad dressings, frozen desserts, ice cream, chocolate milk, beer
vitamin A, thiamine, niacin, riboflavin, ascorbic acid, vitamin D, iron, potassium iodide	wheat flour, bread and biscuits, breakfast cereals, corn meal, macaroni and noodle products, margarine, milk, iodized salt
cloves, ginger, citrus oils, amyl acetate, carvone, benzaldehyde	spice cake, gingerbread, ice cream, candy, soft drinks, fruit-flavored gelatins, fruit-flavored toppings, sausage
potassium acid tartrate, tartaric acid, sodium bicarbonate, citric acid, lactic acid	cakes, cookies, quick breads, crackers, butter, process cheese, cheese spreads, chocolates, soft drinks
propionic acid, sodium and calcium salts of propionic acid, ascorbic acid, butylated hydroxyanisole, butylated hydroxytoluene	bread, cheese, syrup, pie fillings, crackers, fruit juices, frozen and dried fruit, margarine, lard, shortening, potato chips, cake mixes
FDA approved colors, such as: annatto, carotene, cochineal, chlorophyll	confections, bakery goods, soft drinks, cheeses, ice cream, jams and jellies
chlorine dioxide, chlorine, potassium bromate and iodate	wheat flour, certain cheeses
glycerine, magnesium carbonate	coconut, table salt

Source: Manufacturing Chemists Association

Vegetable and fruit juices are refreshing, provide vitamins, especially vitamin C, and stimulate appetites. Fruit juices should be kept cold, covered, and in *opaque* (blocks out light) containers in order to preserve their flavor and vitamin content. Fruit drinks (not juices) and carbonated beverages usually provide only calories in the form of sugar, and sometimes additives.

Coffee and tea have no food value without cream or sugar. Coffee contains the stimulant *caffeine* and tea contains the stimulant *theine*. These stimulants make them inappropriate for children. Boiling makes coffee and tea bitter and increases their strength. *Decaffeinated* coffee products have had 95 percent or more of the caffeine removed. Both coffee and tea should be tightly covered. Coffee should be stored in a cool place to preserve flavor.

MILK AND MILK PRODUCTS

Milk is considered the most nearly perfect food. It is easily digested, and it contains complete protein, carbohydrate, fat, calcium, phosphorus, and vitamins A and B. Milk is low in vitamin C and iron. Most milk sold in the United States has been irradiated with 400 IU of vitamin D per quart, which otherwise is present only in small amounts.

Since *bacteria* (microorganisms) thrive on milk, there are health regulations which must be scrupulously observed by people handling it. Milk that has been handled according to these regulations is *certified*. To assure its safety, most milk is pasteurized. *Pasteurization* is a process named for Louis Pasteur, its originator. In one method of pasteurization, the milk is heated to at least 62.8°C (145°F) for at least 30 minutes and then immediately cooled to 10°C (50°F). Another method is to heat milk very quickly to 71.7°C (161°F) for at least 15 seconds and then cool it immediately. The pasteurization

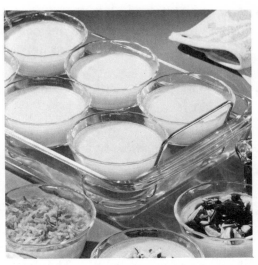

Fig. 10-1 Baked custard is one of the many ways in which milk can be added to the diet. *(Courtesy of the National Dairy Council)*

process kills all harmful bacteria and checks the growth of some harmless bacteria which can cause milk to sour. Milk that has not been pasteurized is called *raw milk*.

Fresh milk is available in one quart, one-half gallon, three quart, and one gallon containers. Usually the larger containers provide the lowest cost, ounce per ounce. These containers will undoubtedly be replaced by liter-sized containers.

Frequently there is a date on the milk container. Milk should not be purchased after the date indicated because it will not remain fresh for more than a day or two. Milk should be refrigerated in clean, covered containers to preserve its nutrient content and inhibit the growth of bacteria. It should be heated at low temperatures because it scorches easily.

Although milk is most often used as a beverage, it is frequently combined with other foods such as soups, gravies, casseroles, baked products, cereals, and desserts. Milk is available in several forms:

• *Whole milk* — milk with all its natural nutrients.

- *Low fat Milk* — milk with fat removed to no more than .5 percent, one percent, 1.5 percent, or two percent, as indicated on the label.

- *Skim milk* — milk with all or nearly all of its fat removed.

- *Chocolate milk* — milk with chocolate added; may be whole or low fat.

- *Dried milk* — milk with all of its water removed.

- *Buttermilk* — skim milk which is a by-product of making butter. Buttermilk is also made artificially by adding special bacteria to skim milk. The bacteria change some of the lactose (milk sugar) to lactic acid. The resulting product is called *cultured buttermilk.*

- *Homogenized milk* — whole milk which has been processed to break the fat into small drops and distribute it evenly throughout the liquid so that it does not separate.

- *Evaporated milk* — whole milk with approximately 60 percent of its water removed.

- *Sweetened condensed milk* — milk which has been evaporated after the addition of sugar.

Cream

Cream is the fat in milk which rises to the surface. It may also be separated from milk by mechanical means. Cream is classified as light or heavy depending upon its fat content. The higher the percentage of fat, the heavier the cream. "Half and half" is equal parts milk and cream. Cream should be kept covered and refrigerated. It is available in one-half pint, pint, and quart containers.

Cheese

When milk coagulates, the curd that results is cheese. The hundreds of types available vary according to the kind of milk used, the amount of moisture, types of seasonings, and the method of ripening. Some cheddar cheese is graded according to quality with Grade AA the best, Grade A nearly as good, and Grade B being the lowest in flavor and cost. Natural cheese is commonly classified according to moisture content: hard, semi-soft and soft, table 10-3. Another popular cheese in the United States is *process cheese.* This is natural cheese which has been blended with additional moisture and sometimes, seasonings, to make cheese spreads.

Cheese is rich in protein, minerals, and vitamins. It is generally easy to digest. The mild-flavored cheeses can usually be served to the patient during convalescence. It is an acceptable meat alternate and is used in sandwiches, casseroles, sauces, salads, and desserts.

Because cheese toughens easily in cooking, low temperatures are recommended. To store cheese, keep it tightly wrapped in a cool place. Since the flavor of cheese is most

TABLE 10-3 Natural Cheese Classification According to Moisture Content

Hard	Semisoft	Soft
Parmesan	Mozzarella	Brie
Cheddar	Roquefort	Camembert
Swiss	Blue	Cream
Edam	Gorgonzola	Cottage
Gouda	Muenster	Ricotta

pronounced at room temperature, it should be removed from the refrigerator an hour before serving.

Butter

Butter might be called a by-product of milk. It is made from the fat in milk. It is an excellent source of fat and vitamin A. It is available as sweet butter, which means it has had no salt added, or as salt or regular butter which has had salt added. The choice depends on taste or specific diet requirements. It is available as Grade AA, A, and B. The best flavored and most expensive is AA. It must be kept refrigerated and covered because it picks up other food odors readily.

EGGS

Eggs are a rich source of protein, minerals, and vitamins and may be considered as a meat alternate. They are inexpensive and easily digested. Because of their high cholesterol content, it may be advisable to limit eggs to four each week.

Eggs are graded according to size and quality. Large eggs usually cost more per dozen than small, but the size has nothing to do with the quality. When an egg is fresh, it sinks in water; an old egg floats because air has seeped into the shell. The freshest, highest quality eggs have a thick white that stays together. The white of eggs which are old or of poor quality is thin and runny. Grade AA and A eggs are excellent and recommended when eggs are to be fried, poached, or presented whole in some manner. Grade B eggs are seldom available at retail level because they are typically dried or frozen. If available, they are quite acceptable for combining with other foods. Because the yolks break quite easily, Grade B eggs are not recommended for use when the whites and yolks must be separated.

Eggs should be stored in their cartons with the small end down as this keeps the air

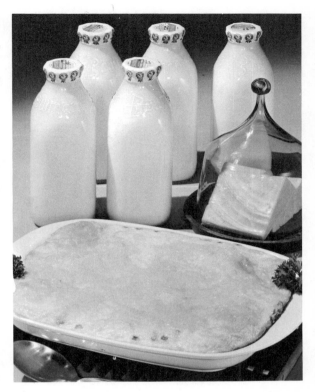

Fig. 10-2   Cheese, milk, and eggs can be combined with other foods to make attractive dishes. *(Courtesy of the National Dairy Council)*

cell at the rounded end and prevents the yolk from slipping out of place. They should be refrigerated until used unless they are to be used in cakes. Because they blend with other cake ingredients better if they are at room temperature, they should be removed from the refrigerator about an hour before the cake is made.

Eggs are a favorite breakfast, lunch, or supper dish and can be prepared in many different ways. They are used in sandwiches, salads, desserts, and baked products. Eggs, like most protein foods, become tough when cooked at high temperatures. They should never be boiled — only simmered.

MEATS, POULTRY, AND FISH

Meats, poultry, and fish provide the greatest source of protein in the diet. They are also rich in minerals and vitamins. Lean meats are easily digested. Some form of these foods should be served daily. Usually they are the foundation of meals. The purple stamp (vegetable dye) on meat is a government seal indicating that the meat is free from disease and has been handled under sanitary conditions.

Meat

The types of meat generally available are beef, veal, lamb, pork, and variety meats. In some places, *venison* (deer meat), *hare* (rabbit meat), and other wild game are available during certain seasons. Meat is graded as prime, choice, good, standard, and commercial. Choice and good are usually the highest grades available in supermarkets; meat markets usually carry prime. Restaurants often use prime meats.

Because the grade of quality is not always marked on packaged meats, one should know how to distinguish good quality meats. Usually, a higher grade meat is more economical than a lower grade because there is less bone, gristle, and fat in the higher grade.

In addition to a pleasant odor, good quality meat should be firm, yet resilient to the touch. Beef should be bright red and marbled with white or creamy fat. Veal should be light pink with some white, brittle fat. Lamb should be reddish pink with creamy white fat. Pork may vary from a grey pink to a deeper rose color with white fat.

Organ meats include liver, kidney, tripe, tongue, sweetbreads, and brains. These are especially good sources of minerals and vitamins and are quite inexpensive because they contain little or no waste.

Meats are available in various cuts, figures 10-3 through 10-7. The muscles which the animal uses most are the least tender. Although the less tender cuts are usually less expensive, the choice of cut should depend on the method of cooking to be used, pages 91, 92, 93, and 94. Tender cuts may be cooked by *dry heat* methods such as roasting, broiling, or frying. Less tender cuts should be cooked covered by *moist heat* methods such as braising or stewing. The nutrient value of meat is not related to its tenderness.

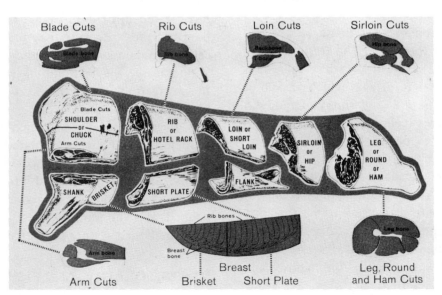

Fig. 10-3   Seven basic retail cuts are used to prepare veal, lamb, beef or pork. *(Courtesy of the National Live Stock and Meat Board)*

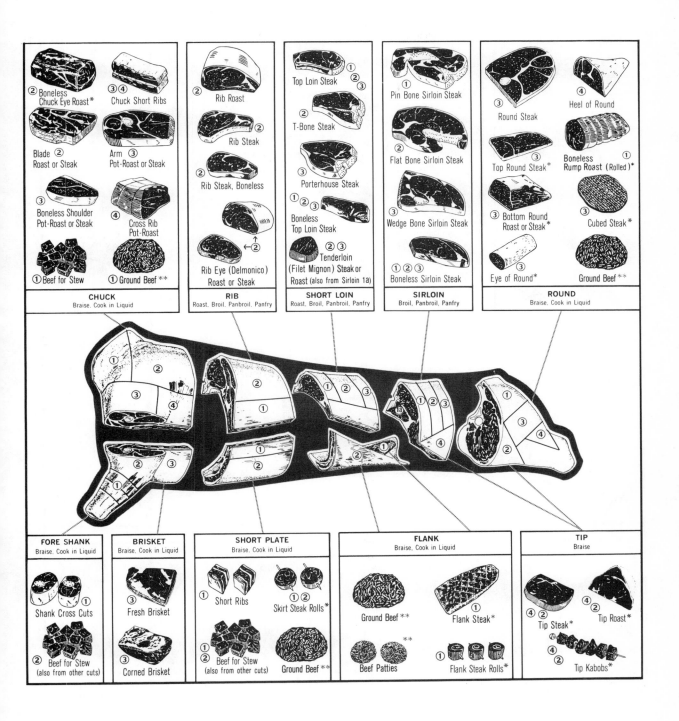

Fig. 10-4 Beef cuts and cooking suggestions *(Courtesy of National Live Stock and Meat Board)*

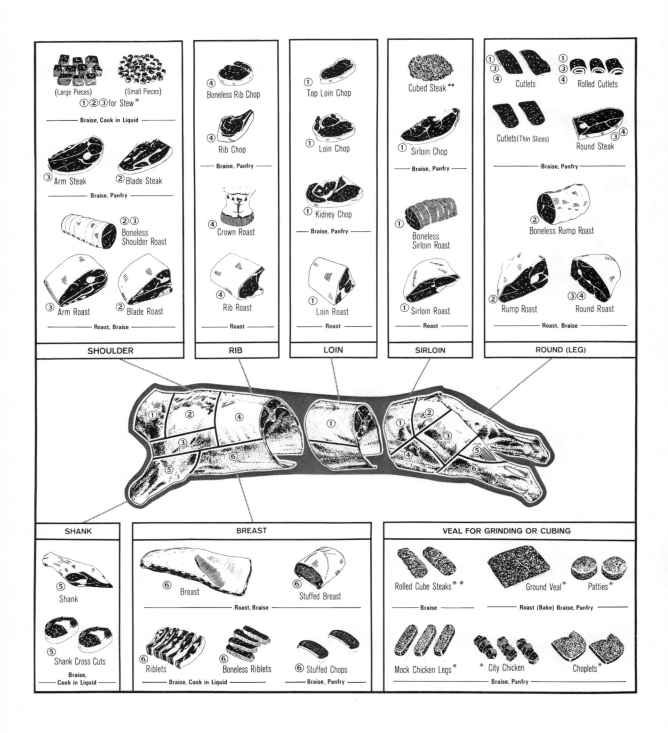

Fig. 10-5   Veal cuts and cooking suggestions *(Courtesy of National Live Stock and Meat Board)*

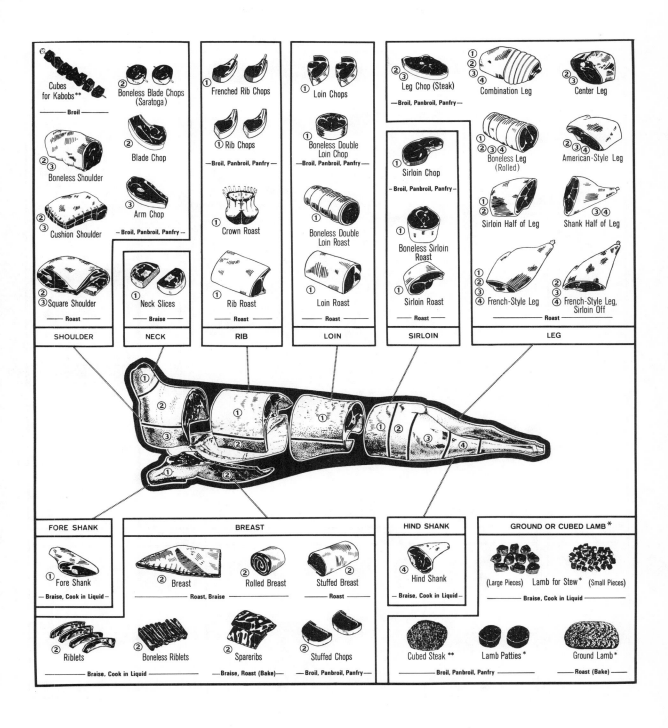

Fig. 10-6 Cuts of lamb and cooking suggestions *(Courtesy of National Live Stock and Meat Board)*

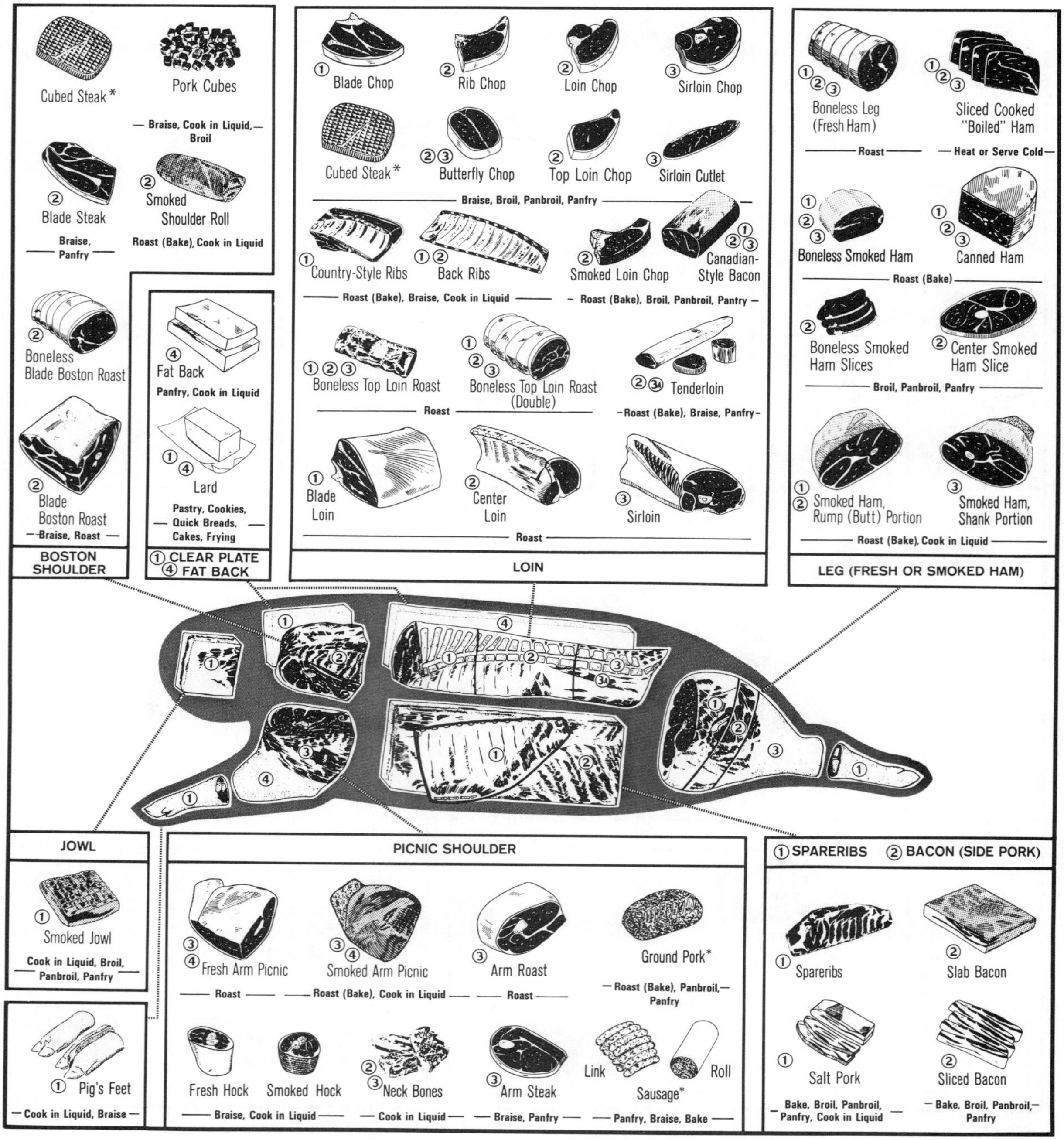

Fig. 10-7 Cuts of pork and cooking suggestions *(Courtesy of National Live Stock and Meat Board)*

Poultry

The common types of poultry available are chicken, turkey, duck, goose, and game hen. Although the modern methods of raising poultry have resulted in a relatively standardized degree of tenderness, young birds are generally more tender and flavorful than old birds. Poultry may be graded *A* (highest quality) or *B* (less attractive, thinner birds) or *C* by government inspectors, but only when the seller pays for the inspection. If the label on the package includes the words "young," "broiler," or "fryer," the birds should be tender. If the label does not specify or says "stewing hen," or "mature turkey," the poultry will probably require moist heat methods of cooking.

Fish

Seafood may be divided into two groups: fish and shellfish. It may be purchased fresh, canned, frozen, and cured or smoked. Seafood is graded according to size and quality, but standards of enforcing the grading are not uniform.

Some of the common fish available are cod, flounder, haddock, trout, salmon, and tuna. When purchased fresh, they should be firm with little slime, have red gills and clear, unsunken eyes. They are packaged as *round* (with head, bones, and scales), *fillets* (long, thin strips of flesh, free of bone, which are cut from the sides of the fish), *steaks* (even, crosswise slices), and various fish sticks and fish balls.

The shellfish usually available include shrimp, oysters, crab, clams, lobsters, scallops, and mussels. They may be purchased raw in the shell, raw without the shell, and cooked, canned, or frozen.

Storage and Cooking of Meats, Poultry and Fish

Because of the additional elements which make up protein, it decomposes more readily than carbohydrate and fat. Therefore, meat, poultry, and fish must be kept in the refrigerator to prevent or delay decomposition. When purchased fresh, poultry and meat should be unwrapped, lightly covered with waxed paper or plastic wrap, and stored in the refrigerator. Fish should be covered well and stored in the refrigerator. Frozen foods should be stored in the freezer and defrosted for use according to package directions. They should never be refrozen before cooking.

Proteins coagulate during cooking. Therefore, most foods containing large amounts of protein should be cooked at low temperatures to prevent them from becoming tough and to prevent shrinkage. Exceptions are tender cuts of meat such as steaks and chops, which, if cooked to a rare or medium state of doneness, may be cooked at a high temperature for a short time in the broiler or on top of the stove. Roasting for a longer period of time at a low temperature is also advisable for tender cuts.

Roasting, broiling, and frying are called dry heat methods of cooking. Less tender

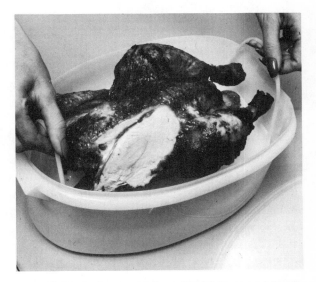

Fig. 10-8. Leftover poultry should be stored in the refrigerator in a container with a tight fitting cover. (*Courtesy of Tupperware*)

TABLE 10-4   Yield of Cooked Meat Per Pound of Raw Meat

Meat as purchased	Meat after Cooking (less drippings)	
	Parts weighed	Approximate weight of cooked parts per pound of raw meat purchased
Chops or steaks for broiling or frying:		ounces
With bone and relatively large amount of fat, such as pork or lamb chops; beef rib, sirloin, or porterhouse steaks	Lean, bone, fat	10-12
	Lean and fat	7-10
	Lean only	5-7
Without bone and with very little fat, such as round of beef	Lean and fat	12-13
veal steaks	Lean only	9-12
Ground meat for broiling or frying, such as beef, lamb, or pork patties	Patties	9-13
Roasts for oven cooking (no liquid added):		
With bone and relatively large amount of fat, such as beef rib, loin, chuck; lamb shoulder, leg; pork, fresh or cured	Lean, bone, fat	10-12
	Lean and fat	8-10
	Lean only	6-9
Without bone	Lean and fat	10-12
	Lean only	7-10
Cuts for pot-roasting, simmering, braising, stewing:		
With bone and relatively large amount of fat, such as beef chuck, pork shoulder	Lean, bone, fat	10-11
	Lean and fat	8-9
	Lean only	6-8
Without bone and with relatively small amount of fat, such as trimmed beef, veal	Lean with adhering fat	9-11

Source: Home and Garden Bulletin no. 72, U.S.D.A., 1971

cuts must be cooked for a longer time by a moist heat method such as stewing or braising. Older fowl should also be cooked by moist heat to insure flavor and tenderness. Larger fowl such as turkey, goose, and roasting chickens must be roasted slowly at a medium-low temperature. Fish is tender and is usually baked in liquid or sauteed to prevent it from drying out.

These foods, when left over, should be refrigerated and, when cold, tightly covered. They may be used advantageously in sandwiches, creamed dishes, salads, and soups.

VEGETABLES

Vegetables are edible plants which provide vitamins, minerals, carbohydrates, and sometimes proteins. Fresh vegetables may be graded U.S. Fancy, U.S. No. 1 and U.S. No. 2. However, some products may have grades above and below these. If a fresh vegetable has a grade mark, it means that the packing of the item was supervised by a U.S. Government grader. Most fresh vegetables are sold according to grades at wholesale markets, but few are marked according to grade in retail stores. Consequently, it is helpful to be able to recognize good quality fresh vegetables. They should be ripe, firm, without *blemishes* (spots) and a good, bright color. Wilted vegetables are old and have lost some of their nutritive value.

Commercially canned, frozen, and dried vegetables are convenient and retain most of their original nutrients. While their cost may be higher than the same product fresh, it must be remembered that these products contain no waste except for the package (s) in which they are packed. They usually contain additives, but their package labels should list them.

These foods are graded as U.S. Grade A (Fancy), U.S. Grade B (Choice or Extra Standard) and U.S. Grade C (Standard). The U.S. grade mark is found on very few of these items. If the label does carry a grade even without the "U.S." preceding it, it must be of the quality marked.

These items are packed and priced according to quality. Grade A is the most attractive, most tender, and most expensive. Grades B and C are less perfect in appearance and less expensive. They may be less tender and have some blemishes. The A grade is best used when appearance is important, but they are all equally nutritious.

Fresh vegetables should be stored in a cool, dry place. They should be served raw whenever possible. When cooked, they retain most nutrients by being cooked in their skins as short a time, and in as little boiling water, as possible. They should be served immediately after cooking. The liquid used in cooking should be added to soups and gravies as this liquid contains minerals and vitamins. Vegetables are commonly baked, boiled, and steamed. Some vegetables, such as potatoes, eggplant, and squash, may be fried for variety. Vegetables may be used as *accompaniment dishes* (food that is served along with the *entree,* or main dish), or in salads and soups. Leftovers should be stored in the refrigerator and covered when cold.

FRUITS

Fruits are the fleshy parts surrounding the seeds of plants. They contribute valuable vitamins and minerals, carbohydrates in the forms of sugar and cellulose, and water. Because they contain cellulose, water, and fruit acids, they have a laxative effect and are useful in overcoming constipation.

There are fresh, canned, frozen, and dried fruits available. When purchased fresh, fruit should be firm, ripe, and unblemished. Both fresh and prepared fruits are graded in the same manner as vegetables.

Fruit keeps best and is often tastiest when stored in the refrigerator. Frozen fruits should be kept frozen until ready for use. Some fruits, such as apples and plums, are more easily digested after cooking. They must be cooked very gently and just until tender. Sugar added at the beginning of the cooking period preserves their shape while sugar added later improves their flavor.

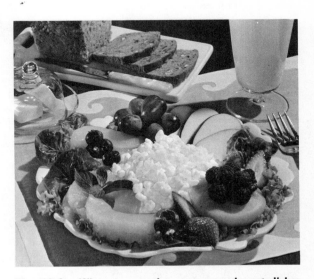

Fig. 10-9 **When appropriate accompaniment dishes are chosen from the Four Basic food groups, a fruit salad may be served as the main course for lunch.** *(Courtesy of the National Dairy Council)*

BREADS AND CEREALS

Cereals are the seeds of grains. As stated previously, these seeds consist of three main parts. The bran contains vitamins, minerals, protein, and cellulose. The endosperm is largely carbohydrate, which is ground and used for refined flour in various baked products. The germ contains the B vitamins and protein. During *milling* (grinding into flour) some of these vitamins and minerals are lost. Manufacturers restore them to their original nutrient value by adding these same nutrients in synthetic form. After this process, they are known as restored cereals. When these nutrients are added in amounts greater than the grain originally contained, the cereal is called enriched or fortified.

Because cereals are easy to grow, transport, and store, they are inexpensive and very popular. Although cereals are easily digested, cooking increases their digestibility. Breakfast cereals, rice, macaroni products, cornmeal, and various flours are the most familiar forms of cereals. Airtight containers preserve their freshness. Soybean flour, because of its fat content, should be stored airtight in a cool dry place to prevent it from becoming rancid.

Essentially, bread is made from flour, water, and yeast with sugar, fat, and flavorings added at the discretion of the baker. It is available in countless shapes and flavors. It must be kept airtight to preserve its freshness, and it may be frozen for long storage.

ORGANIC, NATURAL AND HEALTH FOODS

The terms *organic, natural* and *health food* are of great interest today. In evaluating foods, it is advisable that the consumer understand what these terms mean. Actually, organic materials are chemical compounds of various sorts, which contain the element carbon, in addition to other elements. Nearly all food is organic. Carbohydrates, fats, and proteins all contain carbon; vitamins and minerals are found in association with these nutrients.

Organic food means plants that have been grown without the addition of artificial fertilizers or pesticides, or animal foods from animals raised without treatments of antibiotics or hormones and prepared for market without the use of chemicals.

Natural foods are foods which have not been treated or processed in any way. They may or may not have been organically grown. *Health food* is a general term used to describe foods which some food faddists claim have large quantities of nutrients which prevent, treat and/or cure certain diseases.

Honey, blackstrap molasses, granola and wheat germ are often claimed to be health foods. Honey is considered to be a health food by some because it contains B vitamins, iron and calcium. It does contain these nutrients but only in traces. Blackstrap molasses is an excellent source of calcium and iron if used in large amounts. However, because molasses is strong-flavored and sweet, the amounts used in the everyday diet would not provide any very significant proportion of these nutrients. Some granola cereals provide fewer vitamins and minerals than well-known varieties of the restored or enriched cereals. Among cereals, wheat germ is a good source of protein. It is also a good source of vitamin E, but again the amounts used are relatively small. Consequently, the nutrient intake from it is also small.

Health foods are sometimes overrated in their ability to prevent or cure disease. Many of these so-called health foods are good sources of certain nutrients, but most are nutritionally overrated. Many foods grown or prepared traditionally are equally rich in nutrients. Product labels and prices should be compared before one product is deemed better than another. Most of these organic, natural and health foods are no more nutritious but are far more expensive than traditional foods.

SUMMARY

Beverages are fluids necessary to regulate body processes. Their various forms include water, milk, coffee, tea, fruit juices, and soft drinks. Milk is one of the most valuable foods and is available in many forms. Cheese is the curd which results from milk coagulation. Natural cheese has three basic forms, soft, semisoft, and hard. Eggs, like cheese, are a suitable meat alternate. Meats are graded and cut to aid the consumer in selecting the level of quality desired. The choice of cut depends on the method of cooking to be used. Meat, poultry, fish, or a high-quality meat substitute should be eaten at least once a day. Fruits and vegetables are usually most nutritious when eaten raw. If cooking is necessary, using only small amounts of water helps preserve nutritional quality. Breads and cereals are usually restored or enriched and are inexpensive because they are easy to grow, transport and store. Organic, natural and health foods are usually nutritionally comparable to traditional food products. Many of these foods are expensive and overrated in their overall nutritional value.

DISCUSSION TOPICS

1. Discuss the reasons for cooking vegetables and fruits and the reasons for serving them raw.

2. Discuss the nutritional values of various beverages.

3. Discuss various means of including milk in the diet. Why is milk a wise purchase? Why must it be refrigerated?

4. How does the grade of eggs relate to their use in the menu? Describe 5 ways of using eggs in the diet.

5. Using the meat charts in this chapter, discuss which cuts of meat are tender and which are less tender.

6. Which methods of cooking are advised for the less tender cuts of meat? Why?

7. How does the storage of fruits and vegetables affect their nutrient content?

8. Discuss various organic, natural and health foods. What are their advantages? Disadvantages?

9. Discuss food additives. Are there some that may be unnecessary in terms of nutrition and storage? If so, why are they used?

10. At what general temperature should meat, milk, eggs and cheese usually be cooked? Why?

SUGGESTED ACTIVITIES

a. Organize the class into groups and visit a local supermarket. Each group should make a survey of the various forms and prices of one of the groups of foods discussed in this chapter. Reports should be exchanged and filed for future use in meal preparation.

b. Visit a health food store. Compare the prices of their products with the same products in the supermarket. Are there differences? If so, why?

c. Make a chart of the various forms of milk available and incude a description of each, including cost.

d. Using other sources, prepare a report to the class on the diseases caused by bacteria which may be present in raw milk. Find out what precautions are taken by dairy farmers in the local area to prevent the contamination of milk.

e. Make an appointment and visit a meat market to observe meatcutters at work. Take notes and discuss the visit when you return to class.

WORD STUDY

accompaniment dish	dried milk	process cheese
bacteria	evaporated milk	raw milk
beverage	fillet	skim milk
blemish	food additives	steak
buttermilk	hare	stimulant
caffeine	homogenized milk	sweetened condensed milk
certified milk	milling	theine
coagulate	nutritional value	venison
consumer	opaque	whole milk
decaffeinated	pasteurization	

REVIEW

A. Multiple-multiple Choice. Select the *letter* which precedes the best answer.

1. Milk is an important beverage because it
   1. contains complete protein and calcium
   2. has been pasteurized to increase the amount of vitamin D
   3. contains phosphorus, vitamin A, and riboflavin
   4. contains a stimulant
   5. contains vitamin C and iron
      a) all   b) 1, 3, 4   c) 1, 2, 5   d) 1, 3

2. The following forms of milk have had some of their natural nutrients removed:
    1. homogenized milk
    2. pasteurized milk
    3. skim milk
    4. buttermilk
    5. raw milk
        a) 1, 2, 3, 4   b) 3, 4   c) 2, 3, 5   d) all

3. Good quality beef should have the following characteristics:
    1. a pleasant odor
    2. firm, yet resilient
    3. light pink color with brittle fat
    4. a U.S. Government grade stamp
    5. marbled with white or creamy fat
        a) all   b) 1, 3, 5   c) 1, 2, 4   d) 1, 2, 5

4. To be stored properly, fresh meats should be
    1. unwrapped and uncovered
    2. unwrapped and covered with wax paper
    3. always refrigerated or frozen
    4. refrozen after thawing
    5. never frozen
        a) 2, 3   b) 1, 3, 4   c) 1, 4, 5   d) 1, 2, 4

5. Vegetables are essential to a well-balanced diet because they
    1. contain both fat-soluble and water-soluble vitamins
    2. contain only water-soluble vitamins
    3. contain carbohydrates
    4. are good sources of cellulose
    5. are good sources of complete protein
        a) 1, 3, 4   b) 2, 3, 4   c) 3, 4, 5   d) all

6. Coffee should be
    1. stored in a cool place
    2. tightly covered for storage
    3. diluted by boiling for 2 minutes
    4. given to children only after the theine is removed
    5. added to meals for its food value
        a) 1, 2, 5   b) 1, 2, 4   c) 2, 4, 5   d) 1, 2

7. Food additives can
    1. enrich nutrient content
    2. retard spoilage
    3. enhance flavor
    4. maintain appearance
    5. maintain texture
        a) all   b) 1, 4   c) 2, 3   d) 1, 4, 5

8. Beverages
    1. regulate body processes
    2. provide nourishment
    3. relieve thirst
    4. provide the best source of fat
        a) all   b) 1, 2, 3   c) 2, 3, 4   d) 1, 3, 4

9. A specific cut of beef may be chosen according to its
    1. intended use
    2. protein content
    3. water content
    4. total carbohydrate content
        a) 1, 2, 4   b) 1   c) 1, 4   d) 3, 4

10. Organic foods are
    1. the same as natural foods
    2. only animal foods
    3. those foods produced without the use of any chemicals
    4. generally nutritious if chosen from the Basic Four food groups
    5. generally more expensive than foods from the supermarket
        a) all   b) 1,2   c) 3, 4, 5   d) 1, 2, 3

B.   Match the items in column I to the correct statement in column II.
      Column I   Column II
_____ 1. additives   a. milk with fat removed
_____ 2. caffeine   b. one who buys and uses products
_____ 3. pasteurization   c. microorganisms
_____ 4. skim milk   d. milk with 60% of water removed
_____ 5. consumer   e. stimulant
_____ 6. bacteria   f. grinding into flour
_____ 7. evaporated milk   g. natural cheese with additional moisture
_____ 8. milling   h. may be intentional or incidental
_____ 9. process cheese   i. roquefort cheese
_____10. dried milk   j. process of killing harmful bacteria in milk
                               k. milk with all water removed
                               l. process of breaking up fat in milk

C.   Briefly answer the following questions.
  1. Why are coffee and tea not advisable for children?

  2. How is milk pasteurized?

Chapter 11
Purchasing Food

OBJECTIVES

After studying this chapter, the student should be able to:

- Estimate correct amounts of foods to purchase for a given number of people.
- Identify information commonly given on food labels.
- List guidelines for selecting size and style of food packages.
- Name five considerations which help the consumer maintain a balanced diet on a low food budget.

The appropriate selection of food can be quite challenging. There are countless varieties of foods available in many different styles of preparation and packaging at many different prices. The wise buyer knows that the value of food is measured by its nutritional quality and not by its price. Achieving a well-balanced diet does not depend on a large food budget. A sound knowledge of nutrition is essential for the consumer.

The Basic Four food groups are the foundation upon which all food purchasing plans should be made. It is also necessary to have a basic understanding of how foods are prepared and packaged for consumer use.

LABELING

Reading the label on a food package is the best method of determining the value of the food. Food labeling is somewhat regulated in the United States in order to protect the consumer. The Federal Food, Drug and Cosmetics Act is a law that requires that food shipped from one state to another be pure, safe to eat, and prepared under sanitary conditions. It also requires that containers of food shipped from one state to another have their ingredients and weight printed on the label. Ingredients are listed according to their proportions in the product. The ingredient found in greatest proportion is listed first, the ingredient found in second greatest proportion is listed second and so on. Foods processed and sold within one state are governed by state law.

Labels may also include the number of servings, approximate quantity, size and maturity of the product, recipes and serving suggestions, and other products available from the manufacturer. This information on food labels is particularly important to the consumer who must select foods to be used for special diets.

In an effort to aid the consumer, the United States Food and Drug Administration has issued regulations regarding nutrition labeling. *Nutrition labeling* is the listing of specific nutrition information on packages of foods which are enriched or fortified and/or foods for which a nutritional claim is made. The information required on such

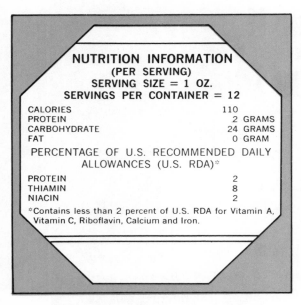

NUTRITION INFORMATION
(PER SERVING)
SERVING SIZE = 1 OZ.
SERVINGS PER CONTAINER = 12

CALORIES	110
PROTEIN	2 GRAMS
CARBOHYDRATE	24 GRAMS
FAT	0 GRAM

PERCENTAGE OF U.S. RECOMMENDED DAILY
ALLOWANCES (U.S. RDA)*

PROTEIN	2
THIAMIN	8
NIACIN	2

*Contains less than 2 percent of U.S. RDA for Vitamin A,
Vitamin C, Riboflavin, Calcium and Iron.

A. Certain labels include only the minimum information required.

NUTRITION INFORMATION
(PER SERVING)
SERVING SIZE = 8 OZ.
SERVINGS PER CONTAINER = 1

CALORIES	560	FAT (PERCENT OF	
PROTEIN	23 G	CALORIES 53%)	33 G
CARBOHYDRATE	43 G	POLYUNSAT-	
		URATED	2 G
		SATURATED	9 G
		CHOLESTEROL*	
		(20 MG/100 G)	40 MG
		SODIUM (365 MG/	
		100 G)	830 MG

PERCENTAGE OF U.S. RECOMMENDED DAILY
ALLOWANCES (U.S. RDA)

PROTEIN	35	RIBOFLAVIN	15
VITAMIN A	35	NIACIN	25
VITAMIN C		CALCIUM	2
(ASCORBIC ACID)	10	IRON	25
THIAMIN (VITAMIN			
B₁)	15		

*Information on fat and cholesterol content is provided
for individuals who, on the advice of a physician, are
modifying their total dietary intake of fat and cholesterol.

B. Some labels include optional lists of nutrients.

Fig. 11-1   Nutritional labeling helps the consumer determine the nutrient value of a product. *(Courtesy of Food and Drug Administration)*

foods must follow a standard format. The label must include serving size, total number of servings, and calories per serving. The following ingredients must also be listed per serving: grams of protein, carbohydrate, and fat, and the percentage of the United States Recommended Daily Allowances (RDAs) for protein, vitamins A and C, thiamine, riboflavin and niacin, and two minerals, calcium and iron, figure 11-1. The listing of cholesterol, fatty acid, sodium content and additional vitamins and minerals may also be included. Additionally, many food manufacturers will, upon request, mail the consumer detailed nutritional information regarding their products.

GRADES

Several foods have United States Department of Agriculture (USDA) grade stamps on them, figure 11-2. The grade varies depending upon the quality of the product. A grade stamp is not mandatory. When food is stamped, the food processor has requested and paid for the service. Foods most commonly graded are beef, lamb, chicken, turkey, butter, and eggs. When a grade stamp is found on a food product, it means that the food has been inspected by a

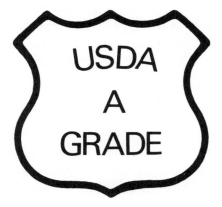

USDA
A
GRADE

Fig. 11-2   A U.S. Government grade stamp shows that the quality of a food item has been evaluated by a federal inspector.

U.S. Government expert and found to conform to specific government standards of quality. The lack of such a stamp does not mean the food is inferior in any way.

PACKAGING

The sizes and styles of food packages purchased depend on several factors. The size of the family and its members' appetites are important considerations as well as the cooking method and the time allowed for cooking. The storage space available also determines the size of the package to be purchased. If there is sufficient storage space and the food keeps well, large packages may be economical even for small families. When there is inadequate storage space, small packages may be more practical. The consumer should select the size of the package needed according to its actual weight or volume. The consumer cannot depend on manufacturers' descriptions such as *jumbo, giant* or *economy* size. All food containers should be checked for breaks or leaks in the packaging and, when appropriate, washed before storing.

CONVENIENCE FOODS

An extremely popular form of food today is the convenience food that requires little or no preparation. The term is used to describe the cake, bread, and dessert mixes; instant puddings; brown-and-serve breads and pastries; frozen TV dinners; and frozen or canned fruits, vegetables, meats, fish and desserts. Most of them are high in quality and save kitchen work. These foods can be expensive for large families but more economical for single or elderly people. Convenience foods reduce waste which often occurs with leftovers. When the cook spends a day away from home, convenience foods are economical in terms of her time. With the addition of a fresh vegetable and milk, the frozen dinner provides a nutritionally balanced meal.

It is wise to keep some of these foods on hand for unexpected situations.

Frozen Foods

It is advisable to buy frozen foods in packages that can be used at one time or in a type of package, usually a plastic bag, that allows the cook to remove only as much food as is needed for a meal. Frozen foods are sold according to weight. The labels usually indicate the number of servings per package. While frozen foods may be more expensive than fresh foods, they are sometimes more economical because they contain no waste and are always in season. Also, when they are fully-cooked foods that require only reheating, they are economical in terms of the cook's time. They do not spoil if stored properly and usually take little time to prepare.

Canned Foods

Because canned foods keep so well, they are popular and especially useful to someone with limited refrigerator space. There are few foods that are not available in cans. Except for certain meats, canned foods are relatively inexpensive. They are sold according to the can sizes shown in table 11-1. Sometimes the weights of two different products in identical cans vary because of the different densities of the foods.

Freeze-Dried Foods

Today, food is being processed by a new method known as *freeze-drying*. In this process, foods are frozen so rapidly that their flavors and textures are not noticeably changed and then they are *dehydrated* (have water removed). The consumer purchases them in small packages that may be kept for long periods of time without refrigeration. Directions for preparing freeze-dried foods usually include a specified period of time for

TABLE 11-1   Common Container Sizes for Canned Foods

CONTAINER				PRINCIPAL PRODUCTS
INDUSTRY TERM	CONSUMER DESCRIPTION APPROX. NET WEIGHT OR FLUID MEASURE (CHECK LABEL)		APPROX. CUPS	
8 oz.	8 oz.		1	Fruits, vegetables, specialties for small families. 2 servings.
Picnic	10 1/2 to 12 oz.		1 1/4	Mainly condensed soups. Some fruits, vegetables, meat, fish, specialties. 2 to 3 servings.
12 oz. (vac.)	12 oz.		1 1/2	Principally for vacuum pack corn. 3 to 4 servings.
No. 300	14 to 16 oz. (14 oz. to 1 lb.)		1 3/4	Pork and beans, baked beans, meat products, cranberry sauce, blueberries, specialties. 3 to 4 servings.
No. 303	16 to 17 oz. (1 lb. to 1 lb. 1 oz.)		2	Principal size for fruits and vegetables. Some meat products, ready-to-serve soups, specialties. 4 servings.
No. 2	20 oz. (1 lb. 4 oz.)	18 fl. oz. (1 pt. 2 fl. oz.)	2 1/2	Juices, ready-to-serve soups, some specialties, pineapple, apple slices. No longer in popular use for most fruits and vegetables. 5 servings.
No. 2 1/2	27 to 29 oz. (1 lb. 11 oz. to 1 lb. 13 oz.)		3 1/2	Fruits, some vegetables (pumpkin, sauerkraut, spinach and other greens, tomatoes). 5 to 7 servings.
No. 3 cyl. or 46 fl. oz.	51 oz. (3 lb. 3 oz.)	46 fl. oz. (1 qt. 14 fl. oz.)	5 3/4	Fruit and vegetable juices, pork and beans. Institutional size for condensed soups, some vegetables. 10 to 12 servings.
No. 10	6 1/2 lb to 7 lb. 5 oz.		12-13	Institutional size for fruits, vegetables and some other foods. 25 servings.

Source: National Canners Association

soaking in a specified amount of liquid. By soaking they regain their original moisture content and appearance. After soaking they are cooked as if they were fresh foods.

ECONOMY IN PURCHASING

Economy is a major goal of the concerned shopper. Careful planning is the key to economical food purchasing. Consideration of the following factors should aid the consumer in planning economical food purchases.

Menu Planning

Careful menu planning is essential if one is to make economical food purchases. In addition, such planning saves time. Meals for the week should be planned at one time around the weekly specials advertised in local newspapers. Planning should also include the appropriate use of leftovers. The food marketing list should be made according to the weekly menu and based on the Basic Four food groups.

Intended Use

Foods should be selected according to their intended use. For example, less-expensive, small fruit is satisfactory for making peach jam, but if peaches are to be served whole or as halves, the larger, more attractive fruit should be purchased. Less tender cuts of meat are as nutritious and, when prepared appropriately, as appealing as tender cuts. However, it must be remembered that the less tender cuts of meat require longer cooking times than the tender cuts. Large cuts of meat are often less expensive per pound than small cuts. Therefore, it is economical to buy large quantities if subsequent meals are planned around leftovers. Leftovers should be properly wrapped and frozen for future use. Sometimes a few portions can be separated from the whole before cooking. The extra portions can then be wrapped and frozen for future use.

Substitutions

Cheaper foods can often be substituted for expensive foods without any loss in nutrition. Some examples include fortified margarine in place of butter, and dried milk instead of fresh milk. Such substitutions can substantially lower food costs. Recipes should be carefully checked and substitutions made whenever appropriate. Table 11-2 shows some common cooking substitutions.

Seasonal Foods

Shipping foods from distant locations is expensive and can increase the amount of food bills. For this reason it is most economical to use foods which are in season. A food's *season* is the period it is normally ripe or ready and hence available in quantity at its lowest price. Fruits, vegetables and certain fish are seasonal and their prices should be considered when planning menus. When a desired food is not locally in season, canned and frozen foods may be more economical than the fresh.

Quantities Needed

It is wise to purchase only as much food as can be used or properly stored. Because

TABLE 11-2 Common Cooking Substitutions

1 square chocolate (ounce)
 3 tablespoons cocoa plus 1 to 3 teaspoons fat

1 cup cake flour
 1 cup all-purpose flour less 2 tablespoons

1 tablespoon cornstarch
 2 tablespoons flour (for thickening)

2/3 teaspoon double-action type baking powder
 1/4 teaspoon baking soda plus 1/2 teaspoon cream of tartar

1 cup fresh milk
 1/2 cup evaporated milk plus 1/2 cup water
 or
 1/2 cup condensed milk plus 1/2 cup water with reduction of sugar used
 or
 1/4 cup powdered whole milk plus 1 cup water
 or
 1/4 cup powdered skim milk plus 2 tablespoons butter plus 1 cup water

fresh fruits, vegetables, meat, fish, poultry, fats, sugar, and many cereal products are sold according to weight, it is advisable to know the number of servings per pound that each of these foods will yield. Table 11-3 can be used as a guide when first preparing market orders.

Selection of the Store or Market

The type of store or market can greatly affect the total cost of the food purchased. Typically, the large cash-and-carry supermarkets have lower prices and offer a wider selection of foods than the small neighborhood markets. Small stores sometimes charge higher prices because they are convenient, allow charge accounts, or because they make home deliveries. Large stores use a great deal of commercial advertising which can ruin the budget of the *impulsive shopper* (one who buys because of a momentary desire). The

TABLE 11-3 Servings per Package or per Pound

Meat, poultry, and fish

The amount of meat, poultry, and fish to buy varies with the amount of bone, fat, and breading.

	Servings per pound[1]
MEAT	
Much bone or gristle	1 or 2
Medium amounts of bone	2 or 3
Little or no bone	3 or 4
POULTRY (READY-TO-COOK)	
Chicken	2 or 3
Turkey	2 or 3
Duck and goose	2
FISH	
Whole	1 or 2
Dressed or pan-dressed	2 or 3
Portions or steaks	3
Fillets	3 or 4

[1] Three ounces of cooked lean meat, poultry, or fish per serving.

CEREAL PRODUCTS

One serving of a cereal may vary from 1/2 cup to 1 1/4 cup. Check package labels.

	Servings per lb.
Flaked corn cereals	18-24
Other flaked cereals	21
Puffed cereals	32-38
Wheat cereals:	
Coarse	12
Fine	16-22
Oatmeal	13
Hominy grits	20
Macaroni, noodles	12
Rice	16
Spaghetti	13

Vegetables and fruits

For this table, a serving of vegetable is 1/2 cup cooked vegetable unless otherwise noted. A serving of fruit is 1/2 cup fruit; 1 medium apple banana, peach, or pear; or 2 apricots or plums. A serving of cooked fresh or dried fruit is 1/2 cup fruit and liquid.

	Servings per pound[1]
FRESH VEGETABLES	
Asparagus	2 or 3
Beans, lima[2]	2
Beans, snap	5 or 6
Beets, diced[3]	3 or 4
Broccoli	3 or 4
Brussels sprouts	4
Cabbage:	
Raw, shredded	9 or 10
Cooked	4 or 5
Carrots:	
Raw, diced or shredded[3]	5 or 6
Cooked[3]	4
Cauliflower	3
Celery:	
Raw, chopped or diced	5 or 6
Cooked	4
Kale[4]	5 or 6
Okra	4 or 5
Onions, cooked	3 or 4
Parsnips[3]	4
Peas[2]	2
Potatoes	4
Spinach[5]	4
Squash, summer	3 or 4
Squash, winter	2 or 3
Sweetpotatoes	3 or 4
Tomatoes, raw, diced or sliced	4

[1] As purchased.
[2] Bought in pod.
[3] Bought without tops.
[4] Bought untrimmed.
[5] Bought prepackaged.

	Servings per package (9 or 10 oz.)
FROZEN VEGETABLES	
Asparagus	2 or 3
Beans, lima	3 or 4
Beans, snap	3 or 4
Broccoli	2 or 3
Brussels sprouts	3
Cauliflower	3
Corn, whole kernel	3
Kale	2 or 3
Peas	3
Spinach	2 or 3

	Servings per can (16 oz.)
CANNED VEGETABLES	
Most vegetables	3 or 4
Greens, such as kale or spinach	2 or 3

	Servings per pound
DRY VEGETABLES	
Dry beans	11
Dry peas, lentils	10 or 11

	Servings per market unit[1]
FRESH FRUIT	
Apples	
Bananas	
Peaches	3 or 4 per pound
Pears	
Plums	
Apricots	
Cherries, sweet	5 or 6 per pound
Grapes, seedless	
Blueberries	
Raspberries	4 or 5 per pint
Strawberries	5 or 6 per unit

[1] As purchased.

	Servings per package (10 or 12 oz.)
FROZEN FRUIT	
Blueberries	3 or 4
Peaches	2 or 3
Raspberries	2 or 3
Strawberries	2 or 3

	Servings per can (16 oz.)
CANNED FRUIT	
Served with liquid	4
Drained	2 or 3

	Servings per package (8 oz.)
DRIED FRUIT	
Apples	8
Apricots	6
Mixed fruits	5
Peaches	6
Pears	4
Prunes unpitted	4 or 5

Source: USDA Home and Garden Bulletin No. 1, 1975

prices of the "super-specials" displayed at prominent places in the markets should be carefully checked against the regular prices of the same article. The actual value of the special should be carefully evaluated by the consumer before the purchase.

SUMMARY

Nutritious meals can be prepared on a small budget as well as on a large budget.

Labels on packaged foods give contents and weight. Consumers who know how a food item will be used can select the appropriate type and size of the package as well as the level of quality needed. Planning menus around weekly specials, buying fresh foods in season, and making nutritionally equal substitutions can reduce food costs. Usually the large supermarkets offer foods at lower prices than the small stores.

DISCUSSION TOPICS

1. Bring grocery advertisements from the newspaper to class.
   a. Compare the prices of the week's specials. Remember to consider the varying qualities of food.
   b. Discuss any new foods that are listed. Ask if anyone in the class has used them.
   c. Discuss the various ways in which one of the meats "on special" can be prepared.
   d. Discuss which foods, if any, are seasonal.
2. What are convenience foods? Name six. Discuss their advantages and disadvantages.
3. Discuss the information found on food packages and how it may or may not affect the purchase and use of some foods. What is nutrition labeling?
4. Discuss quality grade stamps. Has anyone noticed them? What do they indicate?

SUGGESTED ACTIVITIES

a. Plan a week's menu for a family of four who have no special dietary needs. Assume the cost of the week's menu is $80.00.
   1. List some possible changes that would lower the cost, without lowering the nutritional value.
   2. Determine the amounts of food required for the menu. Refer to table 11-3.
   3. Make a market list for this menu, organized according to the Basic Four food groups.
   4. Adapt this menu to suit a single person; to suit a middle-aged couple who have no children.
b. List the fresh fruits and vegetables available at a local supermarket this week. Have the instructor explain the unfamiliar ones. Compare their

costs with the identical frozen products and with canned products. Remember to consider edible portions and waste.

c. List the information printed on the label of a canned food.

d. Check the local supermarkets to see what freeze-dried foods are available. Buy one and prepare it according to package instructions. Compare it with the same frozen food in regard to flavor, appearance, preparation and cost.

e. Visit a supermarket and determine the number of different preparations which are available in each of the following foods (frozen, fresh, canned, etc.): green peas, potatoes, corn, orange juice, bananas, rice, milk, shrimp. Evaluate ease of home preparation and cost of each.

WORD STUDY

convenience food	freeze-dried	nutrition labeling
dehydrated	grade stamps	seasonal
Food, Drug and Cosmetic Act	impulsive shopper	

REVIEW

A.   Multiple Choice. Select the *letter* which precedes the best answer.

1.   The value of food is determined by its
   a. cost
   b. nutritional quality
   c. ease in preparation
   d. all of these

2.   The foundation of all good food purchasing plans is
   a. the Basic Four food groups
   b. nutritional labeling
   c. the federal Food, Drug and Cosmetic Act
   d. quality grading

3.   A substitute for one cup of fresh milk is
   a. 1/4 cup dried milk plus 1 cup water
   b. 1/2 cup evaporated milk plus 1/2 cup water
   c. both a and b
   d. none of the above

4.   The quality of a food
   a. may be shown by a USDA grade stamp
   b. is always indicated on food labels
   c. is never determined by the federal government
   d. is always determined by the food manufacturer

5.   The size of the food package purchased depends on
   a. family size
   b. size of appetites
   c. available storage space
   d. all of these

6. It is advisable to plan meals for a period of
   a. one day   c. two weeks
   b. one week   d. one month

7. A fresh fruit or vegetable which is in season is usually
   a. tastiest   c. available at its lowest cost
   b. available in quantity   d. all of these

8. An example of a convenience food is
   a. frozen dinners   c. bagged coffee beans
   b. fresh picked vegetables   d. Grade AA eggs

9. Under the nutrition labeling regulation, specific nutrition information must be listed on packages for
   a. all foods
   b. enriched and fortified foods
   c. foods making a nutritional claim
   d. both b and c

10. The nutrition labeling regulation was issued by the
    a. Food and Drug Administration
    b. United States Department of Agriculture
    c. National Research Council
    d. Food and Nutrition Board

B. Complete the following sentences.
 1. The law requiring that food shipped from one state to another be un-contaminated, safe to eat, and prepared under sanitary conditions, is the _____ .

 2. This same law requires that labels on food containers list ingredients and _____ .

 3. An RDA is a nutrient's _____ .

 4. Foods which are very easy to serve because they are partially prepared are called _____ .

 5. Freeze-dried foods have the nutrient _____ removed.

 6. The amount of chicken needed to serve six people would be _____ pounds.

 7. The amount of fresh winter squash needed to serve six people would be _____ pounds.

 8. Large cuts of meat usually cost _____ (less, more) per pound than small cuts.

 9. A person who buys foods because of a momentary desire is a (an) _____ shopper.

10. A satisfactory substitute for butter is margarine which is _____ .

C. Briefly answer the following questions.

1. Name at least five considerations which help the consumer maintain a well-balanced diet on a low food budget.

2. What factors determine the size and style of food package to be purchased?

3. Why are frozen or canned foods sometimes more economical than fresh foods?

SECTION EVALUATION 2 MEAL PLANNING

A. Complete the following statements.

1. A balanced diet is one that includes all six _____ .

2. The Basic Four food groups are _____ ,
_____ , _____ ,
and _____ .

3. The edible portion of food is only that part of the food that can be
_____ .

4. When a food provides a feeling of satisfaction after a meal, it has
_____ value.

5. In addition to being used as a beverage, milk may be included in the
diet in _____ , _____ , or _____
_____ .

6. Fruits and vegetables should be eaten _____ times a day.

7. A green, leafy vegetable is especially rich in vitamins _____
and _____ .

8. Yogurt and cottage cheese are included in the _____ group.

9. Milk and milk products provide rich sources of _____ ,
_____ , _____ , _____ ,
and _____ .

10. Breads and cereals are rich sources of the energy nutrient _____ .

11. In addition to providing numerous minerals and vitamins, foods from
the Meat Group are especially rich in _____ .

12. Frozen dinners, brown and serve rolls and instant puddings are all
examples of _____ .

13. Grits, spaghetti and rice are examples of foods in the _____
_____ food group.

14. Changing a menu to meet the special needs of a family member is
called _____ the menu.

15. Foods that have mild flavors are called _____ foods.

16. Food customs refer to a person's eating _____ .

17. The basis for food customs may be _____ ,
_____ , or _____ .

18. Eating habits may change because of _____
or _____ .

19. Diet during childhood directly influences the individual's _____
and _____ development.

20. Nutritional value refers to a food's _____ content.

21. Protein foods should generally be cooked at _____
temperatures.

22. Vegetables are essential to a well-balanced diet because, in addition to vitamins, minerals, water, and digestible carbohydrates, they contain an indigestible carbohydrate called _____ .

23. The law that requires that food shipped from one state to another be pure, safe to eat, and prepared under sanitary conditions is the _____ .

24. The foundation of all meal planning is the _____ .

25. The USDA grade stamp indicates the _____ of a food.

B. Match the terms listed in column I with their proper definitions in column II.

Column I

_____ 1. whole milk
_____ 2. caffeine
_____ 3. irradiated milk
_____ 4. pasteurized milk
_____ 5. skim milk
_____ 6. dried milk
_____ 7. evaporated milk
_____ 8. sweetened condensed milk
_____ 9. raw milk
_____ 10. buttermilk

Column II

a. milk with all water removed
b. unpasteurized milk
c. milk with fat removed
d. milk with harmful organisms removed
e. whole milk with 60% of its water removed
f. stimulant in coffee
g. milk processed to remove harmful organisms
h. milk with sugar added and part of the water removed
i. milk with vitamin D added
j. cultured skim milk
k. major ingredient in decaffeinated coffee

C. Briefly answer the following questions.

1. What are the Basic Four food groups? What is the number of daily servings recommended for each group?

2. How do food customs originate?

3. What is the best method to cook tender cuts of meat? To cook less tender cuts.

4. Name 5 things to be considered when planning nutritious, appetizing meals.

Section 3
MEAL PREPARATION

Chapter 12
Using Kitchen Equipment Efficiently

OBJECTIVES

After studying this chapter, the student should be able to:

- State the criteria for selecting kitchen equipment.
- Describe ways to wash and care for kitchen equipment.
- Name three practices which can reduce accidents in the kitchen.
- Explain how to smother a grease fire.

Kitchen work is complicated because it involves so many different processes. Efficiency is attained when the cook learns to perform the necessary tasks quickly and well. To do this, a good deal of practice is necessary and laborsaving methods must be employed.

Before beginning any *culinary* (relating to the kitchen or cookery) task, one should collect the necessary equipment and ingredients and arrange them conveniently. Cleanup should be considered during the preparation of food. Equipment which has been used should be set apart from ingredients which have been used. To save dishwashing after meals, the equipment used during the preparation of a meal should be washed and stored before the meal whenever possible. It is especially important to keep the school and hospital kitchens clean and orderly.

Order helps prevent accidents and mistakes in the preparation of food, and increases efficiency. Cleanliness reduces the spread of disease.

DISHWASHING

Scrape off food scraps and rinse the dishes just as soon as possible after meals. Those dishes or cooking pans containing sticky starch or protein foods may require soaking in cold water. When a cooking pan is very sticky, it is usually helpful to add a small amount of water, cover the pan and place over direct heat just until the liquid comes to a boil. Remove it from the heat and allow to cool enough so that it may be handled. Then drain, rinse, and wash with hot, soapy water.

To prepare for washing, sort dishes according to type after they have been rinsed.

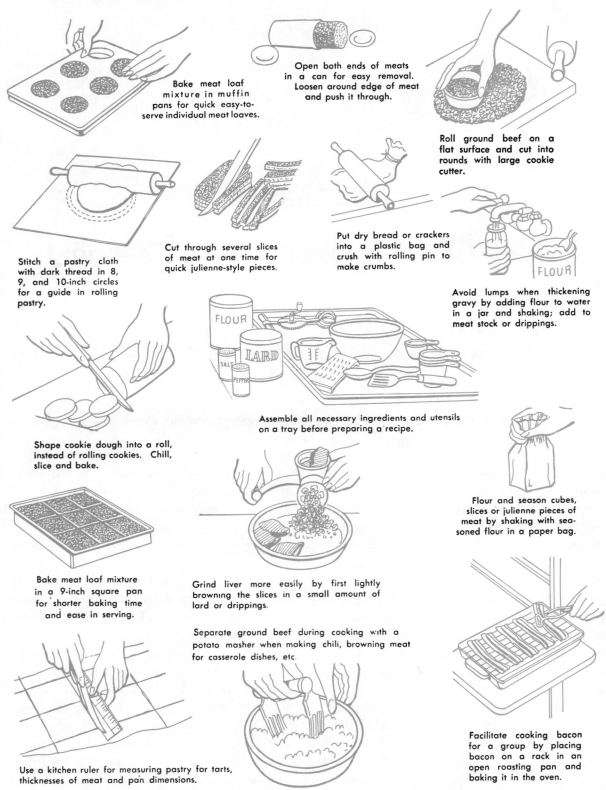

Bake meat loaf mixture in muffin pans for quick easy-to-serve individual meat loaves.

Open both ends of meats in a can for easy removal. Loosen around edge of meat and push it through.

Roll ground beef on a flat surface and cut into rounds with large cookie cutter.

Stitch a pastry cloth with dark thread in 8, 9, and 10-inch circles for a guide in rolling pastry.

Cut through several slices of meat at one time for quick julienne-style pieces.

Put dry bread or crackers into a plastic bag and crush with rolling pin to make crumbs.

Avoid lumps when thickening gravy by adding flour to water in a jar and shaking; add to meat stock or drippings.

Shape cookie dough into a roll, instead of rolling cookies. Chill, slice and bake.

Assemble all necessary ingredients and utensils on a tray before preparing a recipe.

Flour and season cubes, slices or julienne pieces of meat by shaking with sea-soned flour in a paper bag.

Bake meat loaf mixture in a 9-inch square pan for shorter baking time and ease in serving.

Grind liver more easily by first lightly browning the slices in a small amount of lard or drippings.

Separate ground beef during cooking with a potato masher when making chili, browning meat for casserole dishes, etc.

Use a kitchen ruler for measuring pastry for tarts, thicknesses of meat and pan dimensions.

Facilitate cooking bacon for a group by placing bacon on a rack in an open roasting pan and baking it in the oven.

Fig. 12-1 Timesaving techniques for quick and easy cooking. *(Courtesy of the National Live Stock and Meat Board)*

Wash glassware first, then *flatware*, (knives, forks and spoons), dishes, and finally the pots and pans. Rinse in hot water and let the dishes and glassware drain and air-dry, covered with a clean towel. Air-drying is a sanitary method of drying dishes. The use of a dish towel can sometimes spread germs. A towel may be needed to dry some metal equipment to prevent water spots and rust. Store them in their proper places when they are thoroughly dry.

SELECTION OF EQUIPMENT

Equipment is chosen for its durability, efficiency, ease with which it can be maintained and price in relation to these considerations. The student is probably familiar with small equipment or utensils such as skillets, saucepans, double boilers and various spatulas, spoons and hand blenders.

The use of larger equipment and appliances such as pressure pans, mixers, electric blenders, steamers, and dishwashers should be carefully explained and demonstrated. Gas, electric, and microwave cooking equipment have varying types of controls and will require special instructions before use. Observe the demonstration and care of all equipment carefully in order to use it efficiently and safely. When purchasing kitchen equipment, ask the salesperson to demonstrate the use of it. Read the manufacturer's instructions carefully before using any piece of equipment.

CLEANING EQUIPMENT AND KITCHEN SURFACES

The stove should be cleaned after each use. When a spot is too sticky to be removed easily with soap and water, let a small amount of soapy water stand on the sticky area for a few minutes. Then wash again and, if necessary, use a plastic cleaning pad or soap pad to remove the residue. Some cleaning pads are abrasive and should be used cautiously to prevent scratching the surface of equipment. Some surfaces such as stainless steel and enamel are dried and polished to prevent water spots. The oven and broiler should be cleaned regularly and always after food has been spilled in them. There are commercial cleaners available for this purpose. Package directions must be followed carefully because these cleaners can be dangerous when misused.

Only food in clean, covered containers should be placed in the refrigerator. Any spills inside or outside should be removed. The refrigerator should be cleaned regularly and deodorized by washing with a baking soda solution.

The sink should be scoured and washed with hot soapy water after each use. Grease should not be poured in the sink because it increases the difficulty of cleaning and may clog the drain. If the drain should clog, there are commercial products available to clear it. However, they should be used with caution and should never come in contact with the hands or the porcelain of the sink.

Tables and countertops should be washed and dried after each use. Cupboards and storage spaces should be kept orderly and clean.

KITCHEN SAFETY

Each year people are injured or killed as a result of careless habits in the kitchen. All of these incidents are labeled *accidents*, which means they might have been avoided.

Grease and water spilled on the floor should be wiped up immediately to prevent slips and falls. A stepladder should be used to reach articles stored on high shelves or cabinets. Knives should be washed separately and stored apart from other utensils and out of the reach of small children. Pot holders should be used for handling hot utensils but stored a safe distance from the stove burners. The handles of cooking pans should be turned

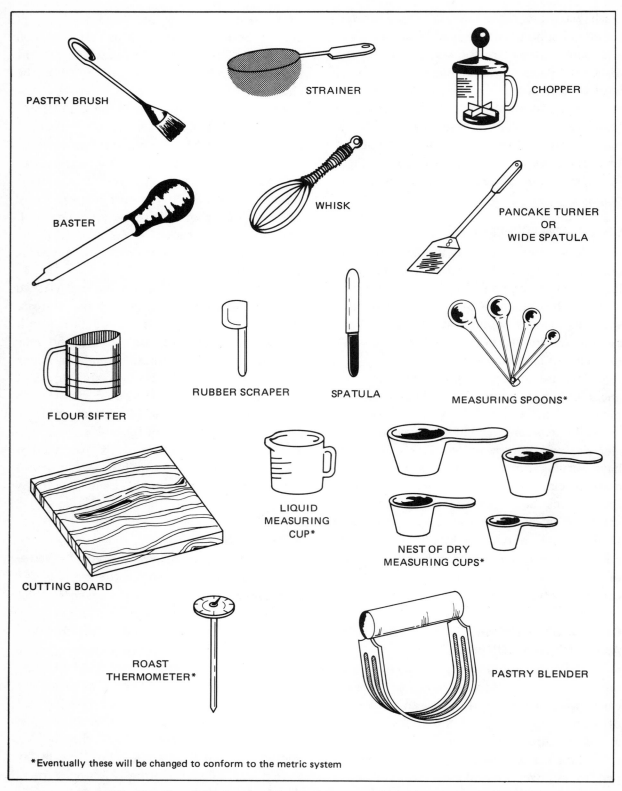

PASTRY BRUSH

STRAINER

CHOPPER

BASTER

WHISK

PANCAKE TURNER
OR
WIDE SPATULA

FLOUR SIFTER

RUBBER SCRAPER

SPATULA

MEASURING SPOONS*

CUTTING BOARD

LIQUID
MEASURING
CUP*

NEST OF DRY
MEASURING CUPS*

ROAST
THERMOMETER*

PASTRY BLENDER

*Eventually these will be changed to conform to the metric system

Fig. 12-2 Use of small kitchen utensils greatly increases efficiency in food preparation.

inward on the stove to prevent burns. Ovens should be kept clean to prevent grease fires. Gas stoves should be turned on only after the match box is closed and one match has been lit. Matches and poisons should be kept out of reach of children. Should a grease fire develop, it must be smothered with salt, baking soda, a tight lid, or a fire blanket. **CAUTION**: Do not throw water on a stove fire since water spreads grease fires.

SUMMARY

Good planning is important in working efficiently in the kitchen. Kitchen equipment is chosen for durability, efficiency, and ease in cleaning. Equipment can only be used effectively when it is used and cleaned properly. All equipment should be washed, dried, and properly stored after use.

DISCUSSION TOPICS

1. Why is it important to keep the kitchen clean?

2. Why is it especially important to keep the school and hospital kitchens clean?

3. Describe how the kitchen should be cleaned efficiently after preparing a meal.

4. Discuss the uses of the various pieces of kitchen appliances and equipment.

5. Ask if students are familiar with the following types of cookware: cast iron, Pyrex, Teflon-coated, copper-bottom, stainless steel, and enamel. Discuss the advantages and disadvantages of this equipment. Discuss their proper care.

SUGGESTED ACTIVITIES

a. Observe a demonstration of the use and care of kitchen equipment.

b. Visit the school cafeteria kitchen. Observe the equipment and ask for demonstrations.

c. Visit a hospital kitchen and observe the use of the equipment.

d. Visit a hotel dining room kitchen and observe the use of the equipment.

e. Make a list of the special cleaning products available at the local supermarket for specific surfaces such as stainless steel, copper, silver, porcelain, enamel, and wood.

f. Visit a store that sells cooking equipment such as crockpots, electric fry pans and so on. List the types available. Discuss the actual value of these items in terms of everyday home use.

g. Give demonstrations of proper dishwashing; oven cleaning; refrigerator cleaning; stove cleaning.

WORD STUDY

abrasive	deodorize	equipment
appliance	durability	meat thermometer
culinary	efficiency	pastry blender

REVIEW

A.   Briefly answer the following questions.

1.   What factors should be considered when purchasing kitchen equipment?

2.   How can sticky substances be removed from the stove?

3.   Why is it unwise to pour grease in the sink?

4.   Why is it especially important to keep the storage spaces in excellent order at all times in the school or hospital kitchen?

5.   List three ways the cook can increase the efficiency of food preparation?

6.   If a protein food such as milk or egg is stuck to a pan, what is the best method of removal?

7.   In what order should dishes be washed?

8. Name three practices which can reduce accidents in the kitchen.

9. Explain how to smother a grease fire.

B.   Identify the kitchen utensils sketched below.

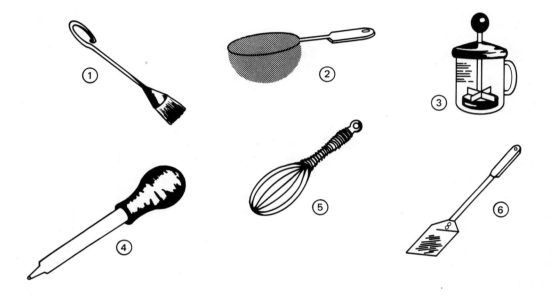

1.

2.

3.

4.

5.

6.

Chapter 13
Preventing Food-Related Illness

OBJECTIVES

After studying this chapter, the student should be able to:

- Identify diseases caused by contaminated food, their symptoms, and the means by which they are spread.
- List signs of food contamination.
- State precautions for protecting food from contamination.

The most nutritious food can cause illness if it is contaminated with harmful *microorganisms* (microscopic plants and animals such as bacteria, viruses, worms, and molds), or chemical poisons. Fortunately, in the United States there are strict federal, state, and local laws regulating the commercial production of food. Dairies, canneries, bakeries, and meat-packing houses are all subject to government inspection. The commercial processing of foods is regularly checked so that these foods are wholesome and safe to eat. Nevertheless, people do sometimes become sick because of something they ate. With few exceptions, such illnesses occur because of the ignorance or carelessness of people who handle food in the kitchen.

There are always microorganisms in the *environment* (surroundings). Sometimes they are present in the food because its animal-source contained them. When foods are undercooked these microbes may be carried to consumers and make them sick. Microorganisms may be introduced to food by a carrier. A *carrier* is a person (or animal) capable of transmitting an *infectious* (disease-causing) organism. Very often the carrier suffers no effects from the organism and

therefore is unaware of the danger. A food handler may have a cut on the hand, a cold, or a skin infection and microorganisms from this person may very easily spread to the food. Insects, dust, and animals may contaminate the food if it is improperly stored. Foods are generally moist and soft and provide an excellent place for microorganisms to grow. When foods are not stored at proper temperatures, these microorganisms multiply very rapidly. Foods should be handled and stored in such ways as to best control the growth of these organisms.

ILLNESSES CAUSED BY MICROORGANISMS IN FOOD

Salmonellosis (commonly called Salmonella) is an infection caused by the Salmonella bacteria. Salmonella may be found in raw meats, poultry, fish, milk, and eggs. It is transmitted by eating contaminated food or by contact with a carrier. Salmonellosis is characterized by headache, vomiting, diarrhea, abdominal cramps, and fever. In very severe cases it may even result in death. Those who suffer the most severe cases are typically the very young, the very old, and the weak or incapacitated.

Refrigeration at 7.2°C (45°F) or below inhibits the growth of these bacteria. However, bacteria can remain alive in the freezer and in dried foods. Salmonella bacteria are destroyed by heating to at least 60°C (140°F) for a minimum of ten minutes. One species of Salmonella causes typhoid fever.

Perfringens poisoning is caused by the *Clostridium perfringens* bacteria. It is commonly found in soil, on food, and in the intestinal tracts of warm-blooded animals. It is transmitted by eating heavily contaminated food. It is characterized by nausea, diarrhea, and inflammation of the stomach and intestines. These are spore-forming bacteria that grow without oxygen and are very difficult to destroy. The spores can survive most cooking temperatures. The best method of controlling them is to refrigerate meats quickly at 4.4°C (40°F) or below.

Staphylococcal poisoning, commonly called *Staph*, is caused by the *Staphylococcus aureus* bacteria. These bacteria are found on the skin and in the respiratory passages. They grow in meats, poultry, fish and egg dishes, and in salads such as potato, egg, macaroni and tuna and in cream-filled pastries. This poisoning is transmitted by carriers and by eating food that contains the toxin. It is characterized by vomiting, diarrhea, and abdominal cramps. It is considered a relatively mild illness. The growth of these bacteria is inhibited if foods are kept at temperatures above 60°C (140°F) or below 4.4°C (40°F). The toxin can be destroyed by boiling the food for several hours, or by heating it in a pressure cooker at 115.6°C (240°F) for 30 minutes. In most cases, long periods of high temperature cooking would reduce the appeal and nutritional value of food. Practically speaking, it would be better to discard foods suspected of being contaminated.

Botulism is caused by the toxin produced by the *Clostridium botulinum* bacteria. This is perhaps the rarest but most deadly of all the food poisonings. It is characterized by double vision, speech difficulties, inability to swallow, respiratory paralysis and sometimes death. The fatality rate in the United States is about 65 percent. The spores of this bacteria can divide and produce toxin without oxygen. This means that toxin can be produced in sealed containers such as cans and jars. The spores are extremely heat resistant. They must be boiled for six hours before they will be destroyed. The toxin, however, may be destroyed by boiling for twenty minutes.

Great care must be taken when canning foods at home in order to prevent botulism. The FDA and USDA report five deaths from botulism traced to commercially canned foods in the United States between 1925 and 1974, and 700 deaths from home-canned foods during that same time period.

Trichinosis is a disease caused by the parasite *Trichinella spiralis*. A *parasite* is a life form that depends completely on another life form without making any contribution towards the needs of the host. Trichinosis is transmitted by eating inadequately cooked pork from pigs that are infected with the *Trichinella spiralis* parasite. Symptoms include vomiting, fever, chills, and muscle pain. Cooking all pork to an internal temperature of at least 58.3°C (137°F) kills the organism and prevents this disease. The parasite may also be destroyed by freezing.

Dysentery is a disease caused by a *protozoa* (a tiny, one-celled animal). The protozoa is transmitted through food by carriers or by contaminated water. It causes severe diarrhea which may occur intermittently until the patient is properly treated.

PREVENTION OF FOOD CONTAMINATION

All of the foregoing illnesses are caused by contaminated food or water. Food becomes contaminated because of poor sanitation

TABLE 13-1 Bacterial Foodborne Illnesses: Causes, Symptoms, and Prevention

Name of Illness	What Causes It	Symptoms	Characteristics of Illness	Preventive Measures
Salmonellosis Examples of foods involved: Poultry, red meats, eggs, dried foods, dairy products.	**Salmonellae.** Bacteria widespread in nature, live and grow in intestinal tracts of human beings and animals.	Severe headache, followed by vomiting, diarrhea, abdominal cramps, and fever. Infants, elderly, and persons with low resistance are most susceptible. Severe infections cause high fever and may even cause death.	Transmitted by eating contaminated food, or by contact with infected persons or carriers of the infection. Also transmitted by insects, rodents, and pets. Onset: Usually within 12 to 36 hours. Duration: 2 to 7 days	Salmonellae in food are destroyed by heating the food to 140°F and holding for 10 minutes or to higher temperatures for less time, for instance, 155°F for a few seconds. Refrigeration at 40°F inhibits the increase of Salmonellae, but they remain alive in foods in the refrigerator or freezer, and even in dried foods.
Perfringens poisoning Examples of foods involved: Stews, soups or gravies made from poultry or red meat.	**Clostridium perfringens.** Spore-forming bacteria that grow in the absence of oxygen. Temperatures reached in thorough cooking of most foods are sufficient to destroy vegetative cells, but heat-resistant spores can survive.	Nausea (without vomiting), diarrhea, acute inflammation of the stomach and intestines.	Transmitted by eating food contaminated with abnormally large numbers of the bacteria. Onset: Usually within 8 to 20 hours. Duration: May persist for 24 hours.	To prevent growth of surviving bacteria in cooked meats, gravies, and meat casseroles that are to be eaten later, cool foods rapidly and refrigerate promptly at 40°F or below or hold them above 140°F.
Staphylococcal poisoning (frequently called staph) Examples of foods involved: Custards, egg salad, potato salad, chicken salad, macaroni salad, ham, salami, cheese	**Staphylococcus aureus.** Bacteria fairly resistant to heat. Bacteria growing in food produce a toxin that is extremely resistant to heat.	Vomiting, diarrhea, prostration, abdominal cramps. Generally mild and often attributed to other causes.	Transmitted by food handlers who carry the bacteria and by eating food containing the toxin. Onset: Usually within 3 to 8 hours. Duration: 1 or 2 days.	Growth of bacteria that produce toxin is inhibited by keeping hot foods above 140°F and cold foods at or below 40°F. Toxin is destroyed by boiling for several hours or heating the food in a pressure cooker at 240°F for 30 minutes.
Botulism Examples of foods involved: Canned low-acid foods, smoked fish	**Clostridium botulinum.** Spore-forming organisms that grow and produce toxin in the absence of oxygen, such as in a sealed container.	Double vision, inability to swallow, speech difficulty, progressive respiratory paralysis. Fatality rate is high, in the United States about 65 percent.	Transmitted by eating food containing the toxin. Onset: Usually within 12 to 36 hours or longer. Duration: 3 to 6 days.	Bacterial spores in food are destroyed by high temperatures obtained only in the pressure canner. More than 6 hours is needed to kill the spores at boiling temperature (212°F). The toxin is destroyed by boiling for 10 to 20 minutes; time required depends on kind of food.

Source: USDA Home and Garden Bulletin No. 162, 1975

on the part of the food handler or from improper storage.

To prevent contamination, persons preparing food must have clean hands that are not cut or infected in any way, clean clothes, and clean cooking equipment. They should touch the food as little as possible. After handling uncooked food, people should wash their hands and any knives or cutting boards used. Tests should be made regularly of

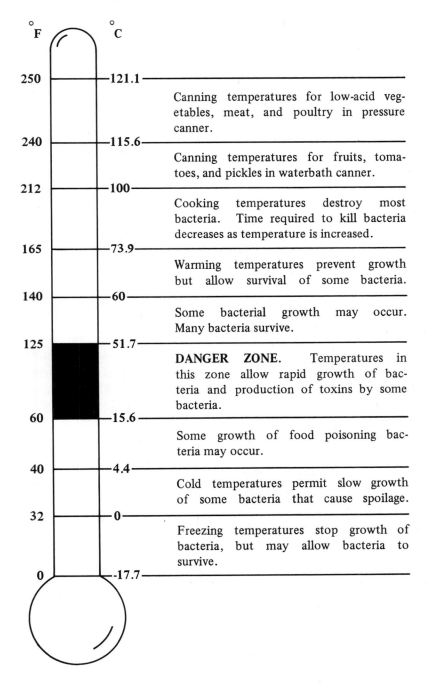

Fig. 13-1 Temperatures of food for control of bacteria. *(USDA Home and Garden Bulletin, No. 162, 1975)*

people working as professional food handlers in order to ascertain that they are not carriers of infectious organisms.

Food poisons cannot be seen, but there are sometimes telltale signs of their existence. If a can bulges, if its contents appear different than usual, or if the food has an unusual odor, it should be discarded in a place where animals and children cannot reach it. **CAUTION**: The food should never be tasted in these circumstances because Clostridium botulinum may be present and can be fatal.

Food Storage

Proper food storage is very important in inhibiting the growth of bacteria. Because bacteria grow best at temperatures between 15.6° and 51.7°C (60° and 125°F) it is important to keep food refrigerated, that is, below 15.6°C (60°F) or to keep it hot, above 51.7°C (125°F). Leftover food should always be refrigerated just as soon as the meal is finished and covered after it is cold. It should not be allowed to cool at room temperature before being refrigerated. Frozen foods should either be cooked from the frozen state or thawed in the refrigerator. (When cooked from the frozen state, cooking time will be increased by at least 50 percent.) Frozen foods should not be thawed at room temperature. Food must always be protected from dust, insects, and animals since all of these can spread contamination.

Miscellaneous Food Poisonings

Occasionally food poisoning is termed natural. This means it is caused by ingesting certain plants or animals which contain poison. Examples are plants such as poisonous mushrooms and rhubarb leaves, and fish from polluted water.

Individuals may develop *allergies* (hypersensitivities) to certain foods. If these foods are eaten, they may cause temporary reactions. Symptoms may include nausea, diarrhea, dizziness, and sometimes serious breathing difficulties.

Poisoning also may result from ingesting cleaning agents, insecticides or excessive amounts of a drug. Children may swallow cleaning agents or medicines. The cook may mistakenly use a poison instead of a cooking ingredient. Sometimes insecticides cling to fresh fruits and vegetables. It is essential that all potential poisons be kept out of the reach of young children and kept separate from all food supplies. Fresh fruits and vegetables should be thoroughly washed before being stored.

SUMMARY

Infection or poisoning traced to food is usually caused by human ignorance or carelessness. The serving of safe meals is essentially the responsibility of the cook. Food should not be prepared by anyone who has or carries a contagious disease. All fresh fruits and vegetables should be washed before being eaten. Meats, poultry, fish, eggs, and dairy products should be refrigerated. Pork should always be cooked to the well-done stage. Foods should be covered to prevent contamination by dust, insects, or animals. Garbage should also be covered so that it does not attract insects. Hands that prepare foods should be clean and free of cuts or wounds. Kitchen equipment should be spotless. Finally, the food itself should be safe. People should avoid foods containing natural poisons.

DISCUSSION TOPICS

1. Name four types of food poisoning. If any class member has suffered from food poisoning, ask the person to describe the symptoms.
2. How may food become contaminated?
3. How may food be kept free of insect and animal contamination?
4. Why should foods be refrigerated?
5. Discuss appropriate storage of cleaning agents in a home with young children.

SUGGESTED ACTIVITIES

a. Using outside sources, present a committee report on diseases that can be carried in food. Include the agent of transmission, mode of transmission, symptoms, and treatment.

b. Visit a restaurant kitchen. Look for practices which may lead to potential food poisoning. Note the practices and uses of equipment designed to prevent food poisoning.

WORD STUDY

botulism	insecticide	protozoa
carrier	microorganisms	Salmonella
diarrhea	nausea	sanitation
dysentery	parasite	Staphylococcus
environment	Perfringens	toxin
infectious	polluted water	trichinosis

REVIEW

A. Multiple Choice. Select the *letter* which precedes the best answer.

1. A microorganism is a (an)
   a. unit of measurement
   b. tiny animal or plant
   c. component of a microscope
   d. individual human cell

2. Salmonella bacteria are destroyed by heating foods to 60°C (140°F) for a minimum of
   a. 2 minutes
   b. 10 minutes
   c. 30 minutes
   d. 2 hours

3. Someone who is capable of spreading an infectious organism but is not sick himself is called a
   a. food handler
   b. carrier
   c. transport
   d. fomite

4. When an organism is infectious, it is
   a. disease-causing
   b. prone to infections
   c. not contagious
   d. always fatal

5. Most cases of food poisoning in the United States are caused by
   a. careless processing in commercial factories
   b. lack of government inspection
   c. careless handling of food in the kitchen
   d. house pets

6. Generally, food poisoning symptoms include
   a. headache   c. abdominal upset
   b. nausea   d. all of these

7. Salmonella infection and staphylococcal poisoning are caused by
   a. virus   c. protozoa
   b. bacteria   d. worms

8. The deadliest of the bacterial food poisonings is
   a. Staphylococcus   c. botulism
   b. Salmonella   d. perfringens poisoning

9. The disease caused by a parasite sometimes found in pork is
   a. tularemia   c. avitaminosis
   b. dysentery   d. trichinosis

10. The disease caused by a protozoa and characterized by severe diarrhea is
    a. Salmonella   c. dysentery
    b. botulism   d. infectious hepatitis

11. Foods may be contaminated by
    a. people   c. animals
    b. insects   d. all of these

12. The temperatures in the danger zone which encourage bacterial growth are between
    a. 0° to 32°F (-18° to 0°C)   c. 60° to 125°F (16° to 52°C)
    b. 32° to 60°F (0° to 16°C)   d. 125° to 212°F (52° to 100°C)

13. A telltale sign of spoiled food may be
    a. a bulging can   c. an unusual appearance
    b. a peculiar odor   d. all of these

14. Leftover foods should be
    a. put in the refrigerator immediately after meals
    b. cooled to room temperature before refrigerating
    c. cooled in the refrigerator for at least an hour before freezing
    d. stored unwrapped in the refrigerator

15. Frozen foods should be
    a. thawed at room temperature
    b. refrozen if not used immediately after thawing
    c. thawed in the refrigerator
    d. any of the above

Chapter 14
Reading Recipes

OBJECTIVES

After studying this chapter, the student should be able to:

- Define cookery terms commonly used in recipes.
- Demonstrate the processes involved in various cookery terms.

Tested recipes list specific amounts of ingredients and include directions for combining them in order to produce satisfactory and predictable food products. Since the preparation of meals involves the use of recipes, it is important to understand the terms used in them.

In order to use cookery terms and follow recipes correctly, the student should learn the definitions of these terms, observe demonstrations of the techniques defined, and practice the techniques when following recipes. It is always wise to use tested recipes to avoid disappointing results and waste. A knowledge of the following terms should prove useful.

a la king: served in a white sauce with bits of green pepper and pimiento. A common example is chicken a la king.

aspic: highly seasoned jelly made from broth, stock, or tomato juice. An example is tomato aspic.

au gratin: prepared in white sauce with cheese added. Potatoes au gratin are an example.

bake: cook in the oven as is done with cakes and cookies

barbecue: to bake or to roast over coals or on a spit, basting with spicy sauce, as is done with chicken and pork ribs

baste: to brush or pour hot fat on cooking foods, as is done with roasting poultry

beat: to combine with air by mixing vigorously; this is often done with eggs.

blanch: to plunge into boiling water and then into cold water. This may be done with almonds to remove their brown skins.

blend: to mix thoroughly, as is done when combining ingredients for cakes and cookies

boil: to cook in liquid at 100°C (212°F) as is indicated when bubbles break on the surface of the liquid

braise: to cook in a covered container with a small amount of liquid, as is done with less tender cuts of meat

broil: to cook under or over direct heat. Tender meats can be broiled.

brush: to spread a thin amount of sauce, oil, or egg over food as is commonly done with yeast breads

casserole: a meal in one dish; sometimes the dish itself is called a casserole

chop: to cut into small, irregular pieces, as is done with onions, celery, hard-cooked eggs, and nuts

combine: to mix together

compote: fruit in syrup; also, the long-stemmed dish in which it may be served *cream:* to mix with beaters or the back of a spoon until food is smooth and creamy in consistency; done to mix shortening and sugar for cakes and cookies

croquette: combination of finely chopped food and white sauce shaped in a ball or cone, rolled in egg and crumbs, and fried in deep fat. An example might be chicken croquettes.

cube: to dice or cut into small, regular squares, as may be done with cheese

cut in: to blend shortening with flour using two knives or a pastry blender

deviled: highly seasoned. An example might be deviled eggs.

dice: to cube or cut into very small, regular squares

dredge: to coat heavily with flour, as is sometimes done before browning meat; or to coat with sugar, as may be done with some cookie dough just before baking

dust: to sprinkle lightly with flour or sugar, as may be done to the top of baked products.

flake: to separate gently with a fork, as may be done to fish

fold: to blend very gently with a down, across, up and over motion to retain air in a mixture, as is done when combining heavy mixtures with light, whipped ingredients

fry: to cook in hot fat, as may be done with potatoes or chicken

garnish: to trim or decorate food; the trimmings. Such trimmings should harmonize in color, flavor, and shape with the dish it decorates. Examples are parsley, egg slices, pickles, carrot curls.

grate: to rub on a rough surface, producing small particles, as is done with onions, lemons, and oranges

grill: to broil

julienne: to cut into thin strips, as may be done with meat used in salads

knead: to mix by folding and squeezing with the hands, as in mixing yeast bread doughs

marinade: distinctive liquid or sauce in which some foods are kept for a specified time to alter their original flavors

marinate: to let stand in a marinade

mince: to chop as finely as possible, as may be done with celery, onions, or parsley

mocha: combination of coffee and chocolate flavors. An example is mocha icing.

pan-broil: to fry, pouring off fat as it accumulates, as may be done when cooking bacon

parboil: to partially cook by boiling or simmering, as may be done to julienne potatoes before frying

poach: to cook in liquid just below the boiling point, as may be done with eggs, fish, or chicken

puree: to press through a strainer to remove cellulose; the food which has been pressed through the strainer. An example is puree of spinach.

saute: to fry slowly in a small amount of fat, as may be done with onions, peppers, or eggs

scald: to bring a liquid just to the boiling point and immediately remove it from the heat, as may be done with milk

score: to make shallow, even cuts on the surface; often done with ham that is to be baked

sear: to brown quickly at a high temperature, as is sometimes done with meat

shred: to tear or rub or cut into thin pieces, as is done with lettuce and cabbage

sift: to put dry ingredients through a sieve to remove lumps, as is done with flour

simmer: to cook in liquid just below the boiling point; indicated by tiny bubbles breaking just beneath the surface of the liquid

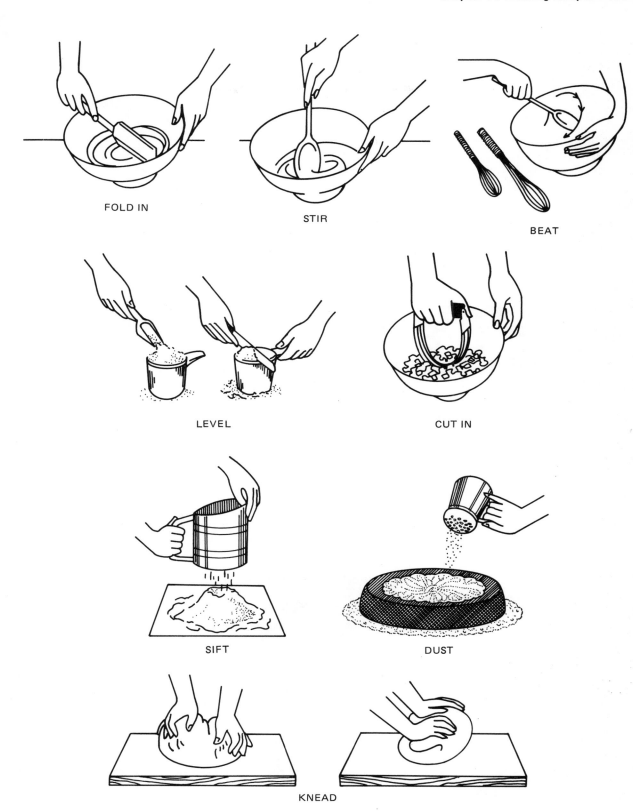

FOLD IN

STIR

BEAT

LEVEL

CUT IN

SIFT

DUST

KNEAD

Fig. 14-1 Baking instructions must be carefully followed.

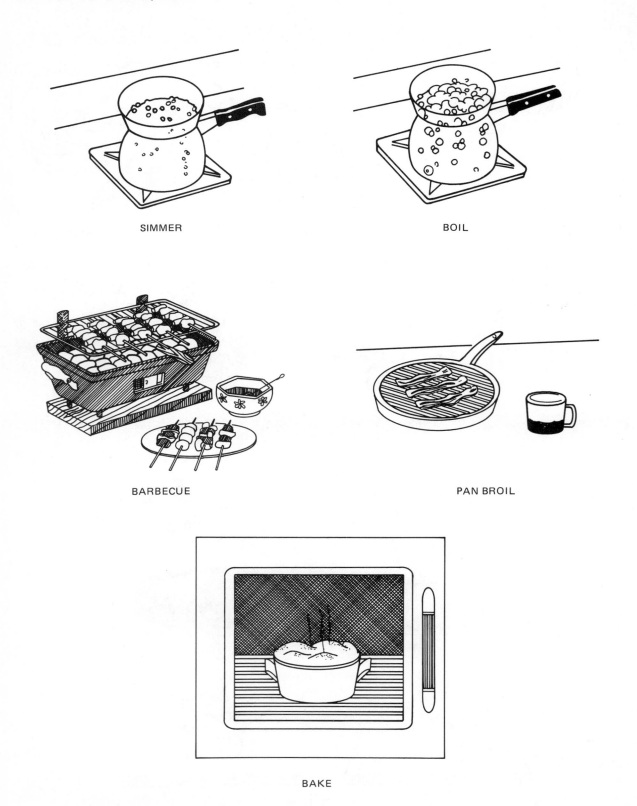

SIMMER

BOIL

BARBECUE

PAN BROIL

BAKE

Fig. 14-2 Different cooking methods are used according to type and quality of food.

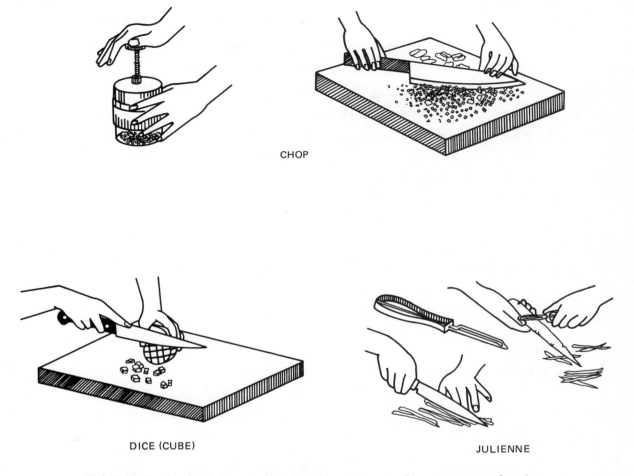

CHOP

DICE (CUBE)

JULIENNE

Fig. 14-3. Cutting foods into smaller pieces is a process used in many types of cookery.

skewer: a metal or wooden pick for fastening foods, or to fasten foods with such a pick

souffle: light, fluffly dish having eggs as the main ingredient. Examples are cheese and chocolate souffles.

steam: to cook in covered container over but not touching boiling water; done with vegetables and some quick breads

steep: to let stand in hot liquid for a specified time, as is done with tea

stew: to cook slowly in liquid or a mixture of meat and vegetables cooked by this method. An example is beef and vegetable stew.

stock: liquid in which foods have been cooked. Examples are meat or vegetable stocks.

timbale: finely chopped foods combined with eggs and baked in a mold. Examples are chicken timbales.

whip: to beat rapidly, introducing air, as may be done to egg whites or heavy cream

SUMMARY

A thorough knowledge of the meanings of cookery terms and the ability to use them correctly is essential for efficient meal preparation. Using appropriate equipment is also necessary in applying the techniques described.

DISCUSSION TOPICS

1. Why is it important for a cook to know the meaning of cooking terms?

2. Why is it wise to use tested recipes rather than untried recipes?

3. Discuss how casseroles can be prepared from leftover foods.

4. How can a chocolate frosting be changed into a mocha frosting?

5. Of what use are the words "serves two" in a recipe?

6. What is beef stock? Chicken stock?

7. Name five foods frequently used as garnishes. What are some attractive garnishes suitable for egg salad?

8. Why are purees frequently included in hospital menus?

9. Name two ingredients which are frequently folded into other ingredients.

10. What is the difference between:
    - fry and pan-broil
    - a la king and au gratin
    - dice and julienne
    - marinate and steep
    - mince and grate
    - whip and fold

SUGGESTED ACTIVITIES

a. Identify the cookery terms in the following recipe and explain them.

Egg Salad

3 eggs
1 tbsp. grated onion
1/2 tsp. salt
1/4 tsp. paprika
1/4 c. chopped celery
1/4 c. mayonnaise

Simmer the eggs 15 minutes. Cool and shell them. Chop the celery and grate the onion. Cube the eggs and add the celery, mayonnaise, salt, paprika and onion. Combine gently. Serve on greens and garnish with tomato wedges. Serves two.

b. Organize two teams and have a "spell-down" on the cookery terms and their definitions.

c. Plan a menu that includes an aspic, a dish a la king, and a compote. Use cookbooks for reference.

d. Plan a menu that includes a casserole, a puree, and a souffle.

e. Divide the class into groups and have each group demonstrate one or more of the cooking terms discussed in this chapter.

f. Browse through a cookbook and look for directions which include some of the following terms. Name the recipe in which each is found.

baste	cream	fold	sear
beat	cut in	marinate	sift
blend	deviled	simmer	steam
braise	dredge	saute	whip

g. Prepare a class cookbook composed of favorite recipes from students and teacher. Include sections on appetizers, soups, fish, poultry, meats, vegetables, breads, and desserts. Allow space for additions.

REVIEW

A. Match the foods listed in column I with the cookery terms commonly used in preparing them, listed in column II. Some choices can be used more than once.

Column I

_____ 1. egg whites
_____ 2. almonds
_____ 3. pot roast
_____ 4. lemon rind
_____ 5. sirloin steak
_____ 6. cookies
_____ 7. milk
_____ 8. flour
_____ 9. bread
_____ 10. parsley

Column II

a. sift
b. braise
c. blanch
d. mince
e. scald
f. puree
g. grate
h. whip
i. poach
j. broil
k. bake
l. knead
m. dice

B. Read the following recipe. In the space provided below the recipe, write definitions of the italicized cookery terms.

Braised Beef

5 pounds top round of beef
3 cups red wine
1/2 cup chopped onion
1/2 cup diced celery
1 tablespoon minced parsley
1/2 cup flour
3 tablespoons margarine
1 cup beef stock

Put the meat in a large bowl. (1) *Chop* the onions, (2) *dice* the celery, (3) *mince* the parsley, and (4) *combine* the vegetables. Place the vegetables on top of and around the meat. Add the wine. Cover and (5) *marinate* in the refrigerator 24 hours. Discard the (6) *marinade*. Dry the meat and (7) *dredge* with the flour. Melt the margarine in a heavy skillet. Add meat and (8) *sear*, turning as the meat browns. Place the browned meat in a casserole with a tight-fitting cover. Add the (9) beef *stock*. Cover and (10) *braise* over low heat 3 hours or until tender. 1 1/4 hours before serving, add 12 medium white potatoes. Bring to a (11) *boil*. Reduce heat and (12) *simmer* 1 hour. Slice meat

Serve with the potatoes and buttered carrots (13) *julienne.* (14) *Garnish* with parsley.

1.   8.

2.   9.

3.   10.

4.   11.

5.   12.

6.   13.

7.   14.

Chapter 15
Measuring and Weighing Ingredients

OBJECTIVES

After studying this chapter, the student should be able to:

- State metric equivalents of common household measures.
- Compare weight and volume of cooking ingredients.
- Convert measurements from the English to the metric system and from the metric to the English system.
- Measure and weigh foods accurately.

Accuracy in weighing and measuring ingredients is essential in order to prepare dishes consistent in quality and to follow the physician's orders when therapeutic diets are prescribed. One must be familiar with the systems of weights and measures and know how to use the measuring devices and scales.

SYSTEMS OF WEIGHTS AND MEASURES

The two systems of weights and measures commonly used are the *English* and the *metric*. The English is most commonly used in the United States. The units of measurement within it originated in various cultures. The English system includes many different measuring units such as pints, quarts, and gallons, as well as inch, foot and yard.

The metric system is an international system of weights and measures based on the number ten. Because a power of ten is common to all measuring units, conversion within the metric system is quite simple. In this system, the basic unit of weight or mass is the *gram*. Length is measured in *meters* and volume is measured in *liters*. The metric units in weight, length, or volume all use the same *prefixes* (beginnings of words), table 15-2.

page 138. Although the metric system is used in many parts of the world, the United States has been slow to accept it. However, it will soon be widely used throughout the country and students must learn how to apply the metric system. Since so many measurements are given in the household and the apothecaries systems, conversion to the metric system must be learned by students and consumers. Learning to convert from one system of measurement to the other is not difficult but it requires practice; quick reference and ways to convert are illustrated in tables, 15-3 and 15-4, page 139.

MEASURING DEVICES AND THEIR CORRECT USE

The measuring devices commonly available in the United States are still based on the English system. Measuring spoon sets include 1/4 teaspoon, 1/2 teaspoon, 1 teaspoon and 1 tablespoon. Measuring cups for solid and dry ingredients include: 1/4 cup, 1/3 cup, 1/2 cup, and 1 cup. To use these for dry ingredients, fill them gently, without shaking, and remove the excess with a flat spatula so they are level across the top.

TABLE 15-1   Metric Equivalents of Common Household Measures*

	Household	Metric
dash	less than 1/8 teaspoon	—
few grains (f. g.)	less than 1/8 teaspoon	—
drop	—	0.060 milliliter (ml)
15 drops	—	1 milliliter (same as one cubic centimeter)
1 teaspoon (tsp)	1/3 tablespoon	5 milliliters (ml)
1 tablespoon (tbsp)	3 teaspoons	15 milliliters (ml)
1 fluid ounce (oz)	2 tablespoons	30 milliliters (ml)
1 cup (c)	8 fluid ounces or 16 tablespoons	240 milliliters or 0.24 liters
1 pint (pt)	2 cups	470 milliliters or 0.47 liters
1 quart (qt)	2 pints or 4 cups	950 milliliters or 0.95 liters
1 gallon (gal)	4 quarts	3.8 liters
1 peck (pk)	2 gallons	7.6 liters
1 bushel (bu)	4 pecks	30.4 liters
1 pound (lb)	16 ounces	.454 kilograms (kg)

*The above equivalents are presented only as a guide to familiarize the user with metric measures. It is recommended that the size of rounded metric measures be learned and used.

TABLE 15-2   Unit Relationships Within the Metric System

Weight	Length	Volume
1000 grams = 1 *kilo*gram	1000 meters = 1 *kilo*meter	1000 liters = 1 *kilo*liter*
100 grams = 1 *hekto*gram*	100 meters = 1 *hekto*meter*	100 liters = 1 *hecto*liter*
10 grams = 1 *deka*gram*	10 meters = 1 *deka*meter*	10 liters = 1 *deka*liter*
1 gram	1 meter	1 liter
.1 gram = 1 *deci*gram*	.1 meter = 1 *deci*meter*	.1 liter = 1 *deci*liter*
.01 gram = 1 *centi*gram*	.01 meter = 1 *centi*meter	.01 liter = 1 *centi*liter*
.001 gram = 1 *milli*gram	.001 meter = 1 *milli*meter	.001 liter = 1 *milli*liter
.000001 gram = 1 *micro*gram*	.000001 meter = 1 *micro*meter*	.000001 liter = 1 *micro*liter*

* units not commonly used

TABLE 15-3 Converting from the English System to the Metric System

CONVERT TO METRIC	WHEN YOU KNOW	MULTIPLY BY	TO FIND
WEIGHT	ounces (oz)	28	grams (g)
	pounds (lb)	0.45	kilograms (kg)
VOLUME	teaspoons (tsp)	5	milliliters (ml)
	tablespoons (Tbsp)	15	milliliters
	fluid ounces (fl oz)	30	milliliters
	cups (c)	0.24	liters (l)
	pints (pt)	0.47	liters
	quarts (qt)	0.95	liters
	gallons (gal)	3.8	liters
	cubic feet (ft^3)	0.03	cubic meters (m^3)
	cubic yards (yd^3)	0.76	cubic meters
TEMPERATURE	Fahrenheit ($^\circ$F) temperature	5/9 (after subtracting 32)	Celsius ($^\circ$C) temperature

Source: Adapted from "Some References on Metric Information" by US Dept of Commerce, National Bureau of Standards, 1975

TABLE 15-4 Converting from the Metric System to the English System

CONVERT TO ENGLISH	WHEN YOU KNOW	MULTIPLY BY	TO FIND
WEIGHT	grams (g)	0.035	ounces (oz)
	kilograms (kg)	2.2	pounds (lb)
	metric tons (1000 kg)	1.1	short tons
VOLUME	milliliters (ml)	0.03	fluid ounces (fl oz)
	liters (l)	2.1	pints (pt)
	liters	1.06	quarts (qt)
	liters	0.26	gallons (gal)
	cubic meters (m^3)	35	cubic feet (ft^3)
	cubic meters	1.3	cubic yards (yd^3)
TEMPERATURE	Celsius ($^\circ$C) temperature	9/5 (then add 32)	Fahrenheit ($^\circ$F) temperature

Source: Adapted from "Some References on Metric Information" by US Dept. of Commerce, National Bureau of Standards, 1975

TABLE 15-5   Equivalent Weights and Measures

Weight Equivalents

	Milligram	Gram	Kilogram	Grain	Ounce	Pound
1 microgram (μg)	.001	.000001				
1 milligram (mg)	1.	.001		.0154		
1 gram (g)	1,000.	1.	.001	15.4	.035	.0022
1 kilogram (kg)	1,000,000.	1,000.	1.	15,400.	35.2	2.2
1 grain (gr)	64.8	.065		1.		
1 ounce (oz)		28.3		437.5	1.	.063
1 pound (lb)		453.6	.454		16.	1.

Volume Equivalents

	Cubic Millimeter	Cubic Centimeter	Liter	Fluid Ounce	Pint	Quart
1 cubic millimeter (mm^3)	1.	.001				
1 cubic centimeter (cm^3)	1,000.	1.	.001			
1 liter (l)	1,000,000.	1,000.	1.	33.8	2.1	1.06
1 fluid ounce (fl oz)		30. (29.57)	.03	1.		
1 pint (pt)		473.	.473	16.	1.	
1 quart (qt)		946.	.946	32	2.	1.

Shaking the measuring cup packs the dry ingredients and results in an excess of the ingredient. When a solid ingredient such as shortening must be measured or when brown sugar is packed into a cup, air pockets should be pushed out with a slender knife. The measurement is leveled by pressing down firmly and then cutting across the top of the cup with a flat spatula.

Liquids are measured in a cup which has marks indicating 1/4 cup, 1/3 cup, 1/2 cup, 2/3 cup, 3/4 cup, and 1 cup and sometimes two cups, figure 15-1. There is a spill area above the one-cup or two-cup mark and a pouring spout. To use the cup accurately, it must be on a level surface at eye level and the liquid being measured should come exactly to the line of measurement specified. This equipment is inexpensive and is available at most supermarkets or variety stores.

Most food scales measure weight in grams or ounces. It is helpful to remember that one ounce equals approximately 30 grams.

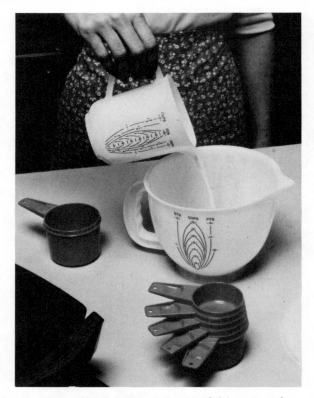

Fig. 15-1   Measuring cups are useful in many sizes. *(Courtesy of Tupperware).*

Measuring foods and weighing them with the scales should be practiced until it can be done quickly and accurately. Learning weights and measurements, their equivalents, and their abbreviations becomes easier with practice.

Weight and volume of food depends on its density. Therefore, two foods of equal weight may differ in volume. For example, one pound of butter equals 2 cups, but one pound of powdered sugar equals 3 3/4 cups. When the cook is comparing amounts of food, both weight and volume must be considered, table 15-6.

SUMMARY

Foods must be weighed and measured accurately to maintain quality in cooking and to conform to the physician's prescription when special diets are ordered. There are convenient devices for measuring and weighing foods. The common weights and measures in both the English and metric systems should be learned.

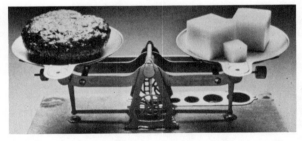

Fig. 15-2 Equal weights of meat and cheese can best be determined on a scale. *(Courtesy of Tupperware)*

TABLE 15-6 Cooking Ingredients Compared in Weight and Volume

Breadcrumbs	
4 ounces	3/4 cup less 1 tablespoon
100 grams	1/2 cup
Currants and Raisins	
1 pound	2 3/8 cups
100 grams	1/2 cup plus 1 tablespoon
Nuts	
4 ounces	2/3 cup, chopped
100 grams	1/2 cup plus 1 tablespoon (chopped)
Brown sugar	
1 pound	2 1/4 cup
100 grams	1/2 cup plus 2 tablespoons
Granulated sugar	
1 pound	2 cups
100 grams	1/2 cup less 1 tablespoon
Butter, margarine, solid fats and cheese	
1 pound	2 cups
1 ounce	2 tablespoons
100 grams	7 tablespoons
Flour	
1 pound	3 1/2 to 4 cups
1 ounce	3 tablespoons
100 grams	3/4 cup less 2 tablespoons
Rice, uncooked	
1 pound	2 cups
Powdered sugar	
1 pound	3 3/4 cups
100 grams	3/4 cup

DISCUSSION TOPICS

1. Why is it important to measure and weigh foods accurately at home? In the hospital kitchen?

2. Why are liquid measuring cups inappropriate for measuring dry ingredients and vice-versa?

3. Discuss the units of measurement in the English and those in the metric systems. Make comparisons of commonly used units in cooking.

4. Why are there 3 1/2 to 4 cups of flour in one pound, but only two cups of granulated sugar in one pound?

5. Which would weigh more, one cup of dry cereal or one cup of cooked cereal? Why?

SUGGESTED ACTIVITIES

a. Observe demonstrations of measuring sugar, flour, and water. Practice measuring these items. Check each other for accuracy.

b. After the use of scales has been demonstrated, practice weighing one cup each of flour, sugar, and water. Remember to subtract the weight of the measuring cup from the total weight to find out the net weight of each item. Write a report of the experiment, listing the items from lightest to heaviest.

c. Weigh a piece of meat with bone before and after cooking. What percentage of the meat is waste? Weigh just the bone. What percentage of the meat was bone? What accounts for the remainder of the waste?

d. Prepare two ground beef patties of equal weight from the same package of ground meat. Fry one patty over medium-low heat until it is cooked through. Fry the second patty over high heat until it has a dark brown crust on the outside. Weigh each again. Is there a difference in the weights of the two patties? If so, which cooking temperature resulted in the lighter-weight patty? Compare the palatability of the two patties.

e. Convert the following recipe to metric measurements:

Meatloaf

2 1/4 pounds ground beef

2 eggs

1/2 cup bread crumbs

2 tbsp. minced onion

1 cup milk

1 tsp. pepper

f. Convert one or more of your favorite recipes to metric measurements. Test one.

g. Convert the following recipe to the English system of measurements

Pound Cake

250 g butter

750 g sugar

6 eggs

250 g flour

5 ml baking soda

250 g sour cream

WORD STUDY

density   kilo   metric system
English system of weights   liter   micro
    and measures   meter   milli
grams

REVIEW

A. Briefly answer the following questions.

1. How many teaspoons are there in one tablespoon?

2. How many ounces are there in 1/2 cup of water?

3. How many cups are there in 1 pint?

4. How many quarts are there in 1 gallon?

5. How many cups are there in 1 pound of butter?

6. How many cups are there in 1 pound of flour?

7. How many cups are there in 5 pounds of granulated sugar?

8. How many grams are there in 2 kilograms?

9. How many grams are there in 3 ounces?

10. How many quarts are there in 1 liter?

11. How many pounds are there in 1 kilogram?

12. How many grams are there in 1 pound?

13. How many kilograms are there in 4 pounds?

14. On what number is the metric system based?

B. Make the alterations indicated in the following measurements for a brownie recipe.

1/4 c. butter	1 oz. chocolate
1 c. sugar	1/4 c. whole milk
1 tsp. vanilla	1 c. all-purpose flour
2 eggs	1 tsp. salt

1. Double the recipe.

2. Convert the measurements to the metric system.

3. How many brownie recipes can be prepared from each of the following ingredients?

a. 1 lb. of sugar   c. 1 qt. of milk
b. 1 lb. of butter   d. 1 doz. eggs

Chapter 16
Preparation of the Patient's Meal

OBJECTIVES

After studying this chapter, the student should be able to:

- Adapt a family menu to suit the needs of the patient.
- Demonstrate correct procedures for feeding a bedridden patient.
- List dietary information that should be included in a patient's chart.

In the home, the family menu should serve as the basis of the patient's meal whenever possible. This usually pleases the patient because he feels more a part of the family. Working from the same basic menu also saves time in preparing additional foods and avoids unnecessary food costs. A review of basic nutrition (Section One) reinforces the need for nutrients and roughage.

Family meals are quite easily adapted to the patient by omitting or adding certain foods or by varying the method of preparation. Suppose the patient was to limit his fat intake and the family menu was:

> Fried Hamburgers
> Mashed Potatoes with Butter
> Buttered Peas
> Lettuce
> with
> French Dressing
> Ice Cream
> with
> Fresh Strawberries
> Whole Milk

Broiling the hamburgers, instead of frying, would help to limit the fat content. The patient's mashed potatoes might be served with little or no butter and the peas with only salt and pepper and perhaps a suitable spice or herb. The patient's lettuce could be served with lemon and he might have plain strawberries for dessert. Skim milk is a simple substitute for whole milk.

SERVING THE MEAL

To serve a meal at the bedside, the tray should be lined with a pretty cloth or paper liner. Attractive dishes which fit the tray conveniently without crowding it should be used. The food should be arranged attractively

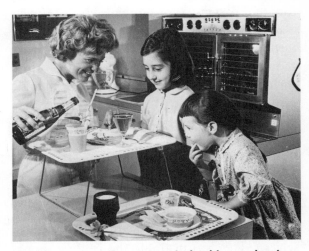

Fig. 16-1 Note how attractively this tray has been prepared for a small patient. *(Courtesy of Parent's Magazine)*

on the plate, with a colorful garnish such as a slice of fruit, parsley, a pickle, or vegetable stick. The garnish must fit into the patient's diet plan. Utensils must be arranged conveniently. Water should be served as well as another beverage (unless it is prohibited by the physician). Foods must be served at proper temperatures.

When the patient is on complete bedrest, special preparations are required before the meal is served. The patient should be given the opportunity to use the bedpan and to wash before the meal is served. The room can be ventilated and the bedcovers straightened. The patient should be helped to a comfortable position and any unpleasant sights removed before the meal is served. Pleasant conversation during the preparations can improve the patient's mood considerably. Certain topics of conversation can help stimulate the patient's interest in eating. The patient might be told that the family is anticipating the same meal. Perhaps the recipes used will interest some patients. Remarks on the patient's progress, whenever possible, are helpful.

When the meal preparations are complete, the tray should be placed so it is easy for the patient to feed himself, or if necessary, convenient for someone else to do the feeding. If the patient needs help, the napkin should be opened and placed, the bread spread, the meat cut, the eggs shelled and the drinking tube offered. The patient should be encouraged to eat and be allowed sufficient time. If the meal is interrupted by the physician, the tray should be removed and the food kept at proper temperatures in the kitchen. It should be served again as soon as the physician leaves.

Some patients are unable to feed themselves. The person doing the feeding should sit near the side of the bed. Small amounts of food should be placed toward the back of

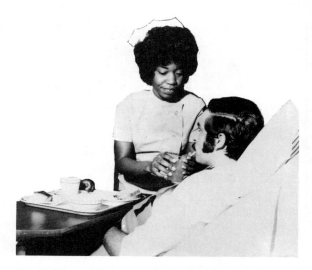

Fig. 16-2　Some patients require assistance with eating.

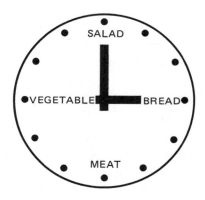

Fig. 16-3　To a blind patient a plate of food can be pictured as the face of a clock.

the mouth with a slight pressure on the tongue with the spoon or fork. If the patient is suffering from one-sided paralysis, the food and drinking straw must be placed in the non-paralyzed side of the mouth. The patient must be allowed to help himself as much as possible. If the patient begins to choke, help him sit up straight. Do not give food or water while the patient is choking. The patient's mouth should be wiped as it is needed.

Special care must be taken in serving a meal for a blind patient. An appetizing description of the meal can help create a desire to eat. To help the blind patient feed himself, arrange the food as if the plate were the face of a clock. The meat might be put at 6 o'clock, vegetables at 9 o'clock, salad at 12 and bread at 3 o'clock. The person who regularly arranges the meal should remember to always use the same pattern. Blind people usually feel better when they can help themselves.

The tray should be removed and the patient helped to brush his teeth when the meal is finished. The kinds and amounts of food refused, the time, the type of diet, and the patient's appetite should be recorded on the patient's chart after each meal. At times, the doctor requests an accurate report of the types and amounts of uneaten food.

SUMMARY

A patient's meal should be adapted from the family's meal whenever possible. This saves time and expense and allows the patient to feel more a part of the family. A patient on bedrest should be given the bedpan and allowed to wash his hands before the meal. Patients should be encouraged to feed themselves. However, help should be offered if it is needed. The blind patient can eat more easily if food is arranged in a set pattern on the plate. Pleasant conversation and cheerfulness on the part of the nurse can improve the patient's appetite. The type of diet, time of meal, patient's appetite and type and amount of food eaten should all be recorded on the patient's chart.

DISCUSSION TOPICS

1. Why is it wise to adapt the family menu to suit the patient's special requirements?

2. Discuss the following menu in terms of nutrient value and attractiveness. Adapt it to a patient on a low-calorie diet:

    Cream of Chicken Soup
    Roast Beef with Gravy
    Baked Potatoes
    Buttered Green Beans
    Rolls and Butter
    Angel Cake
    with
    Chocolate Ice Cream

3. Discuss the importance of proper preparation of the patient and his room before the meal. What can disturb a patient and affect his appetite?

4. How may the appearance of the tray affect the patient's appetite?

5. Why should the patient be encouraged to feed himself?

6. Why is it important to remove the tray as soon as the patient has finished the meal?

7. How can the behavior and attitude of the attending person affect the appetite of the patient?

SUGGESTED ACTIVITIES

a. Plan a family dinner and adapt it to the needs of a patient who should limit his carbohydrate intake.

b. Arrange a tray suitable for serving this meal.

c. Have two students participate in the following role-playing situation. The class should evaluate and discuss the "nurse's tact and skill in dealing with the "patient."

Mrs. Jones is a young, active woman with a family. She is recovering from viral pneumonia. Although she is allowed out of bed, she is not supposed to prepare meals or do housework until her condition improves. Dr. Malcolm has told Miss Wilson that it is important for Mrs. Jones to regain her lost weight. One day before her dinner is served, Mrs. Jones complains to Miss Wilson. She is discouraged about her lack of energy and states that her family needs her. Miss Wilson noted that she ate very little for breakfast and lunch. What should she say to Mrs. Jones?

d. Practice feeding each other. Ask the "nurse" to fill in the "patient's" chart.

e. Practice feeding a blindfolded "patient."

WORD STUDY

adapt	attitude	chart
appetite	bedrest	paralysis

REVIEW

A. A patient on a limited fat intake should avoid foods which are rich in fat. Indicate which foods he may eat on the following list by writing Y (yes). Write N (no) for the foods he should avoid.

_____ 1. fried hamburger   _____ 6. butter

_____ 2. mashed potatoes   _____ 7. ice cream

_____ 3. peas   _____ 8. fresh strawberries

_____ 4. lettuce   _____ 9. whole milk

_____ 5. French dressing

B. Briefly answer the following questions.

1. How may the following menu be adapted for a patient who must avoid foods high in cellulose?

Fresh Fruit Cup

Roast Turkey

Rice with Peas

Mashed Sweet Potatoes with Pecans

Celery and Carrot Sticks

Whole Wheat Bread

Butter

Cherry-Nut Ice Cream

Milk and Coffee

2. What should be done if the patient's meal is interrupted by a visit from the doctor?

3. What dietary information should be recorded on the patient's chart after a meal?

4. Give two examples of a colorful garnish.

SECTION EVALUATION 3: MEAL PREPARATION

A.   Complete the following statements.

1.   An individual who can transmit disease germs although he is not ill himself is a _____ .

2.   A disease caused by eating undercooked, infected pork is _____ .

3.   Salmonella, Staph, perfringens poisoning and botulism are caused by microorganisms known as _____ .

4.   The deadliest of the bacteria-caused food poisonings is _____ .

5.   Bacteria grow best at temperatures between _____ and _____ .

6.   A list of food ingredients with directions for combining and cooking is a _____ .

7.   To plunge foods into boiling water and then immediately into cold water is to _____ them.

8.   To cook food in water just below the boiling point is to _____ .

9.   Using a rough surface to scrape food into small particles is to _____ _____ it.

10.   To press food through a strainer to remove the cellulose is to _____ _____ it.

11.   To put dry ingredients through a sieve to remove lumps is to _____ _____ .

12.   The liquid in which foods have been cooked is _____ .

13.   One ounce equals approximately _____ grams.

14.   Four tablespoons equal _____ cup.

15.   One pound of butter or margarine yields _____ cups.

16.   One kilogram equals _____ pounds.

17.   The number on which the metric system is based is _____ .

18.   There are _____ grams in one pound.

B.   Match the cookery terms in column I with their definitions in column II.

Column I

_____ 1.   a la king
_____ 2.   au gratin
_____ 3.   baste
_____ 4.   blend
_____ 5.   broil
_____ 6.   compote
_____ 7.   cut in
_____ 8.   dust
_____ 9.   fry
_____ 10.   marinate

Column II

a. cook in fat
b. to let stand in a distinctive liquid such as an oil and vinegar mixture
c. fruit in syrup
d. in white sauce
e. combine thoroughly
f. in white sauce with cheese added
g. pour liquid on cooking foods
h. combine flour and shortening using two knives or a pastry blender
i. sprinkle lightly
j. cook over or under direct heat

C.   Briefly answer the following questions.

   1. What is the most efficient way to wash dishes?

   2. Why is it especially important to keep the school and hospital kitchen clean and orderly?

   3. How is a grease fire put out? What must not be used?

   4. What are five foods frequently used as garnishes?

   5. Why is it wiser to adapt the family meal to suit the patient rather than plan a separate menu?

Section 4
FOOD FOR MOTHER AND BABY

Chapter 17
Diet During Pregnancy and Lactation

OBJECTIVES

After studying this chapter, the student should be able to:

- Identify changes in nutritional needs during pregnancy and lactation.
- Modify the normal diet for pregnancy and lactation.

The pregnant woman who follows a well-balanced diet feels better and is more apt to retain her health and bear a healthy infant than one who chooses her food thoughtlessly. Studies have shown a relationship between the mother's diet and the health of the baby at birth. Malnutrition of the mother is believed to cause growth retardation in the *fetus* (infant developing in the mother's uterus). Low birth weight infants have a higher *mortality* (death) rate than those of normal birth weight. A relationship is also suspected between maternal nutrition and the subsequent mental development of the child. It appears that an insufficient amount of protein and energy foods in the diet during pregnancy may reduce the quantity of brain cells in the developing fetus.

Additionally, the occasional complications of pregnancy such as anemia and toxemia may be caused by an inadequate maternal diet. *Toxemia* is a complication of pregnancy characterized by high blood pressure, edema, and the presence of albumin in the urine. Convulsions and coma may occur in severe cases. The cause of toxemia is not known, but it occurs more frequently among pregnant women on inadequate diets than among pregnant women on good diets.

Sometimes *nausea* (the feeling of a need to vomit) may occur during the first *trimester* (3-month period) of pregnancy. This type of nausea is commonly known as *morning sickness*. It typically passes as the pregnancy proceeds to the second trimester. Dry crackers or dry toast eaten before rising, and eliminating some of the fat in the diet may help to reduce it. If nausea persists it should be treated by the doctor.

DIETARY MODIFICATIONS

Although it is often said, "a pregnant woman must eat for two," this is not entirely true. It may have originated because the

TABLE 17-1. Recommended Daily Dietary Allowances for Females Showing Extra Allowances for Pregnancy and Lactation

	Age (years)	Weight (kg)	Weight (lbs)	Height (cm)	Height (in)	Energy (kcal)	Protein (g)	Vitamin A Activity (RE)	Vitamin D (IU)	Vitamin E Activity (IU)	Ascorbic Acid (mg)	Folacin (µg)	Niacin (mg)	Riboflavin (mg)	Thiamine (mg)	Vitamin B6 (mg)	Vitamin B12 (µg)	Calcium (mg)	Phosphorus (mg)	Iodine (µg)	Iron (mg)	Magnesium (mg)	Zinc (mg)
Females	11-14	44	97	155	62	2,400	44	800	4,000	400	12	45	400	16	1.3	1.2	1.6	3.0	1,200	1,200	115	18	300	15
	15-18	54	119	162	65	2,100	48	800	4,000	400	12	45	400	14	1.4	1.1	2.0	3.0	1,200	1,200	115	18	300	15
	19-22	58	128	162	65	2,100	46	800	4,000	400	12	45	400	14	1.4	1.1	2.0	3.0	800	800	100	18	300	15
	23-50	58	128	162	65	2,000	46	800	4,000	400	12	45	400	13	1.2	1.0	2.0	3.0	800	800	100	18	300	15
	51+	58	128	162	65	1,800	46	800	4,000	400	12	45	400	12	1.1	1.0	2.0	3.0	800	800	80	10	300	15
Pregnant						+300	+30	1,000	5,000	400	15	60	800	+2	+0.3	+0.3	2.5	4.0	1,200	1,200	125	18+	450	20
Lactating						+500	+20	1,200	6,000	400	15	80	600	+4	+0.5	+0.3	2.5	4.0	1,200	1,200	150	18	450	25

Source: Food and Nutrition Board, National Academy of Sciences – National Research Council, 1974

TABLE 17-2. Suggested 2400 Calorie Menu for a Pregnant Woman

Breakfast

Orange Juice

Scrambled Egg

Toast
with
Peanut Butter

Skim Milk

Snack
Apple

Lunch

Citrus Fruit Cup

Roast Beef Sandwich
with
Mayonnaise & Lettuce

Vanilla Pudding

Skim Milk

Dinner

Calves Liver

Baked Potato with Butter

Baked Squash

Fresh Spinach Salad
with
Oil and Vinegar

Ice Milk

Skim Milk

Snack
Yogurt

appetite is usually very good during pregnancy. While the *dietary modifications* (changes in the diet) required during pregnancy are of great importance, they do not require doubling one's caloric intake.   The Food and Nutrition Board, National Academy of Sciences — National Research Council has calculated average nutritional requirements for pregnant females of varying ages, table 17-1.   These figures are only estimates; the physician may suggest alternate figures based on specific knowledge of the patient and her activities.

On the average, the pregnant woman only requires an additional 300 calories (1260 joules) per day. It is true that energy needs increase during pregnancy because of the developing fetus and an increased basal metabolism rate.   However, it is also usually true that the pregnant woman reduces her activities as the pregnancy progresses. Decreased activity thereby reduces her energy expenditure.   Consequently the additional energy need is low.

Specific nutrient requirements are increased to meet the needs of the developing fetus. The protein requirement increases substantially — from 46 g to 76 g for the mature pregnant woman and from 48 g to 78 g for the pregnant adolescent. All vitamin and mineral requirements increase for pregnant women of any age. The pregnant adolescent requires more of the essential nutrients than a mature woman because an adolescent is still growing herself.

The diet should, of course, be based on the Basic Four food groups. Special care should be given to the selection of food in order to provide the necessary additional nutrients and not just additional calories.

Additional nutrient requirements may be largely met by drinking an additional 470 ml (one pint) of milk each day (or using appropriate substitutes).   This additional amount brings the total amount of milk required by the mature pregnant woman to 950 milliliters which is about 1 liter (one quart).   The amount required by the pregnant adolescent, then, would be slightly over 1 and 1/2 quarts (1 1/2 liters or 1500 ml).

An additional pint of milk provides 350 calories (1470 joules) if whole milk is used and 190 calories (798 joules) if skim milk is used.   An increase in milk provides added calcium, phosphorus, protein, vitamin A, thiamine, riboflavin and niacin. Except for iron in some cases, the remaining nutrient requirements may be met by eating a protein-rich sandwich at lunch, a yellow or dark green vegetable, and one additional serving of citrus fruit each day. An inexpensive way to include extra protein in the diet is to add dried milk to creamed foods.

Because the need for iron increases to such a degree during pregnancy, there is a danger that the need will not be met in the ordinary diet. Lack of iron can cause anemia. Consequently, the doctor or obstetrician (an obstetrician is a doctor who cares for the mother during pregnancy and helps to deliver the baby) may prescribe an iron supplement in tablet form.

The unusual cravings for certain foods during pregnancy do no harm unless eating them interferes with the normal balanced diet or causes excessive weight gain. *Pica* is the craving for nonfood substances such as starch or clay.   If nonfood substances are eaten in place of nutritious foods, pica becomes an unhealthy practice.

WEIGHT GAIN

Usually there is little weight gain during the first three months of pregnancy. A woman gains about .45 kg (1 pound) a week during the last six months of pregnancy. The average weight gain during pregnancy is 9 to 11 kg (20 to 25 pounds). Adolescents tend to gain more than mature women; women

TABLE 17-3   Suggested 2600 Calorie Menu for a Lactating Woman

Breakfast	Lunch	Dinner
Orange Juice	Creamed Chicken on Toast	Pot Roast of Beef
Poached Egg		Potato
Bacon	Green Salad with	Carrots
Toast	Oil & Vinegar	Coleslaw
Peanut Butter	Baked Apple	Roll & Butter
Skim Milk	Skim Milk	Baked Custard
		Skim Milk

Snack	Snack
Fruit Juice	Milk and Cookie

having their first babies are apt to gain more than women having their second or third babies; and very thin women are inclined to gain more than stout women. Excessive weight gain should be avoided because it may predispose a woman to toxemia, cause complications during delivery, and cause overweight after delivery.

LACTATION

The normal baby consumes about 165 ml (5 1/2 ounces) of milk for every kilogram (2.2 pounds) of body weight. As thirty millilitres of human milk contains 20 calories, an infant weighing 4.5 kg (10 lbs) would require about 500 calories (2100 joules) daily. A woman must have extra calories during *lactation* (the period when the mother nurses her baby) in order to provide the milk for her child. As noted in table 17-1, caloric requirements and some nutrient requirements are greater during lactation than during pregnancy. The estimated average additional caloric requirement during lactation is 500 calories (2100 joules) per day. Extra protein, vitamins, and minerals are needed and should be provided in the foods chosen to fulfill the additional caloric requirement.

It is advisable that the nursing mother have at least 950 ml (one quart) of milk each day. Cheese may be substituted for part of the milk and milk may be included in other foods such as white sauces, custards, and puddings. About 470 ml (2 cups) of milk will provide the additional calories required and many of the additional nutrients required.

The nursing mother should be advised to choose additional foods from the Basic Four food groups and to remember that potato chips, soda, and candy provide little more than calories. It is important that the nursing mother have sufficient fluids to replace those lost in the infant's milk.

SUMMARY

A pregnant woman is more likely to remain healthy and bear a healthy infant if she follows a well-balanced diet. Research has shown that maternal nutrition can affect the subsequent mental and physical health of the child. Anemia and toxemia during pregnancy are two conditions which may result in part from inadequate nutrition. Both caloric and nutrient requirements increase for pregnant women (especially adolescents) and women who are breast feeding. The average weight gain during pregnancy is 9 to 11 kilograms (20 to 25 pounds).

DISCUSSION TOPICS

1. Discuss the truth of the statement, "A pregnant woman must eat for two."
2. Why is it especially important for a pregnant woman to have a highly nutritious diet?
3. Why is an excessive weight gain during pregnancy undesirable?
4. What is morning sickness and how may it be alleviated? If any class member has been pregnant, ask her questions regarding morning sickness.
5. How many servings of each of the Basic Four food groups may be found in the menus in tables 17-2 and 17-3?
6. Why are additional calories needed during lactation?

SUGGESTED ACTIVITIES

a. Using table A-6 in the Appendix, plan a day's menu for a normal pregnant woman.
b. Using table A-6 in the Appendix, plan a day's menu for a normal pregnant woman who dislikes milk.
c. Using table A-6 in the Appendix, plan a lactation diet for a mother who normally requires 2400 calories daily.
d. Ask a physician or a nurse to speak to the class on the importance of adequate nutrition before and during pregnancy. Ask the speaker questions regarding the effects of good or poor nutrition on the health of the mother, prenatal development, infant mortality, and the growth and development of the child.

WORD STUDY

adolescent	morning sickness	pregnancy
dietary modifications	nausea	retardation
fetus	obstetrician	toxemia
lactation	pica	trimester

REVIEW

A. Multiple Choice. Select the *letter* which precedes the best answer.

1. The infant developing in the mother's uterus is called the
   a. sperm
   b. fetus
   c. placenta
   d. ovary
2. Anemia would most likely result from
   a. pica
   b. an excess of vitamin A
   c. a lack of iron
   d. improper cooking of meat
3. High blood pressure, edema, and albumin in the urine are symptoms of
   a. nausea
   b. anemia
   c. pica
   d. toxemia

4. A common name given nausea in early pregnancy is
   a. morning sickness
   b. pica
   c. toxemia
   d. mortality

5. Changes in the diet are also called
   a. diet therapy
   b. dietitian
   c. dietary modifications
   d. dietetic foods

6. The average additional energy requirement for the pregnant woman is
   a. 100 calories
   b. 300 calories
   c. 500 calories
   d. 1000 calories

7. The additional nutrients required during pregnancy are largely met by
   a. eating steak each day
   b. drinking a malted each day
   c. using an additional pint of milk each day
   d. using an iron supplement

8. Craving for nonfood substances during pregnancy is known as
   a. anemia
   b. toxemia
   c. nausea
   d. pica

9. During pregnancy the average weight gain is
   a. 10 to 15 pounds
   b. 15 to 20 pounds
   c. 9 to 11 kilograms
   d. 11 to 15 kilograms

10. The period during which a mother nurses her baby is known as
    a. pregnancy
    b. trimester
    c. lactation
    d. obstetrics

11. A nursing mother should have at least
    a. 1 cup of milk each day
    b. 1 pint of milk each day
    c. 1 and 1/2 pints of milk each day
    d. 1 quart of milk each day

12. Some appropriate substitutes for milk include
    a. orange juice and tomato juice
    b. cheese and custard
    c. breads and cereals
    d. vegetables and fruit juices

13. The average daily additional energy requirement for a nursing mother is
    a. 100 calories
    b. 300 calories
    c. 500 calories
    d. 1000 calories

14. The daily diet during pregnancy and lactation should
    a. be based on the Basic Four food groups
    b. include at least a quart of milk
    c. be limited in hollow calorie foods
    d. all of the above

15. Appropriate snacks for pregnant and lactating women include
    a. fruits and milk
    b. potato chips and pretzels
    c. sodas
    d. hard candies

Chapter 18
Diet During Infancy

OBJECTIVES

After studying this chapter, the student should be able to:

- Identify the ingredients used in infant formulas.
- Explain the aseptic and terminal methods of formula preparation.
- Describe when and how foods are introduced into the baby's diet.
- State the effect inadequate nutrition has on an infant.
- Describe how an infant is fed.

Food and its presentation are extremely important during the baby's first year. Physical and mental development are dependent on the food itself and psychological development is affected by the time and manner in which the food is offered.

The first year of life is a period of very rapid growth. The infant's energy and protein requirements are higher per unit of body weight than are those of older children or adults, table 18-1.

The basis of the infant's diet is milk. It is a highly nutritious, digestible food containing protein, fat, carbohydrate, vitamins, and minerals. It is, however, a poor source of iron and vitamin C. Consequently, these nutrients are usually provided as supplements to the infant's milk diet.

METHODS OF FEEDING

Infants may be breast-fed or bottle-fed. Breast feeding is nature's way of providing a good diet for the baby. It is economical and saves time otherwise spent in formula preparation. Mother's milk gives the baby temporary *immunity* (resistance to) to some infectious diseases. Since it is sterile and so easy to digest, it usually does not cause gastrointestinal disturbances. Additionally, it helps to establish an emotional bond between mother and child that is beneficial to both.

Many mothers prefer to bottle feed their babies. Certain women are unable to produce enough breast milk; others who are employed or involved in many activities outside the home, find bottle feeding more convenient. Still others simply prefer not to breast feed. Either way is acceptable provided the infant is given love and attention during the feeding.

It is important for parents to know that infants react to their parents' emotions. If food is forced on a child or withheld until the child is uncomfortable, or if the food is presented in a tense manner, the child reacts with tension and unhappiness. The infant should be cuddled and kept comfortable and warm during the feeding. During and after the feeding the infant should be *bubbled* (burped) to release gas in the stomach. Bubbling helps prevent *regurgitation* (spitting up food).

TABLE 18-1 Recommended Daily Dietary Requirements for Infants from Birth to One Year

Age	0–5 mo.	5 mo.–1 yr.
Weight		
(kg)	6	9
(lbs)	14	20
Height		
(cm)	60	71
(in)	24	28
Energy		
(kcal)	kgx117	kgx108
Protein		
(g)	kgx2.2	kgx2.0
Vitamin A Activity		
(RE)	420	400
(IU)	1,400	2,000
Vitamin D		
(IU)	400	400
Vitamin E Activity		
(IU)	4	5
Ascorbic Acid		
(mg)	35	35
Folacin		
(μg)	50	50
Niacin		
(mg)	5	8
Riboflavin		
(mg)	0.4	0.6
Thiamine		
(mg)	0.3	0.5
Vitamin B_6		
(mg)	0.3	0.4
Vitamin B_{12}		
(μg)	0.3	0.3
Calcium		
(mg)	360	540
Phosphorus		
(mg)	240	400
Iodine		
(μg)	35	45
Iron		
(mg)	10	15
Magnesium		
(mg)	60	70
Zinc		
(mg)	3	5

Source: Food and Nutrition Board, National Academy of Sciences, National Research Council, 1974

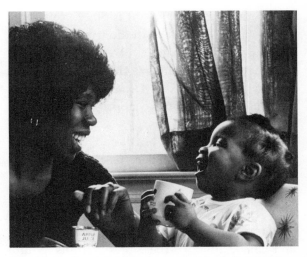

Fig. 18-1 Food is better accepted and digested in a happy and relaxed atmosphere.

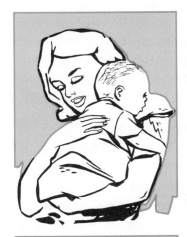

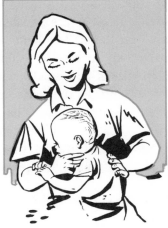

Fig. 18-2 To bubble the baby, hold him in one of the two positions shown and gently stroke his back.

Sometimes the infant is placed on a time schedule for feeding. An alternate method is feeding "on demand." With the demand method, the baby makes the schedule and is fed when hungry. Usually the demand schedule averages out to approximately every four hours.

If the baby is bottle-fed, parents will receive instructions for feeding from the *pediatrician* (baby and children's doctor). One of the convenient, prepared products may be prescribed. There are many ready-to-use formulas available in disposable bottles and cans. Some of these preparations require the addition of water, but many are completely ready to serve. Some have vitamins added and some contain added iron. The cost of milk formula is directly related to the factor of convenience; the most convenient is the most expensive. If parents are more concerned with economy than convenience, the pediatrician can prescribe a homemade formula.

PREPARATION OF
FORMULAS AND STERILIZATION

Normally, cow's milk is used in formulas because it is most abundant and is easily modified to resemble human milk. It is modified because it has more protein and mineral salts and less milk sugar than human milk. Water and sugar are usually added to dilute these nutrients to make the cow's milk more closely resemble mother's milk. When an infant is extremely sensitive or allergic to cow's milk, a *synthetic* (man-made) milk is given. Synthetic milk is commonly made from soybeans. Goat's milk is sometimes used as a substitute for cow's milk in situations where the baby is allergic to cow's milk.

If the infant is to be given a formula prepared at home, it is essential that it be carefully and accurately prepared. Typically, it is made from water, pasteurized cow's milk

and a sweetener. The milk may be fresh, evaporated, dried, whole or skim. The usual forms of sugar used are granulated (sucrose), corn syrup (glucose and maltose), or malt sugar (maltose). The pediatrician prescribes a formula which suits the needs of the baby and adjusts it as the child grows.

The following formula is one recommended by Dr. Spock in his book, *Baby and Child Care* (Pocket Books, Inc., New York, N.Y., 1976).

evaporated milk:	13 oz.
water:	19 oz.
corn syrup:	2 Tbsp.

Two basic methods for preparing formulas are the terminal and the aseptic. The *aseptic* method includes sterilization of each item used in the formula preparation before the formula is poured into the bottles. In the *terminal* method, the bottles and formula are sterilized together. The terminal method is effective and simpler than the aseptic method. Using the terminal method, all equipment is first washed and rinsed. The formula is mixed in a pitcher and poured into the bottles. The bottles are loosely capped and then sterilized by boiling for 25 minutes. The bottles should be allowed to cool in the covered pan until they are lukewarm. The nipples are then tightened, and the bottles refrigerated.

It is essential that all equipment used in preparing formulas be clean. Milk is an excellent medium for the growth of microorganisms. Bottles, caps, and nipples should be thoroughly cleaned after each feeding. The equipment for preparing formulas should consist of a kettle and a wire rack for sterilizing, a long brush for cleaning, measuring cups and spoons, saucepans and a funnel, spoon, can opener, bottles, nipples, nipple caps, and tongs for removing hot bottles.

The formula may be given cold, at room temperature, or warmed, but it should be given at the same temperature consistently. In order to warm formula for feeding, bottles should be placed in a saucepan of warm water or a bottlewarmer. The bottles should be shaken occasionally in order to warm the contents evenly. The temperature of the milk can be tested by shaking a few drops on one's wrist. The milk should feel lukewarm.

Even if the baby is breast-fed, sterile bottles will be needed for water and fruit juices. Sterilization of nipples, rings, and bottles is simple and it is very important in preventing the growth of harmful microorganisms. To sterilize these items, they must be boiled for the number of minutes specified by the pediatrician. The nipple and ring must be attached to the bottle with sterile tongs.

SUPPLEMENTARY FOODS

In addition to milk, an infant is given vitamin drops as early as two weeks, and fruit juice shortly thereafter. However, these should be given only on the advice of the pediatrician. *The age at which new foods are introduced is highly variable.* Some pediatricians encourage early introduction of cereals and fruits whereas others discourage it. Strained cereals and cooked and pureed fruits may be given as early as one month of age. Cooked and pureed vegetables, egg yolk, and finely ground meats may be given soon after one month. At four or five months, toast, zwieback and teething biscuits may be given. By the age of six months, most babies are eating foods from all of the Basic Four food groups. By eight months an infant may have most any food which is easily chewed and digested. The child's few teeth and lack of coordination may limit the types of foods which can be eaten. Gelatin desserts, custards, and ice cream are favorites. It is important that the child be given a well-balanced diet. The Basic Four food groups are an excellent guide. Foods should be selected according to the advice of the pediatrician. New foods should be introduced gradually and in very small amounts.

Weaning (teaching the infant to drink from a cup instead of the breast or bottle) actually begins when the infant is first given

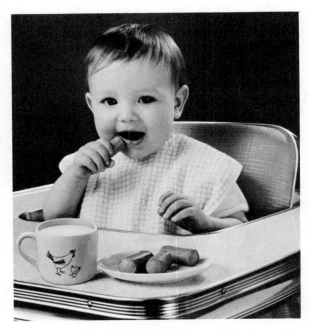

Fig. 18-3   Finger foods encourage self-feeding. This baby is enjoying meat sticks specially manufactured for toddlers. *(Courtesy Gerber Products Company)*

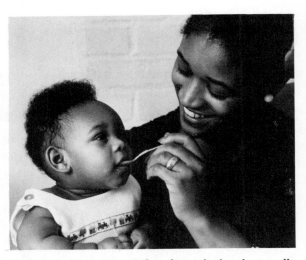

Fig. 18-4   Weaning an infant from the bottle actually begins when food is given with a spoon.

food from a spoon. It progresses as the child shows an interest in and ability to drink from a cup. The child will ultimately discard the bottle. If the child shows great reluctance to discard the bottle, the pediatrician's advice should be sought.

SUMMARY

It is particularly important that babies have adequate diets so their physical and mental development is not impaired. Breast feeding is nature's way of feeding an infant; however, formula feeding is equally acceptable. Cow's milk is usually used in formulas because it is most available and is easily modified to resemble human milk. To modify milk, sugar and water can be added to fresh, evaporated, or dried milk. Two methods of preparing formulas are the aseptic and the terminal methods. The young child's diet is supplemented on the advice of the pediatrician. Added foods should be based on the Basic Four food groups.

DISCUSSION TOPICS

1. Do any of the students know a woman who has breast-fed her baby? What were her reactions to the experience?

2. Why is breast feeding not always possible?

3. Why are some babies not allowed cow's milk? What kind of milk can these children have?

4. Discuss the possible effects of regularly propping the baby's bottle instead of holding the baby during feeding.

5. Why is a rigid time schedule for feeding a baby not advisable?

6. What foods is an 8-month baby usually allowed to eat?

7. How may weaning be accomplished?

SUGGESTED ACTIVITIES

a. Have a panel discussion on the advantages and disadvantages of breast feeding.

b. Observe demonstrations of the preparations of formula by the aseptic and the terminal methods. Practice preparing formula by both methods. Calculate the cost of the ingredients.

c. Observe a demonstration of the actual feeding and bubbling of a baby.

d. Visit a store that carries prepared infant formulas and check prices of these products. Compare the prices of these products with the cost of preparing the formulas yourself.

WORD STUDY

aseptic	sterile	coordination
pediatrician	terminal	synthetic
regurgitation	weaning	immunity

REVIEW

A.   Complete the following statements.

1.   The mother's milk gives the infant temporary _____ to certain diseases.

2.   An infant _____ (does, does not) react to the emotions of the person feeding him.

3.   The doctor who decides what kind of formula to give the baby is the _____ .

4.   Cow's milk has more _____ and _____ than human milk.

5.   Cow's milk has less _____ than human milk.

6.   Usually, the first addition to the infant's milk diet is a _____ .

7.   Because milk contains little vitamin _____ the formula should be supplemented early.

8.   Usually, an infant may have any food which is easily chewed and digested when he is approximately _____ months old.

9.   When an infant is allergic to cow's milk, _____ may be substituted.

10.   Inadequate nutrition during infancy may impair the infant's _____ _____ and _____ development.

B.   Match the items in column I to the correct statement in column II.

Column I

_____ 1. milk
_____ 2. supplement
_____ 3. immunity
_____ 4. regurgitation
_____ 5. bubbling
_____ 6. pediatrician
_____ 7. synthetic
_____ 8. terminal method
_____ 9. aseptic method
_____ 10. weaning

Column II

a. baby doctor
b. teaching the child to drink from a cup instead of a nipple
c. addition
d. basis of the infant's diet
e. burping
f. spitting up of food
g. sterilization of formula equipment before formula is mixed
h. man-made
i. sterilization of formula and equipment together
j. protection from disease
k. doctor who delivers the baby

C.   Briefly answer the following questions.

1. Why should the mother give her baby special attention during feedings?

2. How is a bottle warmed? Is this always necessary?

3. Name two factors which determine the infant's ability to manage solid foods.

SECTION EVALUATION 4: FOOD FOR MOTHER AND BABY

A.   Complete the following statements.

1. High blood pressure, edema, and albumin in the urine are symptoms of a complication in pregnancy called _____ .

2. During pregnancy, a woman's daily protein requirement rises to _____ _____ grams.

3. A mature woman who becomes pregnant requires an additional _____ _____ calories each day.

4. Obstetricians often prescribe a supplement of the mineral _____ _____ for pregnant women.

5. A craving for nonfood substances is called _____ .

6. The average range of weight gain during pregnancy is _____ to _____ kg.

7. A mother who is breast feeding should drink at least _____ ml of milk each day.

8. The basic food in the infant's diet is _____ .

9. A technique used to help an infant release gas trapped in the stomach is called _____ .

10. The technique used to ease infants away from bottle or breast feeding is called _____ .

B.   Briefly answer the following questions.

1. Name one effect that malnutrition of the pregnant mother may have on the fetus.

2. Do low birth weight infants have a higher or lower mortality rate than infants of average weight?

3. Name one symptom of morning sickness.

4. What is the purpose of adding dried milk to cream sauces, baked products or milk beverages?

5. Anemia is a common condition in pregnancy caused by a lack of which trace mineral?

6. What is the meaning of the word *lactation?*

7. Name two essential nutrients which cannot be supplied by a diet of milk alone.

8. Name one way to help an infant avoid regurgitation.

9. Explain the demand method of feeding an infant.

10. Name three types of milk which could be given to an infant who is allergic to cow's milk.

Section 5

SPECIAL DIETS

Chapter 19

Introduction to Diet Therapy

OBJECTIVES

After studying this chapter, the student should be able to:

- Define diet therapy.
- Identify roles of the physician and dietitian in diet therapy.
- Identify standard hospital diets and the ways they can be modified.

Proper nutrition is necessary for maintaining good health and for building good health during and after an illness. Using nutrition to build good health is called *diet therapy*. Diet therapy means modifying or changing the patient's normal diet in order to meet requirements created by disease or injury. Sometimes it is simply a matter of changing a nutritionally inadequate diet to a nutritionally adequate diet. More often, diet therapy means the addition or subtraction of certain nutrients and foods in specified amounts to or from a diet. Such diets are called *therapeutic diets* and must always be prescribed by a physician. A *dietitian* (specialist in planning diets) plans the meals which fit the physician's prescription.

It is often difficult to get the patient to eat meals based on a therapeutic diet. This is because people are often reluctant to eat new foods or familiar foods prepared in unfamiliar ways, especially when they are ill. Weakness, exhaustion, illness, loneliness, and self-pity also discourage appetites.

When serving food to a patient, the tray should be made as attractive as possible. A small flower or a colorful favor often cheers the patient and makes him feel more like eating. The tray and all equipment must be clean and properly arranged. Chipped or cracked dishes should be avoided. Food portions should be appropriately sized as large portions are discouraging to someone with a poor appetite. The tray must be served promptly so the patient receives food at the proper temperatures. Salt, pepper and sugar should be on the tray, if the patient is allowed to have them.

The attitude of the person serving the meal can be an effective means of encouraging the patient to eat. Cheerfulness on the part of the person serving the food can improve the patient's attitude and appetite. At times, an explanation as to the value of the diet motivates the patient to eat. It is useful to explain that the diet will improve health and general well-being. It is important to help the patient learn to select appropriate foods for the diet. The patient should be encouraged to overcome prejudices about certain foods. Elementary facts of nutrition can be explained in simple language. The person serving the meal should see that the patient eats the prescribed diet. Unless the prescribed food is eaten, any diet is useless.

When certain foods are consistently refused, the refusal should be discussed with the dietitian and physician. Sometimes, necessary foods which are disliked can be disguised when combined with other foods. Milk, for example can be included in the diet in pudding, ice cream, cheese, cream sauce, soup or custard. If such measures fail and the patient continues to refuse the needed foods, the physician may prescribe supplements such as calcium and vitamin tablets. Since most people have better appetites when they are rested, it is advisable to serve the most nutritious meals early and to make the evening meals light.

STANDARD HOSPITAL DIETS

Health facilities such as hospitals and nursing homes usually have standard diets which simplify their meal planning. Hospitals typically have *liquid, soft, regular,* and sometimes, *light* diets.

These basic diets may be modified by changing their consistency, energy value, or nutrient content. For example, a low calorie diet or a sodium restricted diet can be prepared as a liquid, soft, light or regular diet.

The person serving a meal should learn to recognize the types of food allowed in each diet. In some facilities it is the duty of the nurse to double-check the meal tray before it is served.

Regular Diet

A regular diet is a nearly normal diet based on the Basic Four food groups. People on the regular diet require nutrients for health maintenance only, and not for therapy. A regular diet includes a great variety of foods. However, the caloric value of this diet is somewhat lower than for normal diets because the people on it are not normally active and consequently require fewer calories than the ordinary person. Some patients on the regular diet are advised to limit or avoid highly seasoned foods, hollow calorie foods, and very rich foods such as pastries, heavy cakes, and fried foods. Such foods may cause digestive disturbances or weight gain in people who are not active. The regular diet is

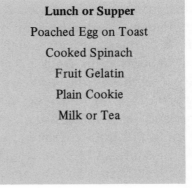

Breakfast	Dinner	Lunch or Supper
Orange Juice	Roast Beef	Poached Egg on Toast
Oatmeal	Mashed Potatoes	Cooked Spinach
Milk-Sugar	Steamed Carrots	Fruit Gelatin
Toast-Butter	Lettuce with French Dressing	Plain Cookie
Coffee or Tea	Bread-Butter	Milk or Tea
	Milk Pudding	
	Milk	

Fig. 19-1 A day's menu with a regular diet can include a wide variety of foods

usually intended for the *ambulatory* patient (one who walks).

SUMMARY

The treatment of disease through diet is called diet therapy. This therapy consists of the addition or subtraction of certain nutrients or foods in the patient's diet. It is difficult to convince people to change their eating habits. The person preparing and serving the meals should be pleasant and be able to explain the value of the special diet to the patient. The standard hospital diets include liquid, soft, regular, and sometimes light. Each diet may be modified by changing its consistency, energy value, or nutrient content. The regular diet is comparable to the average well-balanced diet. A regular diet is sometimes limited in caloric value, hollow calorie foods, highly seasoned foods, and very rich foods.

DISCUSSION TOPICS

1. What is diet therapy?

2. What is a dietitian?

3. What is a regular hospital diet? How can it differ from a well-balanced diet?

4. What are the usual standard hospital diets? If anyone in the class has eaten or seen any hospital diets, ask that person to describe them.

5. Discuss ways in which the nurse may help to solve the problem of friends and relatives bringing food to patients on special diets.

6. What are food prejudices? Name some and discuss how you might attempt to help the patient overcome them.

7. Why is it important to teach the patient about his new diet?

8. Why is the calorie count sometimes lower on the regular hospital diet than on a normal diet?

9. Why do people who are ill frequently experience a decrease in appetite? How can the nurse encourage patients to eat well?

SUGGESTED ACTIVITIES

a. Role play a situation in which a nurse persuades a middle-aged woman who loves sweets that her carbohydrate-controlled diet can be satisfying. The class should evaluate the "nurse's" tact and ingenuity in persuading the "patient."

b. Plan a day's menu for a 40-year-old woman on a regular diet. How might the diet be changed if the patient were a 16-year-old boy with a broken leg?

c. Prepare one of the meals on each of the menus planned in the preceding activity. Make it as attractive as possible. Set up the tray. Evaluate the meal.

d. Plan a visit to a hospital kitchen. If possible, ask the dietitian to explain the various procedures to the class.

WORD STUDY

ambulatory patient	light diet	soft diet
diet therapy	liquid diet	standard diet
dietitian	regular diet	therapeutic diet

REVIEW

A.   Multiple Choice. Select the *letter* which precedes the best answer.

1. The use of diet to build good health during and after illness is called
    a. diet therapy   c. dietitian
    b. dietetics   d. physical therapy

2. Special diets are prescribed by the
    a. nurse   c. physician
    b. dietitian   d. physical therapist

3. The planning of special diets is done by the
    a. nurse   c. dietitian
    b. physician   d. physical therapist

4. Necessary foods which are disliked can be more easily accepted if they are
    a. disguised in a combination with other foods
    b. highly seasoned with spicy sauces
    c. served for lunch rather than for supper
    d. served frequently throughout the week

5. The standard hospital diets are usually
    a. liquid, soft, regular and light
    b. soft, light, and salt-free
    c. low fat, regular, soft and normal
    d. liquid, soft, and diabetic

6. Basic diets may be modified by changing their
    a. color, flavor, or satiety value
    b. consistency, energy value, or nutrient content
    c. temperatures and serving times
    d. cost and efficiency of preparation

7. Regular diets usually limit
    a. pastries and fried foods   c. broiled and boiled foods
    b. all fats   d. meats and meat products

8. Regular diets are based on
    a. individual doctors' prescriptions   c. all-vegetable diets
    b. low calorie foods only   d. the Basic Four food groups

9. The ambulatory patient is one who
    a. cannot walk   c. has no teeth
    b. can walk   d. arrives in an ambulance

10. A therapeutic diet
    a. is always prescribed by a physician
    b. may add certain nutrients and foods in specified amounts
    c. may subtract certain foods from a diet
    d. all of the above

B. In some hospitals, regular diets do not include rich, high calorie foods. Substitute other foods or methods of preparation to make the regular diet which follows more appropriate.

Deep-fried Fish Fillets
French Fried Potatoes
Green Peas
Lettuce with Oil and Vinegar
Bread and Butter
Pecan Pie with Whipped Cream
Milk

Chapter 20
Liquid Diets

OBJECTIVES

After studying this chapter, the student should be able to:

- Identify the types of physical conditions for which liquid diets may be prescribed.
- Identify foods allowed in liquid diets.

A *liquid* diet consists of foods that will pour or are liquid at body temperature. The nutritive value of liquid diets is low and consequently they are usually only used for very limited periods of time. Liquid diets are subdivided into two types: the clear liquid and the full liquid diet. They are standard hospital diets.

CLEAR LIQUID DIET

The clear liquid diet consists of liquids that do not irritate the gastrointestinal tract, cause *flatulence* (gas in the stomach or intestines), or stimulate peristalsis. A clear liquid diet passes through the body easily and does not create residue. Therefore, this diet is used when the amount of *fecal matter* (waste material) in the colon must be kept at a minimum. The clear liquid diet may be used after surgery. The diet may also be ordered to replace fluids lost through vomiting or diarrhea.

TABLE 20-1   Foods allowed in a Clear Liquid Diet

apple and tomato juice

fat-free broths or bouillon (clear soups)

plain gelatin

fruit ice

ginger ale and carbonated water (if permitted by physician)

tea or black coffee with sugar

TABLE 20-2   Sample Menu for a Clear Liquid Diet

Breakfast	10 a.m.	Dinner	3 p.m.	Lunch or Supper	9 p.m.
Apple Juice	Tomato Juice	Beef Bouillon	Grape Juice	Chicken Broth	Beef Bouillon
Tea with Sugar		Gelatin		Fruit Ice	
		Tea with Sugar		Tea with Sugar	

The clear liquid diet is composed mainly of water and carbohydrates. It is only a temporary diet since it is nutritionally inadequate. Its use is typically limited to 24 to 36 hours. The meals which are small and frequent are usually served every two, three, or four hours. It is usually followed by the full liquid diet.

FULL LIQUID DIET

The full liquid diet contains all foods in the clear liquid diet and additional, more nutritious foods as well, table 20-3.

The full liquid diet includes many milk based foods which make this diet more nutritious than the clear liquid diet. Compared to a regular diet, however, the nutritive value of a full liquid diet is low. The caloric value of the full liquid diet may be increased by adding *lactose* (milk sugar) or corn syrup to the beverages. Its protein content may be increased by adding dried milk or commercial protein substitutes to whole milk. In addition, the physician may prescribe a vitamin supplement. A minimum serving of 180 to 240 milliliters (six to eight ounces) is usually given every two or three hours.

This diet may be given to patients who have acute infections; to patients who have difficulty chewing; to those who have had heart attacks; and to patients with gastrointestinal disturbances.

TABLE 20-3   Foods Allowed in a Full Liquid Diet

all clear liquids
fruit and vegetable juices
strained soups (cream or water based)
strained, cooked cereals
custard
ice cream
puddings
junket (sweetened, flavored, thickened milk dessert)
sherbet
milk, cream, buttermilk
cocoa
eggnog
carbonated beverages

TABLE 20-4 Sample Menu for a Full Liquid Diet

Breakfast	10 a.m.	Dinner	3 p.m.	Lunch or Supper	9 p.m.
Strained Orange Juice; Strained Oatmeal Gruel with Cream and Sugar; Coffee or Tea with Cream and Sugar	Tomato Juice	Strained Cream of Chicken Soup; Plain Gelatin with Sweetened Whipped Cream; Milk; Tea with Cream and Sugar	Eggnog	Apple Juice; Beef Broth; Vanilla Ice Cream; Milk; Coffee or Tea with Cream and Sugar	Cocoa

SUMMARY

The clear liquid diet consists only of nonirritating liquids and is nutritionally inadequate. It may be used following surgery. The full liquid diet provides more nourishment than the clear liquid diet, but it is still low in nutritional value. It ordinarily is prescribed to follow the clear liquid diet. It is used for patients who cannot chew, patients with severe infections, for heart attack victims, and for patients with gastrointestinal disturbances.

DISCUSSION TOPICS

1. Why are patients on the clear liquid diet fed so frequently? Why is it only a temporary diet?

2. How does the full liquid diet differ from the clear liquid diet?

3. What is an eggnog? How can calories be added to an eggnog?

4. How can protein be added to cream soup and cocoa?

5. What is bouillon? How is it prepared?

6. What is junket? If anyone in the class has tasted it, ask that person to describe it.

7. Mr. Brown has recently had a stroke which paralyzed his right side. Why do you think a liquid diet has been prescribed for Mr. Brown?

SUGGESTED ACTIVITIES

a. Make a chart of the diets discussed in this chapter and include the foods allowed in each. Compare the charts and correct if necessary. The charts should be kept for reference.

b. Plan a daily menu for each of the diets in this chapter. Compare menus and correct them if necessary.

c. Observe a demonstration of the electric blender. Practice using and caring for it.

d. Prepare one or more of the meals planned in activity b. Evaluate each in terms of nutrient content, flavor, aroma, color, appearance, texture and satiety value.

WORD STUDY

bouillon	eggnog	gastrointestinal
broth	fecal matter	junket
clear liquid diet	flatulence	milliliter
diarrhea	full liquid diet	

REVIEW

A. Match the items in column I to the correct statement in column II.

Column I

_____ 1. clear liquid diet
_____ 2. flatulence
_____ 3. 180 to 240 ml
_____ 4. lactose
_____ 5. fecal matter

Column II

a. accumulation of gas in the digestive tract
b. excessive looseness and frequency of bowel movements
c. replaces body fluids but supplies mainly carbohydrate and water
d. milk sugar
e. form of dextrose
f. waste material in the bowels
g. minimum serving in a full liquid diet

B. Multiple Choice. Select the *letter* which precedes the best answer.

1. The clear liquid diet consists of liquids that do not
    a. irritate   c. stimulate peristalsis
    b. cause flatulence   d. all of these

2. The clear liquid diet
    a. replaces lost body fluids
    b. provides a nutritionally adequate diet
    c. includes any food that pours
    d. is never used after surgery

3. The following group of foods would be allowed on a clear liquid diet:
    a. cream of chicken soup, coffee, and tea
    b. tomato juice, sherbet, and strained cooked cereal
    c. raspberry ice, beef bouillon and apple juice
    d. tea, coffee, and eggnog

4. The full liquid diet
    a. is always nutritionally adequate
    b. is followed by a clear liquid diet
    c. does not include milk in any form
    d. is sometimes given patients with acute infections

5. The full liquid diet
    a. is given all patients on the first day of their hospital stay
    b. includes no protein foods
    c. includes no highly fibrous foods
    d. is commonly given immediately after surgery

6. The caloric value of the full liquid diet
    a. is always adequate
    b. cannot be varied
    c. may be increased by adding lactose or corn syrup
    d. is usually 3000 calories per day

7. The protein content of the full liquid diet
   a. can be increased by adding lactose to beverages
   b. can be increased by adding dried milk to beverages
   c. cannot be varied
   d. is always adequate

8. The clear liquid diet
   a. is given all patients with chewing difficulties
   b. may be used after surgery
   c. includes milk foods
   d. is nutritionally adequate

9. One of the reasons for giving the clear liquid diet is to
   a. rest the teeth and gums
   b. cause weight reduction
   c. activate the colon
   d. reduce peristalsis

10. Eggnog and beef bouillon are
    a. allowed on both liquid diets
    b. not allowed on either liquid diet
    c. allowed only on the clear liquid diet
    d. allowed on the full liquid diet

Chapter 21
The Soft Diet

OBJECTIVES

After studying this chapter, the student should be able to:

- Identify the reasons for using a soft diet.
- Identify foods allowed in the soft diet.
- Adapt a given menu to meet the requirements of a soft diet.

The soft diet is one of the standard diets used in most health care facilities. It is very similar to the regular diet except the texture of the foods has been modified. The soft diet commonly follows a full liquid diet. It may be ordered for *postoperative* (after surgery) cases, for patients with *acute* (severe) infections, gastrointestinal conditions, or chewing problems.

This diet includes liquids and foods that have a soft texture and are easy to digest. The foods allowed are those that contain very little indigestible carbohydrate (cellulose) and no tough connective tissue. As a result, a soft diet leaves little food *residue* (indigestible fiber). Meats in a soft diet are very tender. Sometimes the meats are ground. Most fruits must be cooked, but bananas

TABLE 21-1   Selecting Foods in a Soft Diet

FOODS ALLOWED IN SOFT DIET	FOODS TO BE AVOIDED
milk, cream, butter	meat and shellfish with tough connective tissue
mild cheeses such as cottage or cream cheese	coarse cereals
eggs, except fried	condiments (foods used as seasonings, relishes)
tender chicken, fish, sweetbreads, ground beef and lamb	rich pastries and desserts
soup broth and strained cream soups	foods high in cellulose
tender, cooked vegetables or pureed vegetables	fried foods
fruit juices, cooked fruits, bananas, orange and grapefruit sections with membranes removed	raw vegetables and raw fruits (except bananas and citrus fruits with membranes removed)
refined cereals, cooked cereals, spaghetti, noodles, macaroni, enriched white bread, white crackers	nuts and coconut
tea, coffee, cocoa, carbonated beverages	
sherbet, ices, plain ice cream, custard, pudding, junket, gelatin, plain cookies, angel and sponge cake	
salt and some spices in small amounts as allowed by the physician	

TABLE 21-2 Sample Menu for a Soft Diet

Breakfast	Dinner	Lunch or Supper
Orange Juice	Cream of Tomato Soup	Apple Juice
Cream of Wheat with Milk and Sugar	Broiled Ground Beef Patty	Creamed Chicken with Peas and Noodles
Buttered Toast	Mashed Potatoes with Butter	Baked Squash
Tea or Coffee with Cream and Sugar	Green Beans	Bread and Butter
	Bread and Butter	Custard
	Stewed Peaches	Tea with Cream and Sugar
	Milk	

Note: Between meals the patient may have malted milk, milkshakes, eggnog, or cocoa.

and orange or grapefruit sections (with membranes removed) are sometimes allowed. Usually only young, tender cooked vegetables are served; frequently these are pureed. Cereals are either refined or cooked.

Generally, foods on the soft diet are mild flavored, slightly seasoned or left unseasoned, and are prepared in easily digestible forms. Although this diet nourishes the body, between-meal feedings are sometimes given to increase the energy value.

SUMMARY

The soft diet nourishes the body. It includes foods that are liquid or semisolid with soft textures, very little indigestible carbohydrate, and no tough connective tissue. It may be ordered for postoperative patients, for patients with severe infections, or for patients with gastrointestinal or chewing problems.

DISCUSSION TOPICS

1. Describe a soft diet. Does it nourish the body? When may it be prescribed?

2. What kinds of foods are allowed in the soft diet?

3. Why are between-meal feedings sometimes given to patients on the soft diet?

4. What are condiments and why are they excluded from the soft diet?

5. Name the conditions for which a soft diet may be prescribed.

6. What is indigestible carbohydrate? Why should it be limited in a soft diet? Name several foods that contain a large proportion of indigestible carbohydrate. Name foods containing very little.

7. What are food "membranes?" Why should such membranes be omitted from the soft diet?

8. Review the words: gastrointestinal, cellulose, puree, fiber.

SUGGESTED ACTIVITIES

a. Adapt the following menu to suit the needs of a patient on a soft diet:

> Fresh Fruit Cup
> Oatmeal with Milk and Sugar
> Bran Muffin and Butter
> Tea with Sugar

b. Write your dinner menu for last night. Adapt it to suit a patient on the soft diet.

c. Bring recipes to class. Discuss them and determine why they may or may not be appropriate for a soft diet.

d. Begin a Special Diet Recipe File in which recipes are coded according to the diet in which they are allowed. Code them by using a special color dot in the upper right-hand corner of each recipe or use the initials of the diet. Many of the recipes may be suitable for several different diets.

e. Plan a daily menu for the soft diet. Compare menus and correct them if necessary.

f. Prepare one or more of the meals on the menu. Evaluate each in terms of nutritive content, flavor, aroma, color, shape, appearance, texture, and satiety value.

WORD STUDY

acute   condiment   postoperative

REVIEW

A. Indicate which of the following foods would be allowed on a soft diet by writing Y (yes) and N (no).

_____ 1. banana nut bread   _____ 6. black coffee
_____ 2. roast chicken breast _____ 7. celery sticks
_____ 3. baked halibut   _____ 8. tapioca pudding
_____ 4. french fries   _____ 9. coconut cookies
_____ 5. angel cake   _____ 10. tossed salad

B. Multiple Choice. Select the *letter* which precedes the best answer.

1. The soft diet
    a. is a standard diet in health facilities
    b. is always served to children under 12 years old
    c. is similar to a high-residue diet
    d. does not nourish as well as a full liquid diet

2. A major difference between the regular and the soft diet is the
   a. nutrient content
   b. texture of the foods
   c. energy values
   d. satiety value of the foods

3. It is not unusual for the soft diet to be
   a. ordered to precede the clear liquid diet
   b. ordered to precede the full liquid diet
   c. ordered to succeed the full liquid diet
   d. used in place of the clear liquid diet

4. The soft diet is sometimes ordered for
   a. preoperative patients
   b. postoperative patients
   c. comatose patients
   d. all of these

5. The following would not be included in a soft diet:
   a. ground beef
   b. leg of lamb
   c. roast chicken
   d. baked pork chops

6. Cellulose is
   a. a complete protein
   b. an indigestible carbohydrate
   c. a saturated fat
   d. an essential mineral

7. Texture of food refers to its
   a. color
   b. flavor
   c. consistency
   d. satiety value

8. When a food is pureed, it
   a. loses all nutrients
   b. has sugar added
   c. is baked
   d. has the cellulose broken down

9. A fresh orange is not always permitted in a soft diet because of the
   a. citric acid content
   b. ascorbic acid content
   c. section membranes
   d. tough protein fibers

10. The following group of foods would not be allowed on the soft diet:
    a. coffee, bananas, and sponge cake
    b. salt, sherbet, and scrambled eggs
    c. butter, angel cake, and fried chicken
    d. ginger ale, chocolate ice cream, and cocoa with marshmallows

Chapter 22
The Light Diet

OBJECTIVES

After studying this chapter, the student should be able to:

- Identify the foods included on a light diet.
- Adapt a normal menu to suit the needs of a patient on a light diet.
- Identify the purpose of the light diet.

A light diet is given to a patient who is almost ready for the regular diet. The light diet is an intermediate diet sometimes used between the soft and the regular diets. It is nutritionally adequate.

The light diet is also called the *convalescent diet* because it is primarily used for *convalescent* (recovering from an injury or illness) patients and for those with minor illnesses. The light diet is considered one of the four standard diets. However, some health facilities do not use it because it is so similar to the regular diet.

The important fact to remember concerning the light diet is that the foods must be easy to digest. Foods are simply cooked, with little seasoning, and served without heavy sauces or spicy seasonings. The diet includes all foods allowed on the soft and liquid diets plus those foods listed in table 22-1.

SUMMARY

The light (convalescent) diet is an intermediate diet between the soft and regular diets. It is nutritionally adequate. The light diet is a standard diet but it is not used in all health facilities because it is so similar to the regular diet. It is used for convalescent patients and those with minor illnesses. The light diet contains only foods that are easily digested.

TABLE 22-1 Selecting Foods for a Light Diet

FOODS ALLOWED IN LIGHT DIETS	FOODS TO BE AVOIDED
cheddar cheese	rich pastries
tender cuts of beef, lamb, and veal such as steaks, roasts, and chops	heavy salad dressings
bacon, liver	fried foods
all soups	coarse foods such as some very coarse cereals
cooked vegetables and fruits, citrus fruits, bananas, lettuce and tomato salads	fruits and vegetables that are high in cellulose
enriched and whole wheat bread and crackers	foods that cause flatulence
plain cakes	nuts

TABLE 22-2   Sample Menu for a Light Diet

Breakfast	Dinner	Lunch or Supper
Orange Sections	Vegetable Soup	Tomato Juice
Oatmeal with Cream and Sugar	Roast Lamb	Scrambled Eggs with Cottage Cheese
Buttered Toast	Baked Potato	Asparagus Tips
Jelly	Buttered Carrots	Bread and Butter
Coffee with Cream and Sugar	Lettuce Salad	Orange Sherbet
	Bread and Butter	Tea with Cream and Sugar
	Strawberry Ice Cream	
	Tea with Cream and Sugar	

DISCUSSION TOPICS

1. When is the light diet used? Why is it not included in the diets of all hospitals?

2. What type of foods are included in the light diet?

3. Would the light diet be generally suitable for healthy geriatric patients? For children? Is it nutritionally adequate?

4. Many people have unknowingly been on a self-imposed light diet at home at one time. Under what conditions might this have occurred?

SUGGESTED ACTIVITIES

a. Make a list of the foods eaten yesterday. Circle those foods which would not be allowed on the light diet.

b. Find recipes that are suitable for the light diet. Add them to the special diet recipe file.

c. Adapt the following menu to make it appropriate for a patient on a light diet.

Breakfast	Dinner	Lunch or Supper
Orange Juice	Roast Beef	Pepper Steak
2 Fried Eggs	Mashed Potato	Cooked Spinach
Milk-Sugar	Steamed Carrots	Fruit Gelatin
Danish Pastry	Lettuce with Creamy Garlic Dressing	Pecan Roll
Coffee or Tea	Whole Wheat Bread	Milk or Tea
	Milk Pudding	
	Milk	

d. Plan a day's menu for the light diet. Compare menus and correct them if necessary.

e. Prepare at least one of the meals on the menu. Serve it and evaluate it in terms of nutritive content, flavor, aroma, color, shape, appearance, texture, and satiety value.

WORD STUDY

convalescent   coarse foods   light diet

REVIEW

A.   Indicate which of the following foods are allowed on the light diet by writing Y (yes) in front of foods allowed on the light diet. Write N (no) in front of those foods *not* permitted on a light diet.

_____ 1.	lettuce	_____ 6.	apple pie
_____ 2.	butter and jelly	_____ 7.	applesauce
_____ 3.	fresh tomatoes	_____ 8.	bacon
_____ 4.	baked potato	_____ 9.	stewed prunes
_____ 5.	bran muffins	_____ 10.	broiled lamb chop

B.   Multiple Choice. Select the *letter* which precedes the best answer.

1.   The light diet is also called the
   a. soft diet   c. invalid diet
   b. full liquid diet   d. convalescent diet

2.   The light diet is
   a. always one of the standard hospital diets
   b. more restrictive than the soft diet
   c. very similar to a regular diet in some health facilities
   d. rarely used for obese patients

3.   The light diet, if used, is typically given
   a. after the full liquid diet and before the soft diet
   b. after the regular diet and before the soft diet
   c. after the soft diet and before the regular diet
   d. immediately after surgery

4.   The light diet is given to
   a. newborns
   b. patients recovering from an illness
   c. patients preparing for surgery
   d. all patients over 60

5.   Foods included in the light diet must be
   a. coarse   c. from health food stores
   b. easy to chew   d. easy to digest

6. Of the following diets, the light diet is most similar to the
   a. clear liquid diet   c. soft diet
   b. full liquid diet   d. regular diet

7. The following group of foods would be allowed on a light diet:
   a. cheese, crackers, and rye toast
   b. peanuts, potato chips, and pretzels
   c. hamburgers, french fries, and coke
   d. angel cake, sugar cookies, and apple pie

8. The following menu could *not* be served to patients on the light diet:
   a. apple juice, bran cereal, hard roll, tea
   b. orange juice, rice cereal, plain muffin, coffee
   c. grapefruit half, scrambled egg, bagel, cocoa
   d. stewed prunes, poached egg, rye toast, tea

9. The light diet includes all foods allowed on the
   a. clear liquid diet and the low calorie diet
   b. full liquid diet and the regular diet
   c. regular diet and the clear liquid diets
   d. soft diet and the liquid diet

10. The cooking method that would not be used in preparing the light diet is
    a. poaching   c. baking
    b. broiling   d. deep frying

Chapter 23
The Bland Diet

OBJECTIVES

After studying this chapter, the student should be able to:

- Identify foods allowed on a bland diet.
- State the purpose of the bland diet.
- Identify the type of patient who would use a bland diet.

The definition of *bland* is "mild or soothing." The bland diet includes simply prepared foods that have little connective tissue or fiber. Bland foods do not increase the production of stomach acid, and are mild flavored. Therefore, the bland diet should not irritate the gastrointestinal tract chemically or mechanically. The diet is intended to reduce peristalsis and an excessive flow of gastric juices.

TABLE 23-1   Selecting Foods for a Bland Diet

FOODS ALLOWED IN A BLAND DIET	FOODS TO BE AVOIDED
milk, cream, buttermilk, yogurt	coarse foods
cottage cheese and cream cheese, mild American cheese if combined with another food	fried foods
butter and margarine	usually coffee and tea
eggs, except fried	highly seasoned foods
very tender roast, broiled, and boiled beef, lamb, veal, chicken, fish, liver, and sweetbreads	condiments
refined cereals, macaroni, spaghetti, noodles, white bread, rolls, crackers	pastries and candies
cream soups and broths	raw fruits and vegetables (except bananas, fruit juices, lettuce and tomatoes without seeds)
cooked, mild-flavored vegetables without coarse fibers or strings	alcoholic and carbonated beverages
orange, prune, peach, and pear juice, ripe banana, applesauce, baked apple (no skin), canned fruits including skinless apricots, white cherries, peaches and pears. (Orange juice should be served during or after the meal.)	smoked and salted meats and fish; pork
custard, pudding, gelatin, junket, sponge cake, plain cookies, vanilla ice cream. (The patient should eat ice cream slowly so that it is body temperature when it reaches the stomach.)	avocados, nuts, olives, coconut
decaffeinated coffee, weak tea if permitted by physician	whole grain breads and cereals

TABLE 23-2 Sample Menu for a Bland Diet

Breakfast	Dinner	Lunch or Supper
Cream of Wheat with Apricot Puree and Cream and Sugar	Cream of Tomato Soup	Poached Eggs on White Toast
	Baked Fillet of Sole	Creamed Spinach
	Baked Potato with Butter	Pear Juice
Buttered White Toast	Tender Green Peas	Baked Apple
Orange Juice	White Bread and Butter	Milk
Milk	Canned Peaches	
	Milk	
10 a.m. Eggnog	**3 p.m.** Weak Cocoa	**9 p.m.** Milk

Milk is the basis of the bland diet; other foods are added gradually as tolerated. The bland diet may be a modified liquid or soft diet. It is nutritionally adequate if it is carefully planned. This diet is used in the treatment of some gastrointestinal disturbances.

The foods allowed depend on the type of disturbance being treated and the judgment of the physician. Often the bland diet begins as a full liquid diet and then very soft foods are introduced gradually. The temperatures of the foods served (especially to a patient with a stomach ulcer) should be moderate. The size and frequency of the meals prescribed depend upon the physician's evaluation.

The bland diet is one of the more difficult diets in which to stimulate the patient's interest. It contradicts the basic rules of menu planning because of its monotonous textures and flavors. Encouragement and education of the patient on this diet are especially important.

SUMMARY

The bland diet is intended to be soothing to the gastrointestinal tract. The foods are chemically and mechanically nonirritating. Meal size and frequency vary according to the instructions of the physician. When carefully planned, it is nutritionally adequate.

DISCUSSION TOPICS

1. How does the bland diet differ from the soft diet? From the regular diet? When is it prescribed? Is it nutritionally adequate?

2. Do any of the students know anyone who has been on a soft or a bland diet? If so, have them describe their reaction to the diet.

3. Why is orange juice contraindicated before meals?

4. What foods should be avoided on a bland diet?

5. In what way(s) does the bland diet contradict rules of menu planning?

SUGGESTED ACTIVITIES

a. List 10 of your favorite foods. Circle those foods which would not be allowed in a bland diet.

b. Find recipes suitable for the bland diet and add them to the special diet recipe file.

c. Plan a day's menu for a bland diet. Compare menus and correct them if necessary.

d. Prepare at least one of the meals on the menu. Role play a nurse and serve the bland meal to another student. Ask the patient to evaluate the meal. Discuss how the meal and the service could be improved.

e. Ask a registered nurse to speak to the class regarding the current uses of the bland diet.

REVIEW

A.   Indicate which of the following foods would be allowed on a bland diet by writing Y (yes) or N (no) in the blanks beside the numbers.

_____ 1. baked ham   _____ 6. fried eggs
_____ 2. cream of chicken soup   _____ 7. broiled hamburger
_____ 3. fresh apple   _____ 8. sponge cake with vanilla
_____ 4. coffee   ice cream
_____ 5. white wine   _____ 9. macaroni and cheese
                                          _____ 10. apple pie

B.   Multiple Choice. Select the *letter* which precedes the best answer.

1. The purpose of the bland diet is to reduce
    a. peristalsis   c. both of these
    b. the flow of gastric juices   d. none of these

2. The bland diet may be ordered for
    a. preoperative patients
    b. patients with gastrointestinal disturbances
    c. newborn infants
    d. comatose patients

3. The flavors of foods in the bland diet are generally
    a. spicy   c. mild
    b. highly varied   d. salty

4. If carefully planned, the bland diet
    a. can be colorful but never well-balanced
    b. can be nutritionally adequate
    c. is the equal of the regular diet in all respects
    d. is generally well-liked by patients

5. The bland diet contradicts the basic rules of menu planning because it
    a. does not permit the use of fried foods
    b. must be served as six meals per day instead of three
    c. restricts the use of fruit
    d. is monotonous in texture and flavor

Chapter 24
Diets Modified in Residue Content

OBJECTIVES

After studying this chapter, the student should be able to:

- Describe the restricted residue diet, the minimum residue diet, and the high fiber diet.
- Identify foods allowed on the restricted residue diet, the minimum residue diet, and the high fiber diet.
- Name the conditions for which each of these diets are used.

Occasionally, it is necessary to alter the diet to regulate the amount of food residue remaining after digestion. *Food residue* is that part of food the body cannot digest and, therefore, it is ultimately evacuated in the feces. If there is little food residue, there is little fecal matter for the body to evacuate. If there is a great deal of food residue, the amount of fecal matter is increased.

To increase food residue, the patient is given foods containing large amounts of fiber (roughage). A diet of this type is called a *high fiber diet*. To decrease food residue, patients are given foods believed to leave little residue. Two diets used to reduce food residue are the *restricted residue diet* and the *minimum residue diet*. These diets may be prescribed for patients who have problems involving their gastrointestinal tracts. The specific diet may be prescribed as a medical treatment or as an early preparation for surgery. The specific diet must be ordered by a physician.

THE HIGH FIBER DIET

The high fiber diet is sometimes prescribed as treatment for diverticulosis.

Diverticulosis is an intestinal disorder characterized by little pockets forming in the sides of the intestines. This diet is intended to increase the bulk of the fecal matter and stimulate peristalsis in the intestine. Recommended foods for a high fiber diet are coarse cereals, wheat bran, whole wheat and rye flours, all fruits, raw vegetables, and legumes. This diet is nutritionally adequate.

THE RESTRICTED RESIDUE DIET

The restricted residue diet is intended to reduce the normal work of the intestines by reducing food residue. It consists of foods which contain little fiber, table 24-2. It may be prescribed for postoperative patients. The restricted residue diet may also be used for a period of time by people with *colitis* (inflammation of the colon) or *ileitis* (inflammation of the ileum). It is nutritionally adequate.

THE MINIMUM RESIDUE DIET

The minimum residue diet is extremely restricted. It may be prescribed when the gastrointestinal tract must be as free of undigested

TABLE 24-1 Sample Menu for a High Fiber Diet

Breakfast	Dinner	Lunch or Supper
Stewed Prunes	Baked Pork Chops	Fresh Fruit Cup
Bran Cereal	Baked Potato	Roast Beef Sandwich on
with	Fresh Corn	Cracked Wheat Bread
Milk and Sugar	Green Salad	with
Whole Wheat Toast	with	Lettuce and Tomato
with	Oil and Vinegar	Coleslaw
Marmalade	Dressing	Carrot Cake
Coffee	Whole Grain Bread	Milk
	with Butter	Coffee or Tea
	Fresh Pineapple	
	Milk	
	Tea	

TABLE 24-2 Restricted Residue Foods

FOODS ALLOWED IN RESTRICTED RESIDUE DIET	FOODS TO BE AVOIDED
milk, buttermilk (limited to two cups daily)	fibrous meats
cottage cheese and some mild cheeses as flavoring	fresh fruits and vegetables except as allowed in opposite list
butter and margarine	
eggs, except fried	
tender chicken, fish, sweetbreads, ground beef, and ground lamb (meats must be baked, boiled or broiled)	fried foods
soup broth	coarse breads and
cooked, mild-flavored vegetables without coarse fibers, lettuce, tomatoes (without skins and seeds) vegetable juices, fruit juices, applesauce, canned fruits including white cherries, peaches, and pears; pureed apricots, prunes and plums, citrus fruits without membranes	cereals
	nuts, olives, coconut, garlic, pickles, jams and marmalade
refined breads and cereals, white crackers, macaroni, spaghetti, and noodles	
custard, sherbet, vanilla ice cream, junket, and *cereal puddings* when considered as part of the 2-cup milk allowance; plain gelatin, angel cake, sponge cake, and plain cookies	
coffee, tea, cocoa, carbonated beverage	
salt, sugar, small amount of spices as permitted by the physician	

TABLE 24-3 Sample Menu for a Restricted Residue Diet

Breakfast	Dinner	Supper or Lunch
Strained Orange Juice	Chicken Broth	Tomato Juice
Cream of Rice Cereal	Ground Beef Patty	Macaroni and Cheese
with	Boiled Potato	Green Beans
Milk and Sugar	Baked Squash	White Bread and Butter
White Toast	Lettuce with	Lemon Sherbet
with	Oil and Vinegar	Tea with Milk and Sugar
Butter and Jelly	Gelatin Dessert	
Coffee with	Milk	
Cream and Sugar		

TABLE 24-4   Minimum Residue Foods

FOODS ALLOWED IN A MINIMUM RESIDUE DIET		FOODS TO BE AVOIDED
boiled or evaporated milk, if any milk cottage cheese if tolerated butter and margarine eggs, except fried minced chicken and fish; scraped beef soup broth small amounts of plain, unseasoned vegetable juice strained fruit juice in small amounts	refined breads and cereals, white crackers macaroni, spaghetti, and noodles sherbet, gelatin; plain cake and plain cookies tea, coffee (if physician permits) small amounts of salt and sugar	fruits and vegetables fried foods coarse, whole-grain breads and cereals; quick breads fibrous meats sometimes milk

TABLE 24-5   Sample Menu for a Minimum Residue Diet

Breakfast	Dinner	Supper or Lunch
Strained Orange Juice	Chicken Broth	Tomato Juice
Poached Egg on White Toast	Ground Beef	Minced White Poached Fish
Coffee or Tea	Buttered Noodles	Macaroni with Butter
	Toast with Butter	White Bread and Butter
	Plain Gelatin	Lemon Sherbet
	Tea	Tea

foods as possible. It may be used before or immediately after bowel surgery. Because of the severe limitations of foods allowed, this diet may be inadequate in vitamins and minerals. If this diet must be used for a period of time, the physician may prescribe vitamin and mineral supplements. The modifications made for the minimum residue diet can be seen in table 24-4.

SUMMARY

Diets may be modified in residue content. The high fiber diet includes foods that contain generous amounts of fiber and consequently increase the food residue in the intestines. The restricted residue and the minimum residue diets allow foods with limited amounts of fiber thereby reducing residue in the intestines. The high fiber and the restricted residue diets are nutritionally adequate. The minimum residue diet is inadequate in vitamins and minerals. Modified residue diets are prescribed for specific gastrointestinal problems.

DISCUSSION TOPICS

1. Describe a restricted residue diet.

2. Why is corn on the cob not allowed on a minimum residue diet? Name other foods that are not allowed on this diet. Explain why they are not allowed.

3. For what general type of conditions are low residue diets sometimes ordered?

4. Are the diets discussed in this chapter nutritionally adequate? If not, why not? How can they be made nutritionally adequate?

5. Name 10 foods that are high in fiber content.

SUGGESTED ACTIVITIES

a. Make a list of foods eaten yesterday. Circle the foods that would be allowed on a restricted residue diet.

b. Find recipes for restricted residue and minimum residue diets and add them to the special diet recipe file.

c. Plan a day's menu for a restricted residue diet, another for a minimum residue diet, and another for a high fiber diet. Evaluate the menus for nutritional value, using the Basic Four food groups as a guide. Exchange menu plans with a fellow student and evaluate each other's plans in terms of nutrient content, flavor, aroma, color, shape, appearance, texture, and satiety value.

d. Prepare at least one of the meals on each of the above menus. Evaluate each in terms of nutrient content, flavor, aroma, color, shape, appearance, texture, and satiety value.

e. Adapt the following menu to suit a patient on a minimum residue diet:

> Orange Juice
>
> Fried Egg
>
> Bacon
>
> Whole Wheat Toast
> with
> Butter and Marmalade
>
> Milk
>
> Coffee

WORD STUDY

colitis   minimum residue diet

diverticulosis   restricted residue diet

ileitis

REVIEW

A.   Indicate which of the following foods would be allowed on a minimum residue diet by writing Y (yes) or N (no) in the blanks.

_____ 1. broccoli with hollandaise sauce   _____ 6. fruit cake
_____ 2. bouillon   _____ 7. poached egg
_____ 3. applesauce   _____ 8. macaroni
_____ 4. fresh pears   _____ 9. pecan waffles
_____ 5. sherbet   _____ 10. broiled chicken

B.   Multiple Choice. Select the *letter* which precedes the best answer.

1. Residue is that part of food that
    a. remains longest in the stomach   c. is left uneaten after the meal
    b. is indigestible   d. is inedible

2. Food residue
    a. is ultimately evacuated in the feces
    b. never leaves the stomach
    c. never leaves the intestines
    d. results from incorrect cooking methods

3. Large amounts of food residue cause
    a. a decrease in fecal matter   c. weight gain
    b. an increase in fecal matter   d. diverticulosis

4. Patients requiring low residue diets usually have
    a. heart conditions   c. muscle conditions
    b. lung conditions   d. gastrointestinal conditions

5. The restricted residue diet may be prescribed for patients with
    a. colitis   c. atherosclerosis
    b. measles or mumps   d. congestive heart failure

6. The restricted residue diet
    a. is always very high in calories
    b. is very similar to the full liquid diet
    c. may be inadequate in vitamins and minerals
    d. is nutritionally adequate

7. The minimum residue diet
    a. is always very high in calories
    b. is very similar to the full liquid diet
    c. may be inadequate in vitamins and minerals
    d. is nutritionally adequate

8. The following foods are allowed on a minimum residue diet
    a. milkshake, hamburger, and french fries
    b. tomato juice, scrambled egg, and broiled bacon
    c. chicken sandwich on white bread with butter
    d. corned beef and carrot sticks

9. Three foods which would be included in a high fiber diet are
   a. whole wheat bread, prunes, celery
   b. carrot sticks, bran cereal, apples
   c. coconut bars, pecan rolls, oatmeal
   d. all of the above

10. If the minimum residue diet must be used for a period of time, the physician may
    a. alternate it weekly with the high-iron diet
    b. substitute the full liquid diet
    c. add fresh fruit juices before each meal
    d. prescribe a vitamin and mineral supplement

Chapter 25
High and Low Calorie Diets

OBJECTIVES

After studying this chapter, the student should be able to:

- Identify foods suitable for high calorie diets and those suitable for low calorie diets.
- Name the conditions for which a high calorie diet is prescribed.
- Name the conditions for which a low calorie diet is prescribed.

High and low calorie diets may be any of the standard diets (regular, light, soft, or liquid) modified in energy value.

THE HIGH CALORIE DIET

The high calorie diet is one in which the energy value is increased. This is a highly nutritious diet based on the Basic Four food groups. In this diet, there is an increased intake of foods rich in carbohydrates, some fats, and proteins. Vitamins, and minerals are supplied at least in adequate amounts. Nearly all nutritious foods are allowed in the high calorie diet but easily digested foods (carbohydrates) are recommended. Because an excess of fat can be distasteful and spoil the appetite, fatty foods must be used with discretion. Bulky foods should be used sparingly. Bulk takes up stomach space which could be better used for more concentrated, higher calorie foods.

High calorie meals should be made especially appetizing. They should include the patient's favorite foods to attract the patient's interest. The patient requiring this diet frequently has a poor appetite. It is important to serve small portions to avoid

TABLE 25-1   Foods to be Avoided in a High Calorie Diet

foods which the patient dislikes
fatty foods
bulky low calorie foods

discouraging the patient. Many of the extra calories needed may be consumed as snacks between meals, unless these snacks reduce the patient's appetite for meals and consequently reduce his total calorie intake. In some cases, the patient may consume more calories each day if the number of meals is reduced thereby increasing the appetite for each meal served.

The high calorie diet may be ordered for burn patients, for patients who have fevers or for those who are underweight due to inadequate nutrition such as can be caused by anorexia nervosa. (*Anorexia nervosa* is a self-imposed starvation.) A high calorie diet is also prescribed for patients with *hyperthyroidism,* a condition in which an overactive thyroid gland causes an abnormally high metabolism.

THE LOW CALORIE DIET

The energy value is decreased in the low calorie diet. It may be given to patients who

TABLE 25-2 Sample Menu for a High Calorie Diet — 3000 Calories

Breakfast	Dinner	Lunch or Supper
Orange Juice (1 cup = 110 cal.)	Sirloin Steak (4 oz. = 230 cal.)	Grapefruit Juice (1/2 cup = 50 cal.)
Oatmeal (1 cup = 130 cal.) with Milk and Sugar (1/2 cup milk = 80 cal. +2 tbsp. sugar = 90 cal.)	Baked Potato (90 cal.) with Butter* (1 tbsp. = 100 cal.)	Lamb Chop (150 cal.)
	Lima Beans (1/2 cup = 95 cal.)	Mashed Potatoes (3/4 cup = 145 cal.)
Soft Cooked Egg (80 cal.)	Lettuce and Tomato Salad (1/8 head lettuce = 8 cal. +1/2 tomato at 20 cal.)	Cooked Carrots (1/2 cup = 23 cal.)
Bacon* (2 sl. = 90 cal.)	Salad Dressing* (1 tbsp. commercial "French" type = 65 cal.)	Celery-Apple Salad (1 stalk celery = 5 cal. +1/2 apple at 35 cal. +1 tbsp. mayonnaise at 100 cal.)
Whole Wheat Toast (1 sl. = 60 cal.) with Butter* (2 tsp. = 66 cal.)	Roll and Butter (200 cal.)	Bread and Butter (125 cal.)
Coffee with Milk and Sugar (2 tbsp. milk = 20 cal. +1 tbsp. sugar = 45 cal.)	Chocolate Ice Cream (1/2 cup = 160 cal.) Coffee	Baked Apple (apple = 70 cal. +2 tbsp. sugar at 90 cal.)
		Milk (160 cal.)
		Coffee or Tea

Snack	Snack
1/2 cup Milk (80 cal.) 1 cookie (100 cal.)	1/2 cup Milk (80 cal.) 2 Graham Crackers (55 cal.)

*If patient tolerates the fat

are overweight; to patients with diabetes mellitus; and to some patients with *arthritis* (inflammation of the joints) or *cardiac* (heart) conditions. Although it is low in calories, it is a nutritious diet. It is based on the Basic Four food groups and no nutrient is omitted. The nutrients typically decreased in quantity are fats and carbohydrates but these are supplied in amounts that fulfill the daily dietary requirement. In a low calorie diet, bulky foods such as fresh fruits and vegetables are usually advisable.

The patient on the low calorie diet should be given a reliable calorie chart and taught how to distinguish quickly and easily between high and low calorie foods. It is important that the patient learn to revise former eating habits so that afterward the reduced weight can be maintained.

The doctor may order a low calorie diet ranging from approximately 800 to 2000 calories a day. The number of calories will be determined by the patient's activities, current weight and diet. A proper weight reduction plan will result in a safe, gradual loss of weight ranging from one to three pounds a week. A weight loss plan of one pound per week is typically arranged by eliminating 500 calories per day from the patient's regular diet.

The low calorie, like any special diet, is better accepted if the foods included are familiar and well liked. Some favorite foods can be included in the diet but they may require different methods of preparation in

TABLE 25-3   Selecting Foods for a Low Calorie Diet

FOODS ALLOWED IN A LOW CALORIE DIET	FOODS TO BE AVOIDED
skim milk, buttermilk	fatty meats and gravies
limited butter or margarine	cream, salad dressings
cottage cheese and other skim milk cheeses	nuts, candy, sweet desserts
eggs, except prepared with fat	whole milk and whole milk cheeses
lean beef, lamb, veal, pork, chicken, turkey, fish	alcoholic beverages and sweet sodas
clear soups	
whole grain or enriched bread as allowed by doctor	
vegetables should be low in carbohydrate	
fresh fruits and those canned with little or no sugar	
coffee or tea, without milk and sugar	
salt, pepper, herbs, garlic, and onions	

TABLE 25-4   Sample Menu for a Low Calorie Diet — 1200 Calories

Breakfast	Dinner	Lunch or Supper
Orange Juice (1/2 cup = 55 cal.)	Half Grapefruit (45 cal.)	Sliced Chicken (1/2 breast = 3 oz. at 155 cal.)
Poached Egg (80 cal.)	Lean Roast Beef (3oz. = 125 cal.)	Asparagus on Lettuce (4 spears = 10 cal. + lettuce leaves at 5 cal.) with
Whole Wheat Toast (1 sl. = 60 cal.)	Baked Potato (90 cal.)	Cottage Cheese (2 oz. = 50 cal.)
Butter (1 tsp. = 33 cal.)	Cooked Carrots (1/2 cup = 23 cal.)	Bread (1 sl. = 60 cal.)
Skim Milk (1/2 cup = 45 cal.)	Lettuce and Tomato Salad (1/8 head lettuce = 8 cal. 1/2 tomato = 20 cal.)	Butter (1 tsp. = 33 cal.)
Black Coffee	Bread (1/2 sl. = 30 cal.)	Cantaloupe (1/2 melon = 45 cal.)
	Butter (1 tsp. = 33 cal.)	Black Coffee or Tea
	Strawberries (1 cup fresh = 55 cal.)	
	Skim Milk (1/2 cup = 45 cal.)	
	Black Coffee or Tea	

order to avoid adding calories unnecessarily. For example, fish may be baked, broiled, or poached instead of being fried. Canned tomatoes may be substituted for thickened tomato sauces. Herbs and spices should be used instead of heavy sauces on meats and vegetables. Lemon juice and herbs may be substituted for rich salad dressings.

It is advisable that the low calorie diet be used only on the advice of a physician. There is the danger that a self-imposed low calorie diet will result in a reduction in the intake of essential vitamins, minerals, and proteins as well as calories. If an inadequate diet is maintained over a prolonged period of time, dietary deficiencies can develop and can adversely affect physical development and health. It is especially dangerous for teenagers to undertake self-imposed reducing diets because adolescence is a period of rapid growth and development.

Many of the countless fad reducing diets regulary published in magazines and books are *crash-reducing diets*. This means they are intended to cause a very rapid rate of weight reduction. Often fad diets require the purchase of expensive foods. Others are part of a weight loss plan including exercise with special equipment. Expensive food items and equipment can add to the burden of dieting.

A crash diet usually does result in an initial rapid weight loss. However, the weight loss is thought to be caused by a loss of body water rather than body fat. Sudden weight loss of this type is followed by a plateau period, that is, a period in which weight does not decrease. Disillusionment is apt to occur during this period and this may cause the dieter to go on an "eating binge." This can result in regaining the weight that was lost and sometimes may even add more pounds. Some popular reducing diets severely limit the foods allowed, providing a real danger of nutrient deficiencies over time.

No reducing diet performs magic. Each requires willpower and time. The safest and most economical weight reduction plan is a low calorie diet supervised by a physician. This type of diet is also the most interesting and the easiest to maintain because it does not severely limit the foods allowed.

SUMMARY

The high and low calorie diets may be modifications of any of the four standard diets. The energy value of the diet is increased or decreased as required. The high calorie diet may be used in cases of underweight, hyperthyroidism, burns, or fever. It includes additional high-energy foods. The low calorie diet may be used in cases of obesity, diabetes mellitus, arthritis and some cardiac conditions. It limits the intake of calories. Both diets should be used only under medical supervision.

DISCUSSION TOPICS

1. What may cause underweight? Which of the diets in this chapter may be used to treat this condition? Why?

2. What is obesity? What may cause it? Which of the diets in this chapter may be used to treat this condition?

3. Why may self-imposed diets be especially harmful during adolescence?

4. Describe one or two popular reducing diets. Could such a diet have any effect on the nutrition of those people who subscribe to it? If so, what? Ask if anyone in the class has used such a diet. If so, ask that

person to describe the diet, the physical effects felt during the diet, and the ultimate result.

5. How could the high calorie diet be unpleasant for the patient?

SUGGESTED ACTIVITIES

a. Using table A-6, The Nutritive Values of Foods, in the Appendix, look for caloric values of 10 familiar foods. Make two lists. On the left, list which of the ten foods would be suitable for a high calorie diet. On the right, list those foods suitable for a low calorie diet.

b. Make a list of foods eaten yesterday. Circle those foods which would not be suitable for a low calorie diet.

c. Find recipes that are suitable for the high calorie diet and others that are suitable for the low calorie diet. Add these to the special diet recipe file.

d. Adapt the sample menu for the 1200-calorie diet in this chapter to make it suitable for a regular 2400-calorie diet. Adapt it for a high calorie diet (3000 calories). Use table A-6 for caloric values of foods.

e. Plan a day's menu for a 1200-calorie diet. Compare menus with other class members and correct them if necessary. Repeat for a 3000-calorie diet.

f. Prepare at least one of the meals on the planned menu and evaluate it in terms of nutritive content, flavor, aroma, color, shape, appearance, texture, and satiety value.

WORD STUDY

anorexia nervosa   cardiac

arthritis   crash-reducing diet

REVIEW

A.   Multiple Choice. Select the *letter* which precedes the best answer.

1. The high calorie diet may be a modified
   a. regular diet   c. soft diet
   b. liquid diet   d. any of these

2. The high calorie diet may be prescribed for
   a. obesity   c. arthritic conditions
   b. hyperthyroidism   d. hypothyroidism

3. The general type of foods that should be avoided in the high calorie diet are
   a. fatty foods   c. breads and cereals
   b. foods the patient likes   d. coffee and tea

4. In the high calorie diet, the energy value
   a. is increased
   b. is decreased
   c. is reduced to minimal levels
   d. remains the same as on the regular diet

5. The low calorie diet may be prescribed for
   a. obesity   c. hyperthyroidism
   b. fevers   d. severe allergies

6. In the low calorie diet, the energy value
   a. remains the same as for the regular diet
   b. is decreased
   c. is increased
   d. should equal that of the clear liquid diet

7. On a low calorie diet, the caloric requirement per day may range from
   a. 500 to 800 calories   c. 800 to 2000 calories
   b. 800 to 1000 calories   d. 2000 to 3000 calories

8. A proper weight reduction plan allows for loss of
   a. 1 to 2 pounds per day   c. 3 to 5 pounds per week
   b. 1 to 3 pounds per week   d. 15 to 20 pounds per month

9. Low calorie diets
   a. are prescribed for burn patients
   b. are never nutritionally sound
   c. can be safely self-imposed
   d. should only be used on the advice of a physician

10. Popular crash-reducing diets
   a. are always effective and totally harmless
   b. are very useful for teenagers
   c. result in a slow, even loss of weight
   d. are potentially hazardous

B. Complete the following statements.

1. The high calorie diet is one in which the energy value is _____
   _____ .

2. The patient requiring a _____ calorie diet usually has a poor
   appetite, therefore, serving sizes should be _____ .

3. When the thyroid gland is overactive and raises the metabolism rate,
   the condition is called _____ .

4. The diet ordered for a patient with an overactive thyroid gland is the
   _____ .

5. Bulky foods such as fresh fruits and vegetables are usually advisable for
   _____ calorie diets.

6. Serving snacks between meals may help a patient meet the calorie requirements for a _____ calorie diet.

7. Patients who are overweight and those who suffer from diabetes mellitus, arthritis, and cardiac conditions may be put on the _____ _____ calorie diet.

8. A type of milk recommended for patients on the low calorie diet is _____ or _____ .

9. Steak, lima beans, and ice cream are examples of food allowed on the _____ calorie diet.

10. Lean meat, strawberries, and skim milk are examples of foods recommended for the _____ calorie diet.

Chapter 26
The Diabetic Diet

OBJECTIVES

After studying this chapter, the student should be able to:

- Define diabetes mellitus.
- Name the symptoms of diabetes mellitus.
- State the function of insulin.
- Explain three types of diabetic diets.
- Explain how non-metabolized glucose is excreted.

The diabetic diet is a regular diet modified in nutrient content. It is nutritionally adequate if carefully planned. The energy value should exceed 1000 calories per day. This diet is used in controlling diabetes mellitus. *Diabetes mellitus* is a *chronic* (of long duration) disorder of metabolism which is caused by inadequate production or utilization of insulin. *Insulin* is a hormone secreted by the islets of Langerhans in the pancreas. This hormone enables the body to use glucose, a simple sugar which is the end product of the digestion of carbohydrates. When the supply of insulin is inadequate, the glucose that is not metabolized accumulates in the blood and is subsequently excreted in the urine. Symptoms of untreated diabetes mellitus include: an increase in the output of urine, itching skin, weakness, loss of weight, increased thirst, and increased appetite.

When diabetes develops in individuals over 35, the disease may be less severe than when it occurs in children or young adults. When the condition develops at this age, it is frequently associated with overweight.

Treatment is usually begun when urine and blood tests indicate that sugar is present.

It consists of diet therapy sometimes combined with medication. Patients who require medication are given commercially prepared insulin or oral hypoglycemic agents. *Hypoglycemic agents* are medications which stimulate the pancreas to produce insulin so as to improve glucose utilization. These oral agents are used mainly with adults who tend to have less severe cases of diabetes.

TYPES OF DIABETIC DIETS

The type of diet for the diabetic patient is determined by the physician. The patient may be placed on any of three diets: (1) a weighed diet, (2) an unweighed or so-called "free" diet, or (3) a diet based on exchange lists.

The Weighed Diet

The weighed diet is based on a very conservative approach to the treatment of diabetes. The glucose levels are rigidly controlled by the use of insulin or hypoglycemic agents, carefully weighed food portions, and frequent urine tests during the day. This treatment of diabetes is called the *chemical method of regulation.*

The Unweighed or "Free" Diet

The unweighed diet is based on a very liberal approach to the treatment of diabetes. Patients are allowed to choose their foods (except for sugar and high-sugar foods). If this diet is not successful in controlling the diabetes, they are placed on insulin. Once insulin treatment is begun, it is generally continued throughout the life of the patient. This treatment is known as the *clinical method of regulation.*

Diet Based on Exchange Lists

In the exchange list method of diet therapy, foods are grouped into six major lists. Each list includes measured amounts of foods which contain approximately equal amounts of calories, carbohydrates, proteins, fats, vitamins, and minerals. This means that any one food within a particular list may be substituted for any other food *within that particular list* and still provide the patient with the prescribed types and amounts of nutrients. The types and amounts of nutrients and the number of calories are not the same on different lists.

List 1 contains milk and milk products.

List 2 contains all nonstarchy vegetables.

List 3 contains all fruits and fruit juices.

List 4 contains breads, cereals, pasta, starchy vegetables, and prepared foods such as biscuits, muffins, crackers, french-fried potatoes, potato chips, pancakes, and waffles.

List 5 contains meats.

List 6 contains fats.

When the exchange lists are to be used, the diet is prescribed by the physician who determines the total energy requirement of the patient. This is done by evaluating age, size, sex, and activities. The nurse or physician may then direct the patient to the dietitian who plans the diet.

Diets based on the exchange lists are individualized. The diet is planned in consultation with the patient. Considerations include: (a) where meals will be eaten, (b) the time the meals are usually eaten, (c) personal and family food likes and dislikes, (d) the amount of money typically allotted to food, and (e) the entire life-style of the patient. The plan is carefully devised so that about 50 percent of the total caloric intake will be obtained from the consumption of carbohydrates; 15 percent from proteins, and 35 percent from fats. All of these nutrients are provided by foods which provide sufficient vitamins and minerals as well.

The total energy requirements for adult diabetic patients who are not overweight will be the same as for nondiabetic individuals. When patients are overweight, a reduction in calories will be built into the diet plans. If the total daily intake is 1000 calories or less, vitamin and mineral supplements may be ordered.

The diet is given in terms of exchanges rather than as particular foods. For example, the menu pattern for breakfast may include 1 fruit exchange, 1 meat exchange, 2 bread exchanges, and 2 fat exchanges. The patient may choose the desired foods from the exchange lists for each meal but must adhere to the specific exchange lists named and the specific number of exchanges on each list. In this way, the patient has variety in a simple yet controlled way. Exchange lists form the most commonly used method of diet therapy for diabetic patients. They may also be used to control calories and fats. Note: Diet plans based on the exchange lists must be formed by dietitians or knowledgeable diet counselors so that the diabetic person is certain to get proper nourishment while controlling the diabetes.

Exchange lists have been prepared by the American Diabetes Association and The

American Dietetic Association in cooperation with the United States Public Health Service. Copies may be obtained by writing to the American Diabetes Association, 600 Fifth Avenue, New York, New York 10020, or to the American Dietetic Association, 430 North Michigan Avenue, Chicago, Illinois 60611.

TEACHING THE DIABETIC PATIENT

It is important to point out to the diabetic patient that one can live a near-normal life if the diet is followed, medication is taken as prescribed, and time is allowed for sufficient exercise and rest. The importance of eating all of the prescribed food must be emphasized. It is important for meals to be eaten at regular times so that the insulin-sugar balance may be more easily maintained. It is imperative that the patient learn to read carefully all labels on commercially prepared foods. This is necessary in order to avoid eating or drinking anything that may contain an unknown amount of sugar. It must be explained that prepared foods with unknown amounts of sugar added are not allowed because they will upset the insulin-sugar balance. Adjustments must be made in the shopping, cooking, and eating habits so the diet plan can be followed. Family meals can be simply adapted for the diabetic diet. For example, sugar and flour can be omitted from the patient's portions, and lemon juice, herbs, and spices can be substituted for rich sauces on salads, vegetables, and meats. The American Diabetes Association and the American Dietetics Association in their booklet entitled, "Exchange Lists for Meal Planning," advise against using the food items found in table 26-1 without special permission from the diet counselor. This same booklet advises the diabetic patient that the food items found in table 26-2 may be used freely. The person with

TABLE 26-1   Foods Usually Omitted in Diabetic Diets

sugar	honey
cookies	condensed milk
pies	jam
candy	chewing gum
syrup	jelly
cakes	soft drinks

TABLE 26-2   Foods Usually Allowed in Diabetic Diets

coffee	parsley
tea	nutmeg
bouillon without fat	lemon
unsweetened gelatin	mustard
unsweetened pickles	chili powder
salt	onion salt or powder
pepper	horseradish
red pepper	vinegar
paprika	mint
garlic	cinnamon
celery salt	lime

diabetes will soon learn which exchange lists are to be included at each meal and at snacktimes, and the foods within each exchange list.

SUMMARY

The diabetic diet is used in treating diabetes mellitus, a metabolic disease caused by the improper functioning of the pancreas which results in inadequate production or utilization of insulin. If the condition is left untreated, the body cannot use glucose properly and serious complications leading to death may occur. Treatment includes diet and/or medication. Diabetic diets are prescribed by the physician and planned by a diet counselor after consultation with the patient.

DISCUSSION TOPICS

1. What are the modifications of the diabetic diet?

2. For what glandular condition is the diabetic diet ordered? Why? Is this just a temporary diet? Is it nutritious?

3. What is insulin? What is its use?

4. Does anyone in the class have diabetes mellitus or know anyone who does? If so, ask that person to describe the symptoms, treatment, diet, and reaction to the diet.

SUGGESTED ACTIVITIES

a. Ask a physician or registered nurse to speak to the class on diabetes mellitus and its treatment.

b. Ask a diet counselor to explain and demonstrate the planning of diabetic diets using the exchange lists.
   1. Observe the diet counselor planning a 1200-calorie and a 1500-calorie diabetic diet using the exchange lists.
   2. Observe the diet counselor adapting a normal, 2400-calorie daily menu to suit the needs of the diabetic patient on a 1500-calorie diet.

c. Find recipes suitable for the diabetic diet and add them to the special diet recipe file.

d. Prepare and serve a meal as planned in activity b. Evaluate it in terms of nutritive content, flavor, aroma, color, shape, appearance, texture, and satiety value.

WORD STUDY

diabetes mellitus	insulin	exchange lists
chronic	hypoglycemic agents	

REVIEW

A.   Multiple-multiple Choice. Select the *letter* which precedes the best answer.

1. Diabetes mellitus is a metabolic disorder
    1. caused by malfunction of the pancreas gland
    2. for which a diabetic diet may be ordered
    3. in which sugar accumulates in the blood
    4. for which a regular diet is adequate
    5. which is very contagious
       a) all   b) 1, 2, 3   c) 4, 5   d) 1, 2, 4, 5

2. The metabolism of glucose
    1. depends on insulin secreted by the islets of Langerhans
    2. depends on enzymes present in pancreatic juice
    3. is inefficient if diabetes is left untreated
    4. is directly related to secretions from the thyroid gland
        a) 1,3,4   b) all   c) 2,3   d) 1,3

3. Diabetes mellitus is treated by
    1. administration of insulin
    2. exclusion of foods that contain glucose
    3. administration of thyroxine
    4. use of a diabetic diet
        a) 1,3,4   b) 1,4   c) all   d) 1,2,3

4. When considering diets to be used in the management of diabetes, the doctor may order
    1. unweighed or "free" diet
    2. weighed diet
    3. diet based on exchange lists
    4. elimination diet
        a) 1,2,3   b) 1,3,4   c) 2,3,4   d) all

5. The diabetic diet is
    1. also prescribed for hyperthyroidism
    2. based on age, size, sex, and activity
    3. always a low calorie diet
    4. part of the medical treatment for diabetes mellitus
        a) 1,2,3   b) 2,4   c) 1,3,4   d) all

B. A Question Chain. In order to complete the following set of completion questions, they must be answered in numerical order.

1. The diabetic diet is used to treat a disease called _____
   _____ .

2. The disease named in question 1 is a chronic disorder of _____
   _____ .

3. The chronic disorder named in question 2 is caused by the inadequate production or utilization of the hormone, _____ .

4. The hormone named in question 3 is necessary in order for the body to use the simple sugar, _____ .

5. When the body is unable to use the simple sugar named in question 4, the simple sugar is excreted in the _____ .

6. Symptoms of the disease named in question 1 are _____ ,
   _____ , _____ .

Chapter 27
Fat Controlled Diets

OBJECTIVES

After studying this chapter, the student should be able to:

- State the purposes of fat controlled diets.
- Identify foods suitable for a low fat diet.
- Identify foods suitable for a low cholesterol diet.
- Recognize the characteristics of saturated and polyunsaturated fats.

Fat controlled diets may be ordered for patients with gallbladder disease, *pancreatitis* (inflammation of the pancreas) or heart conditions. These diets are intended to reduce the amount and/or change the type of fat in the diet. Fat controlled diets may be deficient in fat-soluble vitamins as a result of the decreased fat intake. Consequently a vitamin supplement may be prescribed for a patient on a fat controlled diet. The particular diet ordered will depend of course, on the patient's condition and the physician.

LOW FAT DIET

The exact amount of fat contained in the average diet is difficult to determine. However, it is believed by some experts that the average diet contains 155 grams of fat.[1] The low fat (also called fat restricted) diet contains a specific, maximum amount of fat. Such a diet may contain 70 grams of fat, 50 grams of fat, 30 grams of fat, or 20 grams of fat. Obviously, a diet so low in fat will seem very unusual and *unpalatable* (unpleasant tasting) to some patients. Special understanding

[1]Dorothea Turner, Handbook of Diet Therapy. Chicago: University of Chicago Press. 1970

and patience will be required. Information regarding the fat content of foods and methods of preparation that will minimize the amount of fat in the diet should be given. No foods that are high in fat are permitted. Foods must be prepared without the addition of any fat. All visible fat must be removed from meats. Foods must not be fried. Skim milk must be used instead of whole milk. Sometimes such a diet is also somewhat restricted in fiber content.

THE LOW CHOLESTEROL DIET

The low cholesterol diet is modified as to type and amount of fat allowed. It may be prescribed for persons who are risks for coronary heart disease.

Cholesterol is a necessary part of body cells and a component of fats. The human body produces it and it is also found in animal food products. Cholesterol is stored in the liver and is carried by the blood to the cells as it is needed. Evidence indicates that the total fat in the diet and the kinds of fat eaten may have a relationship to the amount of cholesterol in the blood. An excess of cholesterol in the blood is associated with

TABLE 27-1 Selecting Foods for a Low Fat (30 gram) Diet

FOODS ALLOWED IN A LOW FAT DIET	FOODS TO BE AVOIDED
skim milk, buttermilk, and yogurt made from skim milk	cream and whole milk
cottage cheese	cheeses except uncreamed cottage cheese
eggs, but limited in number according to amount of fat allowed in diet	all fats unless a minimum amount of butter or margarine is allowed
butter and margarine — usually limited to 1 Tbsp. or less daily and excluded entirely in very low fat diets	commercially prepared soups or any soups made with whole milk or cream
very lean fish, fowl, and meats — amount limited by physician according to the total amount of fat allowed in diet	fatty meats such as pork, bacon, ham, goose, duck, and fatty fish
fat-free soup broth	desserts except for those on the allowed list
cooked vegetables; lettuce and tomatoes (without skin or seeds); fruit juice; bananas; citrus fruits without membranes	chocolate, nuts, coconut
refined breads and cereals — as desired except for egg noodles	salad dressings, salad oils, gravies
gelatin, angel cake, cereal puddings made with skim milk, ices	fried foods
coffee, tea, carbonated beverages	garlic, pickles
jelly, honey as desired	

TABLE 27-2 Sample Menu for a Low Fat (30 gram) Diet

Breakfast	Dinner	Lunch or Supper
Orange Juice	2 oz. Chicken	Tomato Juice
Cream of Wheat with 1 Tbsp. Sugar and 1 Cup Skim Milk	Boiled Potato	Uncreamed Cottage Cheese on Fruit Salad*
1 Slice Toast	Baked Squash with 1 Tbsp. Honey	2 Slices Toast with 2 Tbsp. Honey
1 Tbsp. Jelly	Lettuce Salad	Angel Cake
Coffee	1 Slice Bread	1 Cup Milk
	1 Tbsp. Jelly	Tea
	Canned Peaches	
	1 Cup Milk	
	Tea	

*No Avocado

TABLE 27-3   Cholesterol Content of Foods.*

Item No.	Item	Amount of cholesterol in —		
		100 grams edible portion	Edible portion of 1 pound as purchased	Refuse from item as purchased
(A)	(B)	(C)	(D)	(E)
		Milligrams	*Milligrams*	*Percent*
1	Beef, raw:			
a	with bone	70	270	15
b	without bone	70	320	0
2	Brains, raw	>2,000	>9,000	0
3	Butter	250	1,135	0
4	Caviar or fish roe	> 300	>1,300	0
	Cheese:			
5	Cheddar	100	455	0
6	Cottage, creamed	15	70	0
7	Cream	120	545	0
8	Other (25% to 30% fat)	85	385	0
9	Cheese spread	65	295	0
10	Chicken, flesh only, raw	60	. . . .	0
11	Crab:			
a	In shell	125	270	52
b	Meat only	125	565	0
12	Egg, whole	550	2,200	12
13	Egg white	0	0	0
	Egg yolk:			
14	Fresh	1,500	6,800	0
15	Frozen	1,280	5,800	0
16	Dried	2,950	13,380	0
17	Fish:			
a	Steak	70	265	16
b	Fillet	70	320	0
18	Heart, raw	150	680	0
19	Ice Cream	45	205	0
20	Kidney, raw	375	1,700	0
21	Lamb, raw:			
a	with bone	70	265	16
b	without bone	70	320	0
22	Lard and other animal fat	95	430	0
23	Liver, raw	300	1,360	0
24	Lobster:			
a	Whole	200	235	74
b	Meat only	200	900	0
	Margarine:			
25	All vegetable fat	0	0	0
26	Two-thirds animal fat, one-third vegetable fat	65	295	0
	Milk:			
27	Fluid, whole	11	50	0
28	Dried, whole	85	385	0
29	Fluid, skim	3	15	0
30	Mutton:			
a	with bone	65	250	16
b	without bone	65	295	0
31	Oysters:			
a	In shell	≥200	≥ 90	90
b	Meat only	≥200	>900	0
32	Pork:			
a	With bone	70	260	18
b	Without bone	70	320	0
33	Shrimp:			
a	In Shell	125	390	31
b	Flesh only	125	565	0
34	Sweetbreads (thymus)	250	1,135	0
35	Veal:			
a	With bone	90	320	21
b	Without bone	90	410	0

*Letters *a* and *b* designate items that have the same chemical composition for the edible portion but differ in the amount of refuse. The data in column C applies to 100 grams of edible portion of the item, although it may be purchased with the refuse indicated in column E and described or implied in column B. Source: U.S. Department of Agriculture *Composition of Foods,* Agriculture Handbook No. 8, 1963 Agricultural Research Service

atherosclerosis, a thickening and narrowing of artery walls due to fatty deposits in their lining. Atherosclerosis may lead to *coronary occlusion* which is a stoppage or blocking of blood flow to the heart.

Saturated fats are thought to raise the level of cholesterol in the blood and polyunsaturated fats are thought to lower it. Most saturated fats are of animal origin and usually solid at room temperature. Unsaturated or polyunsaturated fats are derived from plants and fish and are usually liquid at room temperature.

In the low cholesterol diet, protein requirements are met by lean muscle meats, fish, and skim milk. Other protein-rich foods such as organ meats, eggs, and shellfish are used in very limited quantities because of their high cholesterol content. Skim milk is used instead of whole milk. Desserts containing whole milk, eggs, and cream are avoided. Margarine is substituted for butter, and liquid vegetable oils are used in cooking.

Chapter 3, Carbohydrates and Fats, may be reviewed for additional information.

SUMMARY

Fat controlled diets may be ordered for patients with pancreatitis, gallbladder disturbances, or heart problems. A low fat diet is essentially a regular diet with the fat content (and sometimes fiber content) reduced. There may be a deficiency of the fat-soluble vitamins in this diet. Animal fats, butterfat, and eggs are avoided when cholesterol is restricted.

DISCUSSION TOPICS

1. Name the fat controlled diets discussed in this chapter. For what conditions might these diets be ordered?

2. In what respect are fat controlled diets modified? Is the patient apt to notice these modifications?

3. Are low fat diets nutritious? If not, what nutrient(s) may be lacking? Why?

4. What is cholesterol? Why is it associated with atherosclerosis? What has been published recently in newspapers and magazines concerning cholesterol and heart problems? What is a coronary occlusion?

5. Why is skim milk allowed on low fat diets when whole milk is not?

6. Discuss the differences between saturated and polyunsaturated fats. In what foods are each of these fats predominantly found?

7. Discuss the types of information a patient on a fat controlled diet may need to be given.

SUGGESTED ACITIVITIES

a. Find recipes suitable for low fat diets and for low cholesterol diets. Add them to the special diet recipe file.

b. Make a list of the foods eaten yesterday. Circle those foods that would not be allowed on a low cholesterol diet and suggest substitutions that would be satisfactory.

c. Plan a day's menu for a low fat (70 gram) diet.

d. Plan a day's menu for a low cholesterol diet.

e. Prepare at least one of these meals and evaluate it in terms of nutritive content, flavor, aroma, color, shape, appearance, texture, and satiety value.

WORD STUDY

atherosclerosis	pancreatitis	low cholesterol diet
coronary occlusion	low fat diet	unpalatable

REVIEW

A.   Match the terms in column I with the phrases in column II.

Column I

_____ 1. low fat diet
_____ 2. low cholesterol diet
_____ 3. pancreatitis
_____ 4. supplement
_____ 5. fatty meats
_____ 6. cholesterol
_____ 7. atherosclerosis
_____ 8. saturated fat
_____ 9. unsaturated fat
_____ 10. coronary occlusion

Column II

a. inflammation of the pancreas
b. pork, ham, bacon
c. chicken, turkey
d. fatty accumulations in artery walls
e. sometimes used in treating atherosclerosis
f. butter
g. may be used in gallbladder disease
h. liquid corn oil
i. blockage of blood vessel to heart
j. an addition
k. necessary component of body cells

B.   Multiple-multiple Choice.   Select the *letter* which precedes the best answer.

1. Fat controlled diets may be ordered for patients with
    1. pancreatitis
    2. gallbladder disease
    3. heart conditions
    4. bladder infections
        a) 1,2,3   b) 2,3,4   c) 1,3,4   d) all

2. Fat controlled diets may be
    1. deficient in fat-soluble vitamins
    2. deficient in fiber content
    3. modified in nutrient content
    4. unpalatable to the patient
        a) 1,2,3   b) 1,3,4   c) 1,2,4   d) all

3. In a low cholesterol diet
   1. eggs are used freely
   2. skim milk is used instead of whole milk
   3. lean muscle meats and fish are permitted
   4. vegetable oils are permitted
      a) 1,2,3   b) 2,3,4   c) 1,3,4   d) all

4. The amount of fat allowed in the low fat diet is
   1. reduced   3. eliminated completely
   2. increased   4. the same as in a regular diet
      a) 1,3   b) 1 only   c) 2 only   d) all

5. Persons on a low fat diet will
   1. need information regarding the fat content of foods
   2. need information regarding cooking methods for their diets
   3. never be allowed butter or margarine
   4. probably find the diet somewhat unpalatable
      a) 1,3,4   b) 1,2,3   c) 1,2,4   d) all

6. Foods allowed in a low fat diet include
   1. all cheeses
   2. cooked vegetables
   3. refined cereals
   4. limited amounts of lean meats
      a) 1,3,4   b) 2,3,4   c) 1,3,4   d) all

7. When preparing foods for the low fat diet,
   1. very small amounts of fat may be added
   2. visible fats must be removed from meats
   3. skim milk is never used
   4. no frying is permitted
      a) 1,4   b) 2,3,4   c) 2,4   d) all

8. On the low cholesterol diet, saturated fats are
   1. reduced
   2. eliminated
   3. increased
   4. unchanged from that of the regular diet
      a) 1,2   b) 2 only   c) 1 only   d) all

9. Saturated fats are usually
   1. solid at room temperature   3. found in animal foods
   2. liquid at room temperature   4. derived from plants
      a) 1,3   b) 2,3   c) 1,4   d) all

10. Polyunsaturated fats are usually
    1. solid at room temperature   3. found in animal foods
    2. liquid at room temperature   4. derived from plants
       a) 1,3   b) 2,4   c) 1,4   d) all

Chapter 28
Protein Diets

OBJECTIVES

After studying this chapter, the student should be able to:

- Identify foods allowed in a high protein diet.
- Identify foods suitable for both high and low protein diets.
- List conditions that would require a high protein diet.
- List conditions that would require a low protein diet.

The high protein diet is sometimes prescribed for children and adolescents who need extra protein for growth, for women during pregnancy, for patients following surgery, and for those with illnesses resulting in protein loss. A regular diet which stresses protein-rich foods is usually ordered. The amount of protein in the diet may be further increased by adding dried skim milk to soups and baked products and by adding wheat germ to cereal and baked products. It is a highly nutritious diet. Table 28-1 lists foods that are included in a high protein diet, provided the patient does not need to modify other nutrients such as fat or sodium.

TABLE 28-1 Foods Included in a High Protein Diet

milk: 3 to 4 cups

cheeses

eggs

lean meats, fish, and poultry

vegetables

fruits

cereals (whole grain or enriched) and breads
    as desired

TABLE 28-2 Sample Menu for a High Protein Diet

Breakfast	Dinner	Lunch or Supper
Orange Juice	Roast Chicken	Ground Round Steak
Scrambled Eggs	Baked Potato	Asparagus
Bacon	Green Peas	Tomatoes on Lettuce
Toast with Butter and Jelly	Lettuce Salad	Bread and Butter
Milk	Bread and Butter	Fresh Fruit Cup
Coffee with Cream and Sugar	Custard	Milk
	Milk	Tea with Cream and Sugar

TABLE 28-3 Selecting Foods for a Low Protein (30 Gram) Diet

FOODS ALLOWED IN A LOW PROTEIN (30 GRAM) DIET	FOODS NOT ALLOWED IN A LOW PROTEIN (30 GRAM) DIET
milk: 1/2 cup per day	milk, other than the 1/2 cup allowance (or its equivalent)
soups: permitted if made from allowed foods	high protein cereals
meats, fish, poultry, cheese: 2 oz	legumes
1 egg	baked products containing eggs and milk
vegetables: any except corn, lima beans, peas	
fruits: any	
bread: one serving of cereal, bread, potato, or potato substitute	
butter, margarine, cooking oils, salad dressings	
coffee, tea, carbonated beverages	
fruit ice, plain hard candy	
salt, herbs, spices, pickles	

TABLE 28-4 Sample Menu for a Low Protein (30 Gram) Diet

Breakfast	Dinner	Lunch or Supper
Orange Juice	Pineapple Juice	Apple Juice
Soft Cooked Egg	1 oz. Roast Beef	1 oz. Roast Chicken
Rice Cereal with 1/2 Cup Milk and Sugar	Baked Squash with Butter	Asparagus with Butter
Coffee	Baked Apple with Sugar	Sliced Tomatoes
	Tea	Fruit Cup
		Tea with Sugar

LOW PROTEIN DIET

Sometimes a low protein diet may be prescribed in certain kidney or liver conditions. A low sodium diet may also be prescribed in kidney disease, resulting in a double modification. In some cases the protein may be restricted to 30 grams daily.

It is important to distribute the protein equally among three meals in the low protein diet. The low protein diet contains insufficient protein, minerals, vitamins and in some cases, calories.

SUMMARY

The high protein diet may be prescribed for growing children and adolescents, pregnant women, and for patients with illnesses that cause the loss of protein. It is a regular, nutritious diet that stresses protein-rich foods. The low protein diet may be prescribed in certain liver or kidney conditions. This diet is deficient in protein, minerals, vitamins, and sometimes calories.

DISCUSSION TOPICS

1. How does the high protein diet differ from the regular diet?
2. How can the protein be increased in the following foods: milkshake, eggnog, cocoa, cream soup, and cream of wheat cereal?
3. Is the low protein diet nutritious? Why or why not?
4. Why are beans and peas not allowed on the low protein diet?

SUGGESTED ACTIVITIES

a. Using outside sources, prepare a short report on the functions of the circulatory system, the liver, and the kidneys in eliminating nitrogenous waste products from the body.

b. Find recipes that are suitable for high protein and low protein diets. Add these to the special recipe file.

c. List the foods eaten yesterday. Compute the protein by using table A-6 in the Appendix. Compare the total proteins with the total given for someone your age and sex in table 4-2 on page 33. Would such a diet meet the requirements of the low protein diet? The high protein diet? Does it contain adequate protein for you?

d. Plan a day's menu for a high protein diet. Plan a day's menu for a low protein diet by adapting the high protein menus and correct if necessary.

e. Prepare at least one meal on each of the menus. Evaluate each in terms of nutritive content, flavor, aroma, color, shape, appearance, texture, and satiety value.

f. Using table A-6 in the Appendix, compute the protein in the sample high protein diet menu in this chapter.

REVIEW

A. Before each of the listed foods, insert an *H* for those allowed in high protein diets, and a *B* for those allowed in both high and low protein diets.

_____	1. apple juice	_____	6. ginger ale
_____	2. ice cream	_____	7. coffee
_____	3. two-egg omelet	_____	8. butter
_____	4. cream of tomato soup	_____	9. dill pickles
	5. broiled chicken (half)	_____	10. chocolate pudding

B. Multiple-multiple Choice. Select the *letter* that precedes the best answer.

1. The high protein diet
   1. is nutritious
   2. contains limited amounts of protein
   3. allows fruits and vegetables
   4. may be given during uncomplicated pregnancy

   a) 1,2,3   b) 1,3,4   c) 2,3,4   d) all

2. The high protein diet is
    1. modified in nutrient content
    2. modified in texture
    3. a modified regular diet
    4. always a full liquid diet
        a) 1,2   b) 2,4   c) 1,3   d) all

3. Foods that would be allowed on a high protein diet are
    1. meats
    2. milk
    3. eggs
    4. cheeses
        a) 1,2   b) 1, 2, 3   c) 2, 3, 4   d) all

4. A low protein diet may be given to persons with
    1. diabetes mellitus
    2. certain liver conditions
    3. certain kidney conditions
    4. ulcers
        a) 1, 4   b) 1, 2   c) 2, 3   d) all

5. Foods that would be allowed on a low protein diet are
    1. lettuce
    2. corn
    3. consomme
    4. orange juice
        a) 1, 2, 3   b) 1, 3, 4   c) 2, 3, 4   d) all

Chapter 29
Sodium Restricted Diets

OBJECTIVES

After studying this chapter, the student should be able to:

- Explain why sodium is sometimes restricted in the diet.
- List sodium compounds that are frequently added to food.
- Identify foods not allowed in various sodium restricted diets.

Sodium is a mineral which is essential in regulating the water balance in the body. When it is consumed in normal quantities by healthy people, it is beneficial. Nutritionists estimate that the average person on an unrestricted diet consumes about 6000 milligrams of sodium each day. This amount is much more than the body needs. Healthy people eliminate this excess, however, through perspiration and excretion by the kidneys.

In certain illnesses, particularly kidney and cardiovascular disorders, the body retains water. In such cases sodium is also retained and, in fact, contributes to the water retention. When water and sodium are not normally excreted, they accumulate in body tissues and cause swelling, known as edema. To alleviate this condition, a sodium restricted diet is prescribed. When the sodium content in the diet is reduced, the water and salts in the tissues flow back into the blood to be excreted normally. In this way, the edema is relieved. The amount of sodium to be restricted is determined by the physician on the basis of the patient's condition.

FOODS CONTAINING SODIUM

Nearly all foods contain sodium naturally. Sodium is often added to foods during their processing and/or cooking. The food label usually indicates the addition of sodium to commercial food products. The following sodium compounds are frequently added to foods.[1]

- *Salt* (sodium chloride) — used in cooking or at the table and in canning and processing.
- *Monosodium glutamate* (called MSG, and sold under several brand names) — a seasoning used in home, restaurant and hotel cooking, and in many packaged, canned, and frozen foods.
- *Baking powder* — used to leaven quick breads and cakes.
- *Baking soda* (sodium bicarbonate) — used to leaven breads and cakes; sometimes added to vegetables in cooking or used as an "alkalizer" for indigestion.
- *Brine* (table salt and water) — used in processing foods to inhibit growth of bacteria; in cleaning or blanching vegetables and fruits; in freezing and canning certain foods; and for flavor, as in corned beef, pickles, and sauerkraut.

[1]"Your Mild Sodium-Restricted Diet." American Heart Association (New York, 1969), pp. 8-9

- *Di-sodium phosphate* — present in some quick-cooking cereals and processed cheeses.

- *Sodium alginate* — used in many chocolate milks and ice creams for smooth texture.

- *Sodium benzoate* — used as a preservative in many condiments, such as relishes, sauces, and salad dressings.

- *Sodium hydroxide* — used in food processing to soften and loosen skins of ripe olives, hominy, and certain fruits and vegetables.

- *Sodium propionate* — used in pasteurized cheeses and in some breads and cakes to inhibit growth of mold.

- *Sodium sulfite* — used to bleach certain fruits in which an artificial color is desired, such as maraschino cherries and glazed or crystallized fruit; also used as a preservative in some dried fruit, such as prunes.

Tap water also contains sodium. Since the amount varies in different communities, the local department of health or heart association should be consulted if this information is needed.

Some medicines contain sodium. A patient on a sodium restricted diet should always get his doctor's permission before using any medication.

SODIUM RESTRICTED DIETS

The sodium restricted diet is a regular diet in which the amount of sodium is limited. Foods that are relatively low in sodium are used. They are prepared and served without salt or with very little salt added because ordinary table salt is over 40 percent sodium. Foods that contain relatively large amounts of sodium are allowed in very limited quantities or omitted entirely. It is not possible to have

TABLE 29-1   Sodium Restricted Diet Lists

Lists 1 and 1A: Milk
List 2: Vegetables
List 3: Fruits
List 4: Bread
List 5: Meat
List 6: Fat
List 7: Free Choice

a diet totally free of salt since foods and water contain sodium.

The American Heart Association has devised three sodium restricted diets: (1) the mild sodium restricted diet, (2) the 1000 milligram sodium diet and (3) the 500 milligram sodium diet. In these diets, foods are divided into seven lists. Each list includes a specific group of foods as shown in table 29-1. The foods on each of these lists are listed as units, as are the foods allowed on the diabetic diet lists discussed in chapter 26. In any particular diet, a specified number of units is allowed from each list and arranged into personally planned menus. The units are carefully calculated so that each unit in any specific list has the same number of calories and the same amounts of carbohydrates, fats, and proteins as any other unit in that list. It is important that the patient use the exact number of units from each list on the diet that his physician prescribes.

Each of the low sodium diets planned by the American Heart Association is further subdivided into: the 1200-calorie diet, the 1800-calorie diet, and the unrestricted calorie diet. The doctor decides which one of these diets is best suited for the patient.

The Mild Sodium Restricted Diet

On the mild sodium restricted diet, the patient may use approximately half the salt previously used. Salt may not be added to canned or processed foods which have

TABLE 29-2   Sample Menu for the 1800-Calorie, Mild Sodium Restricted Diet

Breakfast	Lunch	Dinner
2 Medium Prunes with 2 tbsp. Juice	2 oz. Broiled Liver	Baked Casserole of Beef with Whipped Potato
3/4 cup Puffed Wheat	Baked Acorn Squash with 1 small pat Butter	Topping made with 3 oz. cooked Beef, 1/2 cup broth from Beef, 1/2 cup Potato
1 cup Milk	Cabbage Slaw with Caraway Seeds, Green Pepper and Vinegar	Green Beans
1 slice Toast	2 medium Muffins	Tomato and Cucumber Salad on Lettuce Leaf with 1 Tbsp. French Dressing*
1 small pat Butter	1 small pat Butter	2 medium Rolls
Coffee or Tea as desired	Apricot Bread Pudding made with 1 slice Bread, 1/4 cup Milk, 4 dried Apricot halves, 1 small pat Butter	1 small pat Butter*
	Coffee or Tea as desired	1/2 Grapefruit
		Coffee or Tea as desired
Mid-morning snack	**Mid-afternoon snack**	**Evening snack**
1/2 cup Milk	1 small Orange	1 small sliced Banana* with 1/4 cup Milk

*selected as free choice

already been salted during preparation. Baking soda may be used only in baking and not in cooking vegetables or relieving indigestion. Very salty foods such as pickles, olives, ham, canned soups, and meats should be avoided.

The sample menu in table 29-2 is taken from the booklet, "Your Mild Sodium-Restricted Diet," published by the American Heart Association (1969). Specific information regarding diet plans and food lists for other diets discussed in this chapter may be obtained by requesting the booklets, "Your Mild Sodium-Restricted Diet," "Your 1000 Milligram Sodium Diet," and "Your 500 Milligram Sodium Diet" from your local Heart Association. These booklets are the sources for the recommendations given in this chapter concerning sodium restricted diets.

The 1000 Milligram Sodium Diet

The patient on the 1000 milligram sodium diet may not consume more than 1000 milligrams of sodium daily. The diet is calculated so that half the sodium allowed is found in the foods selected and the other half (1/4 teaspoon) comes from the salt that the patient adds to food. It is important that the sodium content of the drinking water be included in the calculations for this diet.

Canned vegetables and vegetable juices must be low sodium dietetic. The American Heart Association suggests that the patient have an individual salt shaker and that 1/4 teaspoon of salt be measured into it each day.

Baked products must not include regular baking powder or baking soda (sodium bicarbonate). Appropriate substitutions are 1 1/2 teaspoons low sodium baking powder for 1 teaspoon regular baking powder and equal amounts of potassium bicarbonate for baking soda.

The 500 Milligram Sodium Diet

The 500 milligram sodium diet is the most restrictive of the three low sodium diets. In some cases, however, even this diet allows the patient too much sodium. If this is the case, the patient may be advised to follow a 250 milligram sodium diet. When the 250 milligram sodium diet is ordered, the American Heart Association advises using the 500 milligram diet but with the substitution of low sodium milk for regular milk.

Because of the relatively high sodium content of milk and meat, only two milk units and five meat units are allowed daily. Canned vegetables and vegetable juices must be low sodium dietetic. Baked products must not include common baking powder or baking soda. If tap water contains more than 5 milligrams sodium per 8-ounce cup, the patient must use distilled water for cooking and drinking.

ADJUSTMENT TO SODIUM RESTRICTION

Sodium restricted diets range from "different" to "tasteless" because most people are accustomed to salt in their food. It may be difficult to understand the necessity of following such a diet, particularly if it must be followed for the remainder of one's lifetime. Cheerfulness, tact, and understanding are essential in impressing the patient with the importance of the diet. For variety, there are numerous herbs, spices, and flavorings which are allowed on sodium restricted diets. Salt substitutes and low sodium dietetic foods are available. The patient must understand, however, that these should be used only with the approval of the physician.

SUMMARY

The sodium restricted diet is a regular diet in which the sodium content is restricted to a prescribed level. It is ordered for persons with medical problems which include *edema*, the accumulation of water in the tissues.

DISCUSSION TOPICS

1. Discuss the functions of sodium in the body.
2. Discuss the uses of the sodium restricted diet.
3. What is edema? In what kinds of conditions is it likely to occur?
4. Are the sodium restricted diets nutritious? Why or why not?
5. If a class member knows anyone who must follow a sodium restricted diet, discuss that person's initial reaction to this diet. Has this person become accustomed to it?
6. Why is it impossible to prepare a diet absolutely free of salt?
7. Why may a sodium restricted diet be unpleasant for a patient?
8. Why are potato chips and peanuts not allowed on sodium restricted diets?
9. Why is table salt restricted in sodium restricted diets?

SUGGESTED ACTIVITIES

a. Visit a local supermarket. List the foods containing sodium compounds. Suggest substitutes for these foods for patients on sodium restricted diets.

b. Find recipes suitable for sodium restricted diets and add them to the special diet recipe file.

c. List the foods eaten yesterday. Circle those that would not be allowed on the mild sodium restricted diet. Make appropriate substitutions for a patient on a mild sodium restricted diet.

d. Plan a day's menu for a patient on the unrestricted calorie, mild sodium restricted diet. Use Tables A-3 and A-4 in the Appendix.

e. Prepare and evaluate at least one of the meals on the menu and evaluate it in terms of nutritive content, flavor, aroma, color, shape, appearance, and satiety value.

WORD STUDY

monosodium glutamate   sodium   sodium bicarbonate

REVIEW

A.   Multiple-multiple Choice. Select the *letter* that precedes the best answer.

1. Sodium
    1. is an essential vitamin
    2. regulates the water balance in the body
    3. adds flavor to foods
    4. is found in table salt
        a) 1, 2, 3   b) 1, 3, 4   c) 2, 3, 4   d) all

2. Sodium is found in
    1. most foods   3. baking soda and baking powder
    2. water   4. brine
        a) 1, 2, 3   b) 2, 3, 4   c) 1, 3, 4   d) all

3. In the 1000 milligram and 500 milligram sodium diets,
    1. baked products containing baking powder and baking soda cannot be used
    2. canned vegetables and vegetable juices must be low sodium dietetic
    3. the amount of sodium in tap water must be considered
    4. only low sodium milk is allowed
        a) 1, 2   b) 3, 4   c) 2, 3, 4   d) 1, 2, 3

4. Herbs, spices, and flavorings may
    1. sometimes be used in sodium restricted diets
    2. never be used in sodium restricted diets
    3. be used with the permission of the physician
    4. be used only in the mild sodium restricted diet
        a) 1, 3   b) 2   c) 4   d) 3, 4

5. On the mild sodium restricted diet, the patient may
    1. use approximately 1/2 the salt previously used
    2. not add salt to processed food
    3. use baking soda in baked foods
    4. not have pickles and ham
        a) 1, 2, 3   b) 2, 3, 4   c) 1, 4   d) all

6. A sodium restricted diet may be ordered for patients with
    1. kidney disorders
    2. avitaminosis A
    3. pancreatitis
    4. cardiovascular disorders
        a) 1, 2, 3   b) 2, 4   c) 1, 4   d) all

7. When water accumulates in body tissues,
    1. the condition is called edema
    2. a sodium restricted diet may be prescribed
    3. it is a definite symptom of kidney disease
    4. salt is completely eliminated from the diet
        a) 1, 3   b) 2, 3, 4   c) 1, 2   d) all

8. Monosodium glutamate and table salt
    1. are not allowed in any sodium restricted diet
    2. both contain sodium
    3. are commonly used in food processing
    4. occur naturally in all foods
        a) 1, 3, 4   b) 2, 3   c) 3, 4   d) all

9. Table salt
    1. is 100 percent sodium
    2. is over 40 percent sodium
    3. contains only negligible amounts of sodium
    4. must be restricted in sodium restricted diets
        a) 1, 3, 4   b) 2, 3, 4   c) 2, 4   d) 2, 3

10. Foods that would be allowed in limited amounts on a sodium restricted diet are
    1. ham and bacon
    2. pickles and olives
    3. fresh fruits and vegetables
    4. milk and coffee
        a) 1, 3   b) 2, 3   c) 3, 4   d) 2,3

Chapter 30
Allergy Diets

OBJECTIVES

After studying this chapter, the student should be able to:

- Identify given allergens present in common foods.
- Plan a meal for a patient allergic to wheat.
- Adapt a menu to a wheat-free diet, an egg-free diet, and a milk-free diet.
- Prepare and evaluate a meal from one of the adapted menus.

An *allergy* is an altered reaction of the tissues of certain individuals who are exposed to substances which, in similar amounts, are harmless to other persons. The substances causing this *hypersensitivity* (abnormal adverse reactions) are called *allergens*. People may be allergic to various things such as pollen, dust, certain drugs, cosmetics, and foods. The discussion in this chapter will be limited to allergic reactions to foods.

Some of the typical symptoms of food allergies include "hay fever," asthma, gastrointestinal disturbances, *urticaria* (hives), and edema. Because allergies are uncomfortable and can be detrimental to health, they should be treated in order to relieve the symptoms. The simplest treatment is to remove the item that causes the allergic reaction. Finding the cause or causes of an allergy, however, is the most difficult part of treatment. This is because allergic reactions to the same food may differ in two individuals. For example, the fact that someone gets hives from eating strawberries does not mean that an allergic reaction to strawberries will appear as hives in another member of

the family. Allergic reactions may even differ from time to time with the same individual. Children frequently outgrow their sensitivities.

THE ELIMINATION DIET

Skin tests (application of a common allergen to a small area of skin) are frequently used to detect allergies. Because food allergies are rather difficult to determine from skin tests, elimination diets are often prescribed in order to find the food or foods that cause the allergic reaction. *Elimination diets* are diets composed of very few, specific foods which are not common allergens.

The elimination diet identifies specific foods as allergens by their individual and gradual addition to a basic diet composed of relatively nonallergenic foods. Doctors specializing in allergies have found that some of the most common food allergies are to milk, wheat, eggs, oranges, chocolate, fish, tomatoes, and strawberries. Diets are planned that eliminate these foods and include those which seldom cause trouble, such as rice, lamb, sugar, and canned pears.

TABLE 30-1   Elimination Diets

Diet 1	Diet 2	Diet 3	Diet 4
Rice	Corn	Tapioca	Milk†
Tapioca	Rye	White potato	Tapioca
Rice biscuit	Corn pone	Breads made of any	Cane
Rice bread	Corn-rye muffins	combination of	Sugar
	Rye bread	soy, Lima, potato	
	Ry-Krisp	starch and tapioca	
		flours	
Lettuce	Beets	Tomato	
Chard	Squash	Carrot	
Spinach	Asparagus	Lima beans	
Carrot	Artichoke	String beans	
Sweet potato		Peas	
or yam			
Lamb	Chicken (no hens)	Beef	
	Bacon	Bacon	
Lemon	Pineapple	Lemon	
Grapefruit	Peach	Grapefruit	
Pears	Apricot	Peach	
	Prune	Apricot	
Cane sugar	Cane or beet sugar	Cane sugar	
Sesame oil	Mazola	Sesame oil	
Olive oil*	Sesame oil	Soybean oil	
Salt	Salt	Gelatin, plain or	
Gelatin, plain or	Gelatin, plain or	flavored with	
flavored with	flavored with	lime or lemon	
lime or lemon	pineapple	Salt	
Maple syrup or	Karo corn syrup	Maple syrup or	
syrup made	White vinegar	syrup made	
with cane sugar	Royal baking	with cane sugar	
flavored with	powder	flavored with	
maple	Baking soda	maple	
Royal baking	Cream of tartar	Royal baking	
powder	Vanilla extract	powder	
Baking soda		Baking soda	
Cream of tartar		Cream of tartar	
Vanilla extract		Vanilla extract	
Lemon extract		Lemon extract	

*Allergy to it may occur with or without allergy to olive pollen. Mazola may be used if corn allergy is not present.

†Milk should be taken up to 2 or 3 quarts a day. Plain cottage cheese and cream may be used. Tapioca cooked with milk and milk sugar may be taken.

Source: Rowe, A. H. *Elimination Diets and the Patient's Allergies* ed. 2, Philadelphia: Lee & Febiger

Four elimination diets are given in table 30-1. The patient is kept on one of these diets for a week. If allergic reactions continue, another elimination diet is tried for a week, and so on. If the reactions continue even during the fourth diet, then it may be assumed that the allergy is due to something other than food and other treatment is sought.

When and if relief is found from the allergic symptoms while on one of the recommended diets, the patient is continued on it for a second week and then, very gradually, other foods are introduced to the diet. Those foods most likely to produce allergic reactions are added last until an allergic reaction occurs. The allergy can then be traced to one or two foods, and these can be eliminated from the diet. Knowing the cause of the allergy enables the patient to lead a healthy, normal life, provided that eliminating these foods does not affect his nutrition.

If the elimination of the allergen results in a diet deficient in certain nutrients, suitable substitutes for these nutrients must be found. For example, if a patient is allergic to citrus fruits, other foods rich in vitamin C to which the patient is not allergic must be found. If the allergy is to milk, soybean milk may be substituted. When the patient is allergic to foods for which it is extremely difficult to find substitutes, concentrated forms of their essential nutrients may be prescribed.

Sometimes, however, the allergies require such a restriction of foods that the diet does become nutritionally inadequate.

As in all cases of allergy, and particularly in such cases, it is hoped that the patient can become *desensitized* (made less sensitive) to the allergens so that a nutritionally balanced diet can be restored. To desensitize the patient, a minute amount of food allergen is given after a period of complete *abstinence* (avoidance) from it. The amount of the allergen is gradually increased until the patient can tolerate it.

The patient must be taught the food sources of the nutrient or nutrients lacking so that other foods may be substituted which are nutritionally equal to those causing the allergy. It is essential that the patient be taught to read the labels on commercially prepared foods and to check the ingredients of restaurant foods carefully. Baked products, mixes, meatloaf, or pancakes may contain egg, milk, or wheat which may be responsible for the allergic reaction.

SUMMARY

Elimination diets are used in the treatment of food allergies. Some of the most common food allergies are caused by milk, eggs, chocolate, wheat, oranges, fish, tomatoes, and strawberries. Diets must be planned which eliminate these foods and include only those which do not commonly cause allergies. Foods are gradually added to the diet until the allergic reaction occurs, thus indicating the cause of the allergy.

Allergy patients must be educated to make nutritionally adequate substitutes for those foods which must be eliminated from their diets.

DISCUSSION TOPICS

1. What are some common allergic reactions to food?

2. What is the most difficult part of treating food allergies?

3. Study the following menu and discuss how it might be adapted for a person with a sensitivity to milk.

Cream Soup	Baker's Bread
Roast Beef	Butter
Mashed Potatoes	Ice Cream
Buttered Peas	Black Coffee

4. Is an allergy diet always nutritious? Explain.

5. Explain how eggs, wheat, or milk may be hidden in each of the following foods: mayonnaise, bread, rye crackers, potato salad, gravy, meatloaf, breaded veal cutlet, bologna, malted milk.

SUGGESTED ACTIVITIES

a. Visit a local supermarket and look for the ingredients wheat, eggs, and milk, in frozen prepared meals, baked products and baking mixes.

b. Find recipes that are suitable for diets in which eggs, wheat, or milk must be eliminated. Add these recipes to the special diet recipe file.

c. Plan a luncheon for a patient who is allergic to wheat.

d. Ask a doctor or registered nurse to explain skin tests to the class. Discuss these tests after the lecture.

e. Write the menus of the meals eaten yesterday. Adapt one meal to a wheat-free diet. Adapt another to an egg-free diet. Adapt a third meal to a milk-free diet.

f. Prepare at least one of the adapted menus. Evaluate it, stressing its nutrient content.

WORD STUDY

abstinence	desensitize	skin test
allergen	elimination diet	urticaria
allergy	hypersensitivity	

REVIEW

A. Multiple Choice. Select the *letter* which precedes the best answer.

1. An adverse physical reaction to a food is called a food
   a. refusal
   b. allergy
   c. symptom
   d. allergen

2. Substances which cause altered physical reactions are called
   a. symptoms
   b. allergies
   c. allergens
   d. abstinence

3. One of the typical symptoms of food allergies is
   a. diabetes mellitus
   b. colitis
   c. hives
   d. atherosclerosis

4. The simplest treatment for a food allergy is
   a. a skin test
   b. the clear liquid diet
   c. elimination of the allergen
   d. the use of penicillin

5. In cases of food allergy, an elimination diet may be prescribed to
   a. desensitize the patient
   b. avoid medication
   c. avoid surgery
   d. find the allergen

6. Some foods which frequently cause an allergic reaction are
   a. milk, eggs, and wheat
   b. lamb, rice, and sugar
   c. canned pears and tapioca
   d. rice and pears

7. If a person is found to be allergic to milk,
   a. milk of any kind must be eliminated
   b. ordinary cheese may be substituted
   c. soy milk may be substituted
   d. dry milk may be substituted

8. The ultimate goal in treating food allergy is to
   a. find the allergen
   b. eliminate the allergen from the diet
   c. substitute another food for the allergen
   d. desensitize the patient

9. The person on an egg-free diet may not have
   a. cow's milk
   b. ordinary bakery cake
   c. fresh fruits
   d. olives

10. Foods which seldom cause food allergies are
    a. rice, canned pears, and lamb
    b. milk, eggs, and wheat
    c. chocolate, oranges, and tomatoes
    d. strawberries and fish

Chapter 31

Tube Feeding

OBJECTIVES

After studying this chapter, the student should be able to:

- Give three reasons why tube feedings may be necessary.
- State major points to consider in the feeding of patients by funnel or drip methods.
- List precautions to take for prevention of cramps and diarrhea.
- Describe how to test that the tube is in the stomach.

Patients are sometimes given tube feedings because of unconsciousness, accidents, surgery, strokes, severe malnutrition, extensive burns, emotional problems, or obstruction of the esophagus. These feedings are administered by a nasogastric tube through the nose or by a gastrostomy tube directly into the stomach through an abdominal incision. The nasogastric tube is inserted by a doctor or a registered nurse. The gastrostomy tube is inserted by the doctor during surgery. Patients who are tube fed require a great deal of patience and understanding. They have been deprived of a basic pleasure of life—eating. They may also be fearful and apprehensive about the tube itself.

Diets for tube feeding must be liquid in consistency and nutritionally adequate. Tube feedings are usually high in caloric value and often high in protein. Occasionally, a lactose-free feeding may be ordered. A food blender is very useful for converting some foods into liquid form. Baby foods may be used when diluted to liquid consistency. Feedings often need to be strained to remove any lumps that may have formed from poor blending or preparation.

Commercially prepared tube feedings are available. These are nutritionally adequate and convenient because the unopened cans do not require refrigeration and no further preparation is necessary.

The first feedings are small and usually given every hour. If the patient has difficulty in tolerating the feeding and regurgitates it, the person giving the feeding must be especially careful to prevent *aspiration* (breathing in) of the vomitus. First feedings are usually diluted to half strength with equal amounts of water in order to prevent diarrhea. Diarrhea causes the loss of essential nutrients and fluids thereby weakening the patient. Diarrhea can also occur when feedings are too cold, given too rapidly or in too concentrated a form, or are contaminated by bacteria. As the patient tolerates the feedings, they may be gradually increased to full strength, larger feedings, and with a longer time span between feedings.

Tube feedings are a good medium for bacterial growth. At best, tube feeding is a clean procedure and not an absolutely sterile technique. However, precautions must be taken to prevent contamination.

1. Keep the tube clamped off between feedings.

2. Keep the end of the tube covered with sterile gauze between feedings.

3. Cover opened cans with clean plastic covers.

4. Keep opened cans covered tightly and stored in the refrigerator.

5. Flush the tube with water after every feeding.

6. Wash and dry the equipment between feedings.

ADMINISTERING THE TUBE FEEDING

A demonstration of the tube feeding procedure is first given by the instructor. The student must carefully observe and study the procedure before attempting it. The prescribed feeding must first be double checked against the doctor's written order. It should be at room temperature before being administered. A feeding that is too cold may give the patient abdominal cramps or diarrhea.

There are two methods which may be used to administer nutrients to a patient who has had a nasogastric or gastrostomy tube inserted for tube feeding purposes. The funnel method (figure 31-2) or the drip method (figure (31-3) may be used.

The Funnel Method

Supplies should be put on a tray and taken to the bedside:
- A large Asepto syringe (the glass barrel may be used as a funnel)
- Prescribed feeding at room temperature
- 60 ml (2 oz) of lukewarm water (to flush tubing)
- Glass of water (for checking position of tube)
- Sterile 2″ x 2″ gauze sponge
- Rubber band
- Emesis basin

The procedure should be described to the patient beforehand in order to reduce anxiety. Anyone who has a nasogastric tube inserted may be especially afraid of choking. If the patient has a nasogastric tube in place, he should be helped into a semi-Fowler's position. In this position, the patient lies on his back with the head and shoulders elevated to a 45° angle; the knees are slightly flexed and the heels are resting on the bed. This position helps the feeding to flow to the stomach using the force of gravity. If the patient has a gastrostomy tube in place, the head of the bed should be raised to a semi-Fowler's position *only if the patient's condition permits it.* If the patient's condition does not permit a semi-sitting position, the feeding may be given while the patient is lying flat with his head on a pillow.

The doctor may order that the gastrostomy tube be aspirated before the feeding is given. This is done in order to determine if the preceding feeding has passed into the small intestine. If the preceding feeding has not passed into the small intestine, the current feeding may need to be withheld. The doctor's order would indicate how to determine if a feeding is to be withheld.

It is essential that the nurse check to see that the tube is in the stomach before a tube feeding is given. (If the tube is in the lungs or trachea, the patient can aspirate the feeding causing choking, pneumonia, or death.) To check, the clamp on the tube should be opened or removed before testing:

- The open end of the tube should be placed in a glass of water, figure 31-1. If there is bubbling each time the patient breathes, the tube may be in the lungs. If this occurs, the feeding must not be

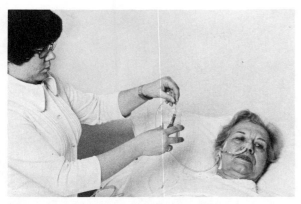

Fig. 31-1 Check to be sure the tube is in the patient's stomach by placing the end of the tube in a glass of water. No bubbles should appear if the tube is in the stomach.

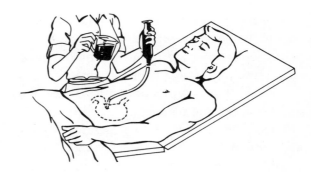

Fig. 31-2 The funnel method may be used to tube feed patients who have a gastrostomy tube or a nasogastric tube. The principles of nursing care are the same. This illustration shows tube feeding through a gastrostomy tube.

given and the doctor or the nurse in charge must be notified. If no bubbles can be seen in the water, the tube is probably in the stomach.

• Another way to check if the tube is in the stomach is to aspirate the tube with a syringe to check for gastric content; an Asepto syringe may be used to gently suck out some of the stomach contents. The rubber bulb should be squeezed *before* it is inserted in the glass part of the Asepto syringe. If a greenish yellow fluid returns, the tube is in the stomach.

The funnel must be attached to the tubing. The tubing must be pinched off or clamped while the funnel is attached. This prevents excess air from entering the stomach. Excess air in the stomach causes gas pains and abdominal distention. Thirty milliliters (1 oz) of warm water should be poured into the funnel before the feeding. The water should be allowed to run in by gravity and not forced. If the water flows through the tube, it indicates the tube is open and the feeding may proceed. If the water does not run in, the nurse in charge should check the tube.

The prescribed feeding should be poured into the funnel and given in an unhurried

manner. More of the solution should be added before the funnel has emptied. This prevents air from entering the stomach. When a feeding is given through a gastrostomy tube, the funnel should be held about two to three inches above the abdomen. The rate of the feeding can be controlled by raising or lowering the funnel, or by slightly pinching the tubing. A typical feeding takes about 20 minutes. An emesis basin should be available in case the patient regurgitates the feeding.

The patient should be carefully observed for signs of distress. **CAUTION:** If the patient with a nasogastric tube is coughing, choking, or becoming *cyanotic* (turning blue), he may be aspirating the fluid because the tube has become displaced. In such a case, the feeding must be stopped immediately and the nurse in charge notified.

After the feeding has been completed, about 30 ml (1 oz) of water should be poured into the tube in order to clear the tubing and prevent it from clogging. The tubing must be clamped just before the funnel empties. This prevents the feeding solution and gastric juices from escaping. After the funnel has been removed, the end of the tube should be covered with a sterile 2 x 2 inch gauze sponge and secured with a rubber band. This prevents bacteria from entering the tube.

The time, type, amount of feeding, and how well the patient tolerated it must be charted. Charting must be accurate, prompt, and complete. If an Intake and Output record is being kept for the patient, record the time, amount, and type of feeding on it also.

The patient's condition should be carefully monitored. A feeling of fullness or nausea after a meal may indicate that the patient is being fed too often or is receiving too much at each feeding. If the patient feels this way, the nurse in charge should be notified as the order for feeding may need to be changed.

The patient should rest for about 20 minutes after the feeding. He may remain in the semi-Fowler's position or he can be turned on the right side with his head elevated. An elevated position and relaxation aids digestion.

The Drip Method

The drip method of tube feeding is often used when the patient has an ulcer of the digestive tract, figure 31-3. Milk and *antacids* (agents which neutralize acidity) are usually the prescribed feedings. They are given by the drip method 24 hours a day in order to neutralize the gastric juices and allow the ulcer to heal. In order to prevent souring of the milk and to help reduce the chance of contamination by bacteria, only a small amount of feeding is placed in the bag at one time. It is important to check the setup often to make sure the fluid is flowing properly.

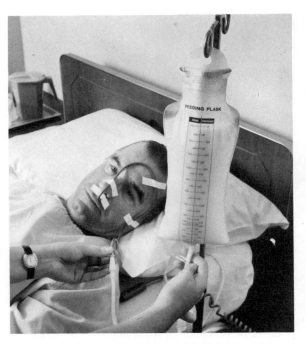

Fig. 31-3 Continuous drip feeding

Supplies should be collected and taken to the patient's bedside:

- Continuous drip feeding set with attached tubing
- IV stand
- Prescribed feeding at room temperature

The procedure should be clearly described to the patient before it is begun. The continuous drip set with the attached tubing should be hung on the IV stand. The tubing on the drip set must be clamped. The plastic bag with the prescribed solution should be filled. The tubing must be unclamped to allow the solution to run through and expel the air which could cause uncomfortable gas pains for the patient. Then the tubing on the drip set must be reclamped.

The gastric tube should be temporarily unclamped to check if the tube is still in the patient's stomach. The drip set tubing must be attached to the gastric tube and the drip regulated according to the doctor's order. The drip set tubing is then unclamped and the procedure charted. This must be checked frequently to be sure the fluid is flowing properly. The tubing and bag should be changed at least every 8 hours. This is necessary in order to prevent the growth of bacteria.

DISCUSSION TOPICS

1. What is a nasogastric tube? A gastrostomy tube? When are they used?
2. Discuss the preparation, nutritional content, and consistency of tube feedings according to the procedures of the affiliated hospital.
3. Why is the positive attitude of the nurse so important for patients on tube feedings?
4. Why is it important to prevent diarrhea? What precautions should be taken?

SUGGESTED ACTIVITIES

a. Observe a demonstration of preparing food for a tube feeding by using an electric blender.
b. Observe a demonstration of the procedure for a tube feeding.
c. Practice setting up the necessary supplies and equipment for a tube feeding.

WORD STUDY

abdominal	esophagus	nasogastric tube
antacid	Fowler's position	semi-Fowler's position
cyanotic	gastric tube	

REVIEW

A. Multiple-multiple Choice. Select the *letter* which precedes the best answer.
1. Patients must occasionally be fed by tube because of
   1. accidents
   2. childbirth
   3. surgery
   4. unconsciousness
      a) 1, 2, 4   b) 1, 2, 3   c) 1, 3, 4   d) all

2. Tube feedings *must* be
   1. colorful
   2. nutritionally balanced meals
   3. liquid
   4. smooth
      a) 1, 2, 4   b) 1, 3, 4   c) 2, 3, 4   d) all

3. For tube feedings, one may use
   1. commercially prepared liquid diets
   2. baby foods
   3. regular diets blended to a liquid consistency
   4. high calorie diets blended to a liquid consistency
      a) 1, 2, 3   b) 2, 3, 4   c) 1, 3, 4   d) all

4. To prevent diarrhea during tube feedings, one should
   1. add iron to the feeding
   2. give feeding very slowly
   3. give feeding very quickly
   4. give feeding at room temperature
      a) 1, 3   b) 2, 4   c) 3   d) all

5. The first tube feedings are usually
   1. small   3. diluted to half strength
   2. given hourly   4. given slowly
      a) 1, 3   b) 2, 4   c) 1, 3, 4   d) all

B. Briefly answer the following questions.

1. What are the advantages of commercially prepared tube feedings?

2. List five precautions to take to avoid contamination of tube feedings.

3. Name two ways of checking that the tube is in the stomach.

4. Name two methods for administering tube feedings.

SECTION EVALUATION 5: SPECIAL DIETS

A.   Complete the following statements.

1.   The treatment of disease through diet is called _____ .

2.   Special diets are prescribed by the _____ .

3.   Hospital diets are planned by the _____ .

4.   The regular hospital diet is comparable to a _____ diet.

5.   The diet which does not nourish and consists only of clear liquids is the _____ diet.

6.   The caloric value of the full liquid diet may be increased by adding _____ .

7.   The protein value of the full liquid diet may be increased by adding _____ .

8.   The light diet is also called the _____ diet.

9.   The diet that normally succeeds the full liquid diet and that contains semisolid foods is the _____ diet.

10.   The diet consisting of only soft-textured and mild-flavored foods is the _____ diet.

11.   Food allergens may be identified by the _____ diet.

12.   The restricted residue diet consists of foods that leave little _____ .

13.   The diet calling for an increase in energy foods is the _____ diet.

14.   The condition resulting from an overactive thyroid gland is known as _____ .

15.   When a patient is overweight, the doctor may prescribe a _____ diet.

B.   Match the items in column I with the appropriate statement in column II

Column I	Column II
_____ 1. regular diet	a. for treatment of allergies
_____ 2. clear liquid diet	b. for overweight patients
_____ 3. bland diet	c. hospital "normal" diet
_____ 4. soft diet	d. consists only of mild and soothing foods
_____ 5. light diet	e. includes mainly polyunsaturated fats
_____ 6. high calorie diet	f. postoperative liquid diet that does not nourish
_____ 7. low calorie diet	
_____ 8. low cholesterol diet	g. consists of liquids and soft, easily digested foods
_____ 9. sodium restricted diet	h. for reducing edema
	i. convalescent diet
_____ 10. elimination diets	j. for underweight patients

C.   Multiple-multiple Choice.   Select the *letter* which precedes the best answer.

1. The clear liquid diet is
    1. only a modification in consistency
    2. a modification in consistency and nutritive value
    3. composed mainly of water and carbohydrates
    4. nutritionally inadequate
        a) 2, 3   b) 1, 3, 4   c) 2, 3, 4   d) all

2. The full liquid diet
    1. supplies minimal nourishment
    2. includes food that is liquid at body temperature
    3. is sometimes given patients who have difficulty chewing
    4. is sometimes used in place of the high protein diet
        a) 1, 2, 3   b) 2, 3, 4   c) 1, 3, 4   d) all

3. The soft diet
    1. includes low residue foods
    2. includes foods that are easily digested
    3. is one of the routine hospital diets
    4. is nutritionally adequate
        a) 1, 2, 3   b) 1, 3, 4   c) 2, 3, 4   d) all

4. The light diet
    1. is also known as the "convalescent diet"
    2. is essential in every hospital's diet plans
    3. contains foods that are easily digested
    4. contains citrus fruits
        a) 1, 2, 4   b) 1, 2   c) 1, 3, 4   d) all

5. The bland diet
    1. includes no fruits of any kind
    2. includes pureed fruits
    3. is intended to avoid any irritation to the digestive tract
    4. is nutritionally adequate
        a) 1, 3   b) 2, 3, 4   c) 1, 3, 4   d) 1

6. The restricted residue diet
    1. consists of foods which leave very little residue in the intestines
    2. is typically low in vitamin content
    3. restricts milk to 2 cups daily
    4. does not include coarse cereals
        a) 1, 2, 3   b) 1, 3, 4   c) 2, 3, 4   d) all

7. The minimum residue diet
    1. is another name for the bland diet
    2. may be nutritionally inadequate
    3. sometimes includes boiled or evaporated milk
    4. always contains regular, homogenized milk
        a) 1, 2, 3   b) 1, 2, 4   c) 2, 3   d) all

8. The low calorie diet
   1. is typically used in cases of diarrhea
   2. is a regular diet with reduced caloric value
   3. is nutritionally adequate
   4. always includes concentrated foods
      a) 1, 2, 3   b) 1, 2   c) 2, 3   d) all

9. Sodium restricted diets may be ordered for patients with
   1. kidney disorders
   2. cardiovascular disorders
   3. colitis
   4. diabetes mellitus
      a) 1, 2, 3   b) 1, 2   c) 3, 4   d) all

10. A high protein diet may be prescribed for
    1. patients following surgery
    2. children
    3. pregnant women
    4. illnesses resulting in a protein loss
       a) 1   b) 1, 2   c) 3, 4   d) all

APPENDIX

Table A-1 Recommended Daily Dietary Allowances. 236
Table A-2 Desirable Weights for Men and Women 25 and Over. 238
Table A-3 Mild Sodium-Restricted Diet Plans 239
Table A-4 Food Lists for the Mild Sodium-Restricted Diet 240
Table A-5 Temperature Conversions from Fahrenheit to Celsius. 248
Table A-6 Nutritive Values of the Edible Part of Foods. 249

TABLE A-1 Recommended Daily Dietary Allowances[a]

AGE (years)	WEIGHT (kg)	(lbs)	HEIGHT (cm)	(in)	ENERGY kcal[b]	PROTEIN (g)	FAT-SOLUBLE VITAMINS Vit. A Activity (I.U.)	Vitamin D (I.U.)	Vit. E Activity (I.U.)
INFANTS									
0.0-0.5	6	14	60	24	kg x 117	kg x 2.2	1,400	400	4
0.5-1.0	9	20	71	28	kg x 108	kg x 2.0	2,000	400	5
CHILDREN									
1-3	13	28	86	34	1,300	23	2,000	400	7
4-6	20	44	110	44	1,800	30	2,500	400	9
7-10	30	66	135	54	2,400	36	3,300	400	10
MALES									
11-14	44	97	158	63	2,800	44	5,000	400	12
15-18	61	134	172	69	3,000	54	5,000	400	15
19-22	67	147	172	69	3,000	54	5,000	400	15
23-50	70	154	172	69	2,700	56	5,000		15
51+	70	154	172	69	2,400	56	5,000		15
FEMALES									
11-14	44	97	155	62	2,400	44	4,000	400	12
15-18	54	119	162	65	2,100	48	4,000	400	12
19-22	58	128	162	65	2,100	46	4,000	400	12
23-50	58	128	162	65	2,000	46	4,000		12
51+	58	128	162	65	1,800	46	4,000		12
PREGNANCY					+300	+30	5,000	400	15
LACTATION					+500	+20	6,000	400	15

[a] The allowance levels are intended to cover individual variations among most normal persons as they live in the United States under usual environmental stresses. The recommended allowances can be attained with a variety of common foods. Such a variety also provides other nutrients for which human requirements have been less well defined.

[b] Kilojoules (kJ) = 4.2 x kcal

TABLE A-1 (continued)

WATER-SOLUBLE VITAMINS							MINERALS					
Ascorbic Acid (mg)	Niacin[c] (mg)	Folacin[d] (μg)	Ribo-flavin (mg)	Thiamine (mg)	Vitamin B_6 (mg)	Vitamin B_{12} (μg)	Calcium (mg)	Phos-phorus (mg)	Iodine (μg)	Iron (mg)	Magnesium (mg)	Zinc (mg)
35	5	50	0.4	0.3	0.3	0.3	360	240	35	10	60	3
35	8	50	0.6	0.5	0.4	0.3	540	400	45	15	70	5
40	9	100	0.8	0.7	0.6	1.0	800	800	60	15	150	10
40	12	200	1.1	0.9	0.9	1.5	800	800	80	10	200	10
40	16	300	1.2	1.2	1.2	2.0	800	800	110	10	250	10
45	18	400	1.5	1.4	1.6	3.0	1,200	1,200	130	18	350	15
45	20	400	1.8	1.5	2.0	3.0	1,200	1,200	150	18	400	15
45	20	400	1.8	1.5	2.0	3.0	800	800	140	10	350	15
45	18	400	1.6	1.4	2.0	3.0	800	800	130	10	350	15
45	16	400	1.5	1.2	2.0	3.0	800	800	110	10	350	15
45	16	400	1.3	1.2	1.6	3.0	1,200	1,200	115	18	300	15
45	14	400	1.4	1.1	2.0	3.0	1,200	1,200	115	18	300	15
45	14	400	1.4	1.1	2.0	3.0	800	800	100	18	300	15
45	13	400	1.2	1.0	2.0	3.0	800	800	100	18	300	15
45	12	400	1.1	1.0	2.0	3.0	800	800	80	10	300	15
60	+2	800	+0.3	+0.3	2.5	4.0	1,200	1,200	125	18+[e]	450	20
80	+4	600	+0.5	+0.3	2.5	4.0	1,200	1,200	150	18	450	25

[c]Although allowances are expressed as niacin, it is recognized that on the average 1 mg of niacin is derived from each 60 mg of dietary tryptophan.

[d]The folacin allowances refer to dietary sources as determined by Lactobacillus casei assay. Pure forms of folacin may be effective in doses less than 1/4 of the RDA.

[e]This increased requirement cannot be met by ordinary diets; therefore, the use of supplemental iron is recommended.

Source: Food and Nutrition Board, the National Academy of Sciences-National Research Council (1974)

Table A-2   Desirable Weights for Men and Women Twenty-Five and Over (Weight in Pounds According to Frame in Indoor Clothing)

MEN

Height (with shoes on) 1-inch heels Feet	Inches	Small Frame	Medium Frame	Large Frame
5	2	112–120	118–129	126–141
5	3	115–123	121–133	129–144
5	4	118–126	124–136	132–148
5	5	121–129	127–139	135–152
5	6	124–133	130–143	138–156
5	7	128–137	134–147	142–161
5	8	132–141	138–152	147–166
5	9	136–145	142–156	151–170
5	10	140–150	146–160	155–174
5	11	144–154	150–165	159–179
6	0	148–158	154–170	164–184
6	1	152–162	158–175	168–189
6	2	156–167	162–180	173–194
6	3	160–171	167–185	178–199
6	4	164–175	172–190	182–204

WOMEN

Height (with shoes on) 2-inch heels Feet	Inches	Small Frame	Medium Frame	Large Frame
4	10	92–98	96–107	104–119
4	11	94–101	98–110	106–122
5	0	96–104	101–113	109–125
5	1	99–107	104–116	112–128
5	2	102–110	107–119	115–131
5	3	105–113	110–122	118–134
5	4	108–116	113–126	121–138
5	5	111–119	116–130	125–142
5	6	114–123	120–135	129–146
5	7	118–127	124–139	133–150
5	8	122–131	128–143	137–154
5	9	126–135	132–147	141–158
5	10	130–140	136–151	145–163
5	11	134–144	140–155	149–168
6	0	138–148	144–159	153–173

(For girls between 18 and 25, subtract 1 pound for each year under 25.)

Source: Metropolitan Life Insurance Company

TABLE A-3   Mild Sodium-Restricted Diet Plans (Based on Daily Number of Calories Allowed)

Food List	1200-Calorie Diet	1800-Calorie Diet	Unrestricted-Calorie Diet
1	Not applicable	2	2 or more
1A	2	Not applicable	Not applicable
2	At least one each from groups A, B, C	At least one each from groups A, B, C	At least one each from groups A, B, C
3	4	4	2 or more
4	5	7	4 or more
5	5	5	5 or more
6	None	4	As desired
7	1	2	As desired

Source: Adapted from "Your Mild Sodium-Restricted Diet" (Revised), American Heart Association

TABLE A-4 Food Lists for the Mild Sodium-Restricted Diet*

LIST 1: MILK

Note: Each unit contains about 170 calories, 8 grams protein, 10 grams fat, and 12 grams carbohydrate. Two units from List 5, Meat, may be substituted for not more than one milk unit a day, or 6 ounces of plain yogurt (3/4 cup)

CAUTION: Do not use any commercial foods made of milk such as ice cream, sherbet, milkshakes, chocolate milk, malted milk, milk mixes, and condensed milk.

Evaporated whole milk, reconstituted	1 cup
Nonfat buttermilk.	2 fat units and 1 cup
Nonfat dry milk, powdered	2 fat units and 3 tablespoons (Use amount specified on package for making one cup of milk.)
Nonfat dry milk, reconstituted or skim milk	2 fat units and 1 cup
Whole milk.	1 cup
Whole milk buttermilk	1 cup

LIST 1A: MILK FOR 1200-CALORIE DIET PLAN

Note: Each unit contains about 85 calories, 8 grams protein, negligible fat, and 12 grams carbohydrate. One unit from List 5, Meat may be substituted for not more than one milk unit a day.

Caution: When milk is used in cooking be sure to count it as part of the day's allowance. Do not use whole milk or any commercial foods made of milk such as ice cream, sherbet, milkshakes, chocolate milk, malted milk, milk mixes, and condensed milk.

Evaporated skim milk, reconstituted	1 cup
Nonfat buttermilk.	1 cup
Nonfat dry milk, powdered	3 tablespoons (Use amount specified on package for making one cup of milk.)
Nonfat dry milk, reconstituted or skim milk	1 cup

*It is important to keep in touch with your physician while on any sodium-restricted diet.

TABLE A-4 (continued)

LIST 2: VEGETABLES

Use fresh, frozen, or canned. Frozen peas and lima beans usually contain a small amount of salt, and often this is enough to season them adequately for the mild sodium-restricted diet. Do not use sauerkraut, pickles, or other vegetables prepared with brine or salted.

Group A

Note: Each unit contains negligible calories, protein, fat and carbohydrate. Each unit is a 1/2-cup serving.

Artichoke	Cucumber	Okra
Asparagus	Dandelion greens	Peppers, green or red
Beet greens	Eggplant	Radishes
Broccoli	Endive	Spinach
Brussels sprouts	Escarole	Squash, summer (yellow, zucchini)
Cabbage	Green beans	Tomato juice
Cauliflower	Kale	Tomatoes
Celery	Lettuce	Turnip greens
Chard, Swiss	Mushrooms	Wax beans
Chicory	Mustard greens	

Group B

Note: Each unit contains about 35 calories, 2 grams protein, negligible fat, and 7 grams carbohydrate. Each unit is a 1/2-cup serving. Two units from Group A may be substituted for one unit from Group B.

Beets	Peas	Squash, winter (acorn, Hubbard)
Carrots	Pumpkin	Turnip, white
Onions	Rutabaga (yellow turnip)	

Group C

Note: Each unit contains about 70 calories, 2 grams protein, negligible fat, and 15 grams carbohydrate. One unit from List 4, Breads, Cereals, and Cereal Products, may be substituted for one unit from Group C.

Beans, lima or navy, fresh, frozen, or dried....	1/2 cup, cooked	Parsnips.............	2/3 cup
Beans, baked (no pork)...	1/4 cup	Peas, dried (split green or yellow, cowpeas).......	1/2 cup, cooked
Corn................	1/3 cup or 1/2 small ear	Potato, white.........	1 small
Hominy.............	1/2 cup	Potatoes, mashed.......	1/2 cup
Lentils, dried	1/2 cup, cooked	Sweet potato	1/4 cup, or 1/2 small

TABLE A-4   (continued)

LIST 3: FRUIT

Use frozen, fresh, canned, or dried. Fresh lemons and limes and their juice, unsweetened cranberries and cranberry juice, and unsweetened rhubarb may be used as desired.

Note: Each unit contains about 40 calories, negligible protein and fat, and 10 grams carbohydrate.

CAUTION: If following the 1200- or 1800-calorie diet plan do not use crystallized or glazed fruit, sweetened fruit, or fruit canned or frozen in sugar syrup.

Apple	1 small	Grape juice	1/4 cup
Apple juice or apple cider	1/3 cup	Honeydew melon	1/8 medium
Applesauce	1/2 cup	Mango	1/2 small
Apricots, dried	4 halves	Orange	1 small
Apricots, fresh	2 medium	Orange juice	1/2 cup
Apricot nectar	1/4 cup	Papaya	1/3 medium
Banana	1/2 small	Peach	1 medium
Blackberries	1 cup	Pear	1 small
Blueberries	2/3 cup	Pineapple	1/2 cup diced or 2
Cantaloupe	1/4 small		small slices
Cherries	10 large	Pineapple juice	1/3 cup
Cranberries, sweetened	1 tablespoon	Plums	2 medium
Cranberry juice,		Prunes	2 medium
sweetened	1/3 cup	Prune juice	1/4 cup
Dates	2	Raisins	2 tablespoons
Fig	1 medium	Raspberries	1 cup
Fruit cup or mixed fruits	1/2 cup	Rhubarb, sweetened	2 tablespoons
Grapefruit	1/2 small	Strawberries	1 cup
Grapefruit juice	1/2 cup	Tangerine	1 large
Grapes	12	Tangerine juice	1/2 cup
		Watermelon	1 cup

LIST 4: BREADS, CEREALS, AND CEREAL PRODUCTS

Note: Each unit contains about 70 calories, 2 grams protein, negligible fat, and 15 grams carbohydrates. One unit from List 2, Vegetables, Group C, may be substituted for one bread unit.

CAUTION: Do not use breads and rolls with salt toppings, potato chips, pretzels, regular salted popcorn, and other heavily salted snack foods. If following the 1200- or 1800-calorie diet plan, do not use sugar-coated cereals.

Breads and Rolls

Bread	1 slice
Melba toast	4 pieces (3 1/2" x 1 1/2" x 1/8")
Roll	1 medium
Biscuit	1 medium
Cornbread	1 cube (1 1/2")
Griddle cakes	two 3-inch
Muffin	1 medium

Cooked Cereals, Lightly Salted: Each unit is a 1/2-cup serving.

Farina	Rolled wheat
Grits	Wheat meal
Oatmeal	

Dry Cereals

Shredded wheat	2/3 biscuit
Other dry cereal	3/4 cup

Cereal Products

Barley	1 1/2 tablespoons, uncooked
Cornmeal	2 tablespoons
Cornstarch	2 1/2 tablespoons
Crackers, preferably with unsalted tops	five 2-inch square
Flour	2 1/2 tablespoons
Graham crackers	2
Macaroni	1/2 cup cooked
Matzo	one 5-inch square
Noodles	1/2 cup, cooked
Popcorn, lightly salted	1 1/2 cups
Rice, brown or white	1/2 cup, cooked
Spaghetti	1/2 cup, cooked
Tapioca	2 tablespoons, uncooked
Waffle	one 3-inch square section

TABLE A-4   (continued)

LIST 5:   MEAT, POULTRY, FISH, EGGS, CHEESE, AND LOW-SODIUM PEANUT BUTTER

Note: Units allowed per day average about 75 calories, 7 grams protein, 5 grams fat, and negligible carbohydrate.

Meat or Poultry, Fresh, Frozen, or Canned

CAUTION: Do not use salty or smoked meat such as bacon, bologna, chipped or corned beef, frankfurters, ham, meats koshered by salting, luncheon meats, salt pork, sausage, and smoked tongue.

One ounce, cooked, of any of the following is one unit.

Beef	Pork
Brain	Quail
Chicken	Rabbit
Duck	Tongue
Kidney	Turkey
Lamb	Veal
Liver (beef, calf, chicken, pork)	

Fish or Fish Fillets (Fresh, Frozen, or Canned)

CAUTION: Do not use salty or smoked fish such as anchovies, caviar, salted and dried cod, herring, and sardines.

One ounce, cooked, of any of the following is one unit.

Bass	Clams	Eels	Lobster	Salmon	Sole
Bluefish	Cod	Flounder	Oyster	Scallops	Trout
Catfish	Crab	Halibut	Rockfish	Shrimp	Tuna

Eggs, Cheese, and Peanut Butter

CAUTION: Do not use processed cheese or cheese spreads unless they are low-sodium dietetic. Do not use any cheese such as Roquefort, Camembert, or Gorgonzola.

American cheddar or Swiss cheese	1 ounce
Cottage cheese (lightly salted)	1/4 cup
Egg	1
Low-sodium dietetic peanut butter	2 tablespoons

LIST 6: FAT

Note: Each unit contains about 45 calories and 5 grams fat.

CAUTION: Do not use salted nuts, olives, bacon and bacon fat, salt pork, and heavily salted snack foods such as potato chips and sticks, and crackers.

Avocado	1/8 of 4-inch fruit
Butter	1 teaspoon (1 small pat)
Cream, heavy (sweet or sour)	1 tablespoon
Cream, light (sweet or sour)	2 tablespoons
Fat or oil for cooking	1 teaspoon
French dressing	1 tablespoon
Margarine	1 teaspoon
Mayonnaise	1 teaspoon
Nuts, unsalted	6 small

LIST 7: FREE CHOICE

Note: Each free choice unit contains about 75 calories. One free choice unit daily is allowed on the 1200-calorie diet, and two free choice units daily are allowed on the 1800-calorie diet. If calories are not restricted, patient may have as many free choice units as desired. The free choice unit may be divided. For example, the patient may have one unit from the fruit list and two teaspoons of sugar as the free choice unit.

List 6, fat	2 units
List 3, fruit	2 units
Sugar, white or brown	4 teaspoons
Syrup, honey, jelly, jam, or marmalade	4 teaspoons
List 2, vegetables, Group C	1 unit
List 4, Breads	1 unit
*Candy made without salted nuts	75 calories

*The following amounts of candy furnish approximately 75 calories:

1 piece (1″ x 1″ x 3/4″) fondant or fudge 24 pieces to a pound)
2 large, or 16 small, gum drops (2/3 ounce)
4 pieces (1″ x 1″ x 1/2″), or 7 - 8 pieces, hard candy (2/3 ounce)
3 marshmallows (2/3 ounce)
10 jelly beans (1 ounce)

TABLE A-4 (continued)

SEASONINGS: FLAVORING EXTRACTS; HERBS, SPICES, AND AROMATIC SEEDS

The following seasonings may be used:

Allspice	Mint
Almond extract	Mustard, dry, or mustard seed
Anise seed	Nutmeg
Basil	Onion, onion juice, or onion powder
Bay leaf	Orange extract
Bouillon cube, low-sodium dietetic	Oregano
Caraway seed	Paprika
Cardamom	Parsley or parsley flakes
Catsup, dietetic	Pepper, fresh green or red
Celery leaves, dried or fresh	Pepper, black, red, or white
Celery seed	Peppermint extract
Chili powder	Pimiento peppers
Chives	Poppy seed
Cinnamon	Poultry seasoning
Cloves	Purslane
Cocoa	Rosemary
Coconut	Saffron
Cumin	Sage
Curry	Salt, used lightly in cooking
Dill	Salt substitutes, if recommended by the physician
Fennel	Savory
Garlic, garlic juice, or garlic powder	Sesame seeds
Ginger	Sorrel
Horseradish	Sugar
Juniper	Tarragon
Lemon juice or extract	Thyme
Mace	Turmeric
Maple extract	Vanilla extract
Marjoram	Vinegar
Meat extract, low-sodium dietetic	Wine, if allowed
Meat tenderizers, low-sodium dietetic	Walnut extract

The following may not be used:

Artificial sweeteners unless recommended by the physician	Mustard, prepared
	Olives
Commercial bouillon in any form	Onion salt, except when used as allowed seasoning
Catsup	Pickles
Celery salt, except when used as allowed seasoning	Relishes
	Salt substitutes unless recommended by the physician
Chili sauce	
Garlic salt except when used as allowed seasoning	Saccharin, unless recommended by the physician
Meat extracts, sauces, and tenderizers if not low-sodium dietetic	Cooking wine (salt has been added)
	Worcestershire sauce

TABLE A-4 (continued)

MISCELLANEOUS FOODS

The following may be used:
Beverages

Alcoholic beverages, if allowed by the physician
Cocoa made with milk from diet
Coffee, instant or regular
Coffee substitute
Fruit juices (must be counted as fruit units)
Lemonade, using sugar allowance from diet
Milk as allowed on Milk List 1 or 1A
Tea

Candy

If calories are restricted, candy may be used as a 75-calorie free choice

Cornstarch

Gelatin

Leavening Agents

Baking powder
Baking soda (for baking only)
Cream of tartar
Potassium bicarbonate
Yeast

Rennet Tablets

Use milk and sugar from the day's allowance

Tapioca

For thickening fruit, or milk tapioca pudding (Be sure to count the tapioca, fruit, milk, and egg from the day's allowance.)

The following may be used unless the patient is on the 1200- or 1800-calorie diet plan:

Baking chocolate
Instant cocoa mixes
Prepared beverage mixes, including fruit-flavored powders
Malted milk and other milk preparations
Fountain beverages
Sugar-sweetened carbonated beverages
Candies, except as free choice
Sugar-sweetened gelatin desserts
Prepared pudding mixes, including rennet powder desserts
Molasses, honey, syrups

Source: "Your Mild Sodium-Restricted Diet (revised)," American Heart Association

Table A-5 Temperature Conversions from Fahrenheit to Celsius

°F	°C	°F	°C	°F	°C	°F	°C
70	21.1	117	47.2	160	71.1	197.6	92
71	21.7	118	47.8	161	71.7	198	92.2
72	22.2	119	48.3	161.6	72	199	92.8
73	22.8	120	48.9	162	72.2	199.4	93
74	23.3	121	49.4	163	72.8	200	93.3
75	23.9	122	50	163.4	73	201	93.9
76	24.4	123	50.6	164	73.3	201.2	94
77	25	124	51.1	165	73.9	202	94.4
78	25.6	125	51.7	165.2	74	203	95
79	26.1	126	52.2	166	74.4	204	95.6
80	26.7	127	52.8	167	75	204.8	96
81	27.2	128	53.3	168	75.6	205	96.1
82	27.8	129	53.9	168.8	76	206	96.7
83	28.3	129.2	54	169	76.1	206.6	97
84	28.9	130	54.4	170	76.7	207	97.2
85	29.4	131	55	170.6	77	208	97.8
86	30	132	55.6	171	77.2	208.4	98
87	30.6	132.8	56	172	77.8	209	98.3
88	31.1	133	56.1	172.4	78	210	98.9
89	31.7	134	56.7	173	78.3	211	99.4
90	32.2	135	57.2	174	78.9	212	100
91	32.8	136	57.8	174.2	79	213	100.6
92	33.3	136.4	58	175	79.4	214	101.1
93	33.9	137	58.3	176	80	215	101.7
94	34.4	138	58.9	177	80.6	215.6	102
95	35	139	59.4	177.8	81	216	102.2
96	35.6	140	60	178	81.1	217	102.8
96.8	36	141	60.6	179	81.7	218	103.3
97	36.1	141.8	61	179.6	82	219	103.9
98	36.7	142	61.1	180	82.2	219.2	104
98.6	37	143	61.7	181	82.8	220	104.4
99	37.2	144	62.2	181.4	83	221	105
100	37.8	145	62.8	182	83.3	225	107.2
100.4	38	145.4	63	183.2	84	230	110
101	38.3	146	63.3	184	84.4	235	112.8
102	38.9	147	63.9	185	85	239	115
102.2	39	147.2	64	186	85.6	240	115.6
103	39.4	148	64.4	186.8	86	245	118.3
104	40	149	65	187	86.1	248	120
105	40.6	150	65.6	188	86.7	250	121.1
105.8	41	150.8	66	188.6	87	255	123.9
106	41.1	151	66.1	189	87.2	257	125
107	41.7	152	66.7	190	87.8	260	126.7
107.6	42	152.6	67	190.4	88	265	129.4
108	42.2	153	67.2	191	88.3	266	130
109	42.8	154	67.8	192	88.9	270	132.2
110	43.3	154.4	68	192.2	89	275	135
111	43.9	155	68.3	193	89.4	280	137.8
112	44.4	156	68.9	194	90	284	140
113	45	156.2	69	195	90.6	285	140.6
114	45.6	157	69.4	195.8	91	290	143.3
115	46.1	158	70	196	91.1	295	146.1
116	46.7	159	70.6	197	91.7	300	148.9
116.6	47	159.8	71				

TABLE A-6 NUTRITIVE VALUES OF THE EDIBLE PART OF FOODS

[Dashes in the columns for nutrients show that no suitable value could be found although there is reason to believe that a measurable amount of the nutrient may be present]

	Food, approximate measure, and weight (in grams)		Water	Food energy	Protein	Fat	Fatty acids			Carbo-hydrate	Calcium	Iron	Vitamin A value	Thiamin	Ribo-flavin	Niacin	Ascorbic acid
							Saturated (total)	Unsaturated Oleic	Unsaturated Linoleic								
		Grams	Per-cent	Calo-ries	Grams	Grams	Grams	Grams	Grams	Grams	Milli-grams	Milli-grams	Inter-national units	Milli-grams	Milli-grams	Milli-grams	Milli-grams
	MILK, CHEESE, CREAM, IMITATION CREAM; RELATED PRODUCTS																
	Milk:																
	Fluid:																
1	Whole, 3.5% fat----- 1 cup------	244	87	160	9	9	5	3	Trace	12	288	0.1	350	0.07	0.41	0.2	2
2	Nonfat (skim)------- 1 cup------	245	90	90	9	Trace				12	296	.1	10	.09	.44	.2	2
3	Partly skimmed, 2% 1 cup------ nonfat milk solids added.	246	87	145	10	5	3	2	Trace	15	352	.1	200	.10	.52	.2	2
	Canned, concentrated, undiluted:																
4	Evaporated, un-sweetened. 1 cup------	252	74	345	18	20	11	7	1	24	635	.3	810	.10	.86	.5	3
5	Condensed, sweet-ened. 1 cup------	306	27	980	25	27	15	9	1	166	802	.3	1,100	.24	1.16	.6	3
	Dry, nonfat instant:																
6	Low-density (1⅓ 1 cup------ cups needed for re-constitution to 1 qt.).	68	4	245	24	Trace				35	879	.4	[1]20	.24	1.21	.6	5
7	High-density (⅞ cup 1 cup------ needed for recon-stitution to 1 qt.).	104	4	375	37	1				54	1,345	.6	[1]30	.36	1.85	.9	7
	Buttermilk:																
8	Fluid, cultured, made 1 cup------ from skim milk.	245	90	90	9	Trace				12	296	.1	10	.10	.44	.2	2
9	Dried, packaged------- 1 cup------	120	3	465	41	6	3	2	Trace	60	1,498	.7	260	.31	2.06	1.1	------
	Cheese:																
	Natural:																
	Blue or Roquefort type:																
10	Ounce----------- 1 oz-----	28	40	105	6	9	5	3	Trace	1	89	.1	350	.01	.17	.3	0
11	Cubic inch-------- 1 cu. in.--	17	40	65	4	5	3	2	Trace	Trace	54	.1	210	.01	.11	.2	0

[1] Value applies to unfortified product; value for fortified low-density product would be 1500 I.U., and the fortified high-density product would be 2290 I.U.

TABLE A-6 NUTRITIVE VALUES OF THE EDIBLE PART OF FOODS — Continued

[Dashes in the columns for nutrients show that no suitable value could be found although there is reason to believe that a measurable amount of the nutrient may be present]

	Food, approximate measure, and weight (in grams)		Water	Food energy	Protein	Fat	Fatty acids			Carbohydrate	Calcium	Iron	Vitamin A value	Thiamin	Riboflavin	Niacin	Ascorbic acid
							Saturated (total)	Unsaturated									
								Oleic	Linoleic								
		Grams	Percent	Calories	Grams	Grams	Grams	Grams	Grams	Grams	Milligrams	Milligrams	International units	Milligrams	Milligrams	Milligrams	Milligrams
	MILK, CHEESE, CREAM, IMITATION CREAM; RELATED PRODUCTS—Con.																
	Cheese—Continued																
	Natural—Continued																
12	Camembert, packaged in 4-oz. pkg. with 3 wedges per pkg. 1 wedge	38	52	115	7	9	5	3	Trace	1	40	0.2	380	0.02	0.29	0.3	0
	Cheddar:																
13	Ounce 1 oz.	28	37	115	7	9	5	3	Trace	1	213	.3	370	.01	.13	Trace	0
14	Cubic inch 1 cu. in.	17	37	70	4	6	3	2	Trace	Trace	129	.2	230	.01	.08	Trace	0
	Cottage, large or small curd:																
	Creamed:																
15	Package of 12-oz., net wt. 1 pkg.	340	78	360	46	14	8	5	Trace	10	320	1.0	580	.10	.85	.3	0
16	Cup, curd pressed down. 1 cup	245	78	260	33	10	6	3	Trace	7	230	.7	420	.07	.61	.2	0
	Uncreamed:																
17	Package of 12-oz., net wt. 1 pkg.	340	79	290	58	1	1	Trace	Trace	9	306	1.4	30	.10	.95	.3	0
18	Cup, curd pressed down. 1 cup	200	79	170	34	1	Trace	Trace	Trace	5	180	.8	20	.06	.56	.2	0
	Cream:																
19	Package of 8-oz., net wt. 1 pkg.	227	51	850	18	86	48	28	3	5	141	.5	3,500	.05	.54	.2	0
20	Package of 3-oz., net wt. 1 pkg.	85	51	320	7	32	18	11	1	2	53	.2	1,310	.02	.20	.1	0
21	Cubic inch 1 cu. in.	16	51	60	1	6	3	2	Trace	Trace	10	Trace	250	Trace	.04	Trace	0
	Parmesan, grated:																
22	Cup, pressed down 1 cup	140	17	655	60	43	24	14	1	5	1,893	.7	1,760	.03	1.22	.3	0
23	Tablespoon 1 tbsp.	5	17	25	2	2	1	Trace	Trace	Trace	68	Trace	60	Trace	.04	Trace	0
24	Ounce 1 oz.	28	17	130	12	9	5	3	Trace	1	383	.1	360	.01	.25	.1	0
	Swiss:																
25	Ounce 1 oz.	28	39	105	8	8	4	3	Trace	1	262	.3	320	Trace	.11	Trace	0
26	Cubic inch 1 cu. in.	15	39	55	4	4	2	1	Trace	Trace	139	.1	170	Trace	.06	Trace	0

No.	Food and measure	Grams	Water (%)	Food energy	Protein (g)	Fat (g)	Saturated fatty acids (g)	Oleic (g)	Linoleic (g)	Carbohydrate (g)	Calcium (mg)	Iron (mg)	Vitamin A (I.U.)	Thiamin (mg)	Riboflavin (mg)	Niacin (mg)	Ascorbic acid (mg)
	Pasteurized processed cheese:																
	American:																
27	Ounce — 1 oz	28	40	105	7	9	5	3	Trace	1	198	.3	350	.01	.12	Trace	0
28	Cubic inch — 1 cu. in.	18	40	65	4	5	3	2	Trace	Trace	122	.2	210	Trace	.07	Trace	0
	Swiss:																
29	Ounce — 1 oz	28	40	100	8	8	4	3	Trace	1	251	.3	310	Trace	.11	Trace	0
30	Cubic inch — 1 cu. in.	18	40	65	5	5	3	2	Trace	Trace	159	.2	200	Trace	.07	Trace	0
	Pasteurized process cheese food, American:																
31	Tablespoon — 1 tbsp.	14	43	45	3	3	2	1	Trace	1	80	.1	140	Trace	.08	Trace	0
32	Cubic inch — 1 cu. in.	18	43	60	4	4	2	1	Trace	1	100	.1	170	Trace	.10	Trace	0
33	Pasteurized process cheese spread, American — 1 oz.	28	49	80	5	6	3	2	Trace	2	160	.2	250	Trace	.15	Trace	0
	Cream:																
34	Half-and-half (cream and milk) — 1 cup	242	80	325	8	28	15	9	1	11	261	.1	1,160	.07	.39	.1	2
35	Light, coffee or table — 1 tbsp.	15	80	20	1	2	1	1	Trace	1	16	Trace	70	Trace	.02	Trace	Trace
36	1 cup	240	72	505	7	49	27	16	1	10	245	.1	2,020	.07	.36	.1	2
37	1 tbsp.	15	72	30	1	3	2	1	Trace	1	15	Trace	130	Trace	.02	Trace	Trace
38	Sour — 1 cup	230	72	485	7	47	26	16	1	10	235	.1	1,930	.07	.35	.1	2
39	1 tbsp.	12	72	25	Trace	2	1	1	Trace	1	12	Trace	100	Trace	.02	Trace	Trace
40	Whipped topping (pressurized) — 1 cup	60	62	155	2	14	8	5	Trace	6	67	----	570	Trace	.04	Trace	Trace
41	1 tbsp.	3	62	10	Trace	1	Trace	Trace	Trace	Trace	3	----	30	----	----	----	----
	Whipping, unwhipped (volume about double when whipped):																
42	Light — 1 cup	239	62	715	6	75	41	25	2	9	203	.1	3,060	.05	.29	.1	2
43	1 tbsp.	15	62	45	Trace	5	3	2	Trace	1	13	Trace	190	Trace	.02	Trace	Trace
44	Heavy — 1 cup	238	57	840	5	90	50	30	3	7	179	.1	3,670	.05	.26	.1	2
45	1 tbsp.	15	57	55	Trace	6	3	2	Trace	1	11	Trace	230	Trace	.02	Trace	Trace
	Imitation cream products (made with vegetable fat):																
	Creamers:																
46	Powdered — 1 cup	94	2	505	4	33	31	1	0	52	21	.6	²200	0	Trace	Trace	Trace
47	1 tsp.	2	2	10	Trace	1	Trace	Trace	0	1	1	Trace	²Trace	0	----	----	----
48	Liquid (frozen) — 1 cup	245	77	345	3	27	25	1	0	25	29	----	²100	0	----	----	----
49	1 tbsp.	15	77	20	Trace	2	Trace	Trace	0	2	2	----	²10	0	----	----	----
50	Sour dressing (imitation sour cream) made with nonfat dry milk. — 1 cup	235	72	440	9	38	35	1	Trace	17	277	.1	10	.07	.38	.2	1
51	1 tbsp.	12	72	20	Trace	2	2	1	Trace	1	14	Trace	Trace	Trace	Trace	Trace	Trace
	Whipped topping:																
52	Pressurized — 1 cup	70	61	190	1	17	15	1	0	9	5	Trace	²340	0	0	Trace	Trace
53	1 tbsp.	4	61	10	Trace	1	1	Trace	0	Trace	Trace	Trace	²20	0	0	Trace	Trace

² Contributed largely from beta-carotene used for coloring.

TABLE A-6. NUTRITIVE VALUES OF THE EDIBLE PART OF FOODS — Continued

[Dashes in the columns for nutrients show that no suitable value could be found although there is reason to believe that a measurable amount of the nutrient may be present]

	Food, approximate measure, and weight (in grams)	Water	Food energy	Protein	Fat	Fatty acids			Carbohydrate	Calcium	Iron	Vitamin A value	Thiamin	Riboflavin	Niacin	Ascorbic acid
						Saturated (total)	Unsaturated Oleic	Unsaturated Linoleic								
		Percent	Calories	Grams	Grams	Grams	Grams	Grams	Grams	Milligrams	Milligrams	International units	Milligrams	Milligrams	Milligrams	Milligrams
	MILK, CHEESE, CREAM, IMITATION CREAM; RELATED PRODUCTS—Con.															
	Whipped topping—Continued															
54	Frozen ------ 1 cup ------ 75	52	230	1	20	18	Trace	0	15	5	-----	[2]560	-----	0	-----	-----
55	1 tbsp ------ 4	52	10	Trace	1	1	Trace	0	1	Trace	-----	[2]30	-----	0	-----	-----
56	Powdered, made with 1 cup whole milk. ------ 75	58	175	3	12	10	1	Trace	15	62	Trace	[2]330	.02	.08	.1	Trace
57	1 tbsp ------ 4	58	10	Trace	1	1	Trace	Trace	1	3	Trace	[2]20	Trace	Trace	Trace	Trace
	Milk beverages:															
58	Cocoa, homemade ------ 1 cup ------ 250	79	245	10	12	7	4	Trace	27	295	1.0	400	.10	.45	.5	3
59	Chocolate-flavored drink made with skim milk and 2% added butterfat. ------ 1 cup ------ 250	83	190	8	6	3	2	Trace	27	270	.5	210	.10	.40	.3	3
	Malted milk:															
60	Dry powder, approx. 1 oz. 3 heaping teaspoons per ounce. ------ 28	3	115	4	2	-----	-----	-----	20	82	.6	290	.09	.15	.1	0
61	Beverage ------ 1 cup ------ 235	78	245	11	10	-----	-----	-----	28	317	.7	590	.14	.49	.2	2
	Milk desserts:															
62	Custard, baked ------ 1 cup ------ 265	77	305	14	15	7	5	1	29	297	1.1	930	.11	.50	.3	1
	Ice cream:															
63	Regular (approx. 10% fat). ½ gal ------ 1,064	63	2,055	48	113	62	37	3	221	1,553	.5	4,680	.43	2.23	1.1	11
64	1 cup ------ 133	63	255	6	14	8	5	Trace	28	194	.1	590	.05	.28	.1	1
65	3 fl. oz. cup ------ 50	63	95	2	5	3	2	Trace	10	73	Trace	220	.02	.11	.1	1
66	Rich (approx. 16% fat). ½ gal ------ 1,188	63	2,635	31	191	105	63	6	214	927	.2	7,840	.24	1.31	1.2	12
67	1 cup ------ 148	63	330	4	24	13	8	1	27	115	Trace	980	.03	.16	.1	1
	Ice milk:															
68	Hardened ------ ½ gal ------ 1,048	67	1,595	50	53	29	17	2	235	1,635	1.0	2,200	.52	2.31	1.0	10
69	1 cup ------ 131	67	200	6	7	4	2	Trace	29	204	.1	280	.07	.29	.1	1
70	Soft-serve ------ 1 cup ------ 175	67	265	8	9	5	3	Trace	39	273	.2	370	.09	.39	.2	2

No.	Food, approximate measure, and weight	Measure	Grams	Water (%)	Food energy (Cal.)	Protein (g)	Fat (g)	Saturated (total) (g)	Oleic (g)	Linoleic (g)	Carbohydrate (g)	Calcium (mg)	Iron (mg)	Vitamin A (I.U.)	Thiamine (mg)	Riboflavin (mg)	Niacin (mg)	Ascorbic acid (mg)
	Yoghurt:																	
71	Made from partially skimmed milk.	1 cup	245	89	125	8	4	2	1	Trace	13	294	.1	170	.10	.44	.2	2
72	Made from whole milk.	1 cup	245	88	150	7	8	5	3	Trace	12	272	.1	340	.07	.39	.2	2
	EGGS																	
	Eggs, large, 24 ounces per dozen:																	
	Raw or cooked in shell or with nothing added:																	
73	Whole, without shell	1 egg	50	74	80	6	6	2	3	Trace	Trace	27	1.1	590	.05	.15	Trace	0
74	White of egg	1 white	33	88	15	4	Trace	---	---	---	Trace	3	Trace	0	Trace	.09	Trace	0
75	Yolk of egg	1 yolk	17	51	60	3	5	2	2	Trace	Trace	24	.9	580	.04	.07	Trace	0
76	Scrambled with milk and fat.	1 egg	64	72	110	7	8	3	3	Trace	1	51	1.1	690	.05	.18	Trace	0
	MEAT, POULTRY, FISH, SHELLFISH; RELATED PRODUCTS																	
77	Bacon, (20 slices per lb. raw), broiled or fried, crisp.	2 slices	15	8	90	5	8	3	4	1	1	2	.5	0	.08	.05	.8	---
	Beef,[3] cooked:																	
	Cuts braised, simmered, or pot-roasted:																	
78	Lean and fat	3 ounces	85	53	245	23	16	8	7	Trace	0	10	2.9	30	.04	.18	3.5	---
79	Lean only	2.5 ounces	72	62	140	22	5	2	2	Trace	0	10	2.7	10	.04	.16	3.3	---
	Hamburger (ground beef), broiled:																	
80	Lean	3 ounces	85	60	185	23	10	5	4	Trace	0	10	3.0	20	.08	.20	5.1	---
81	Regular	3 ounces	85	54	245	21	17	8	8	Trace	0	9	2.7	30	.07	.18	4.6	---
	Roast, oven-cooked, no liquid added:																	
	Relatively fat, such as rib:																	
82	Lean and fat	3 ounces	85	40	375	17	34	16	15	1	0	8	2.2	70	.05	.13	3.1	---
83	Lean only	1.8 ounces	51	57	125	14	7	3	3	Trace	0	6	1.8	10	.04	.11	2.6	---
	Relatively lean, such as heel of round:																	
84	Lean and fat	3 ounces	85	62	165	25	7	3	3	Trace	0	11	3.2	10	.06	.19	4.5	---
85	Lean only	2.7 ounces	78	65	125	24	3	1	1	Trace	0	10	3.0	Trace	.06	.18	4.3	---
	Steak, broiled:																	
	Relatively fat, such as sirloin:																	
86	Lean and fat	3 ounces	85	44	330	20	27	13	12	1	0	9	2.5	50	.05	.16	4.0	---
87	Lean only	2.0 ounces	56	59	115	18	4	2	2	Trace	0	7	2.2	10	.05	.14	3.6	---
	Relatively lean, such as round:																	
88	Lean and fat	3 ounces	85	55	220	24	13	6	6	Trace	0	10	3.0	20	.07	.19	4.8	---
89	Lean only	2.4 ounces	68	61	130	21	4	2	2	Trace	0	9	2.5	10	.06	.16	4.1	---
	Beef, canned:																	
90	Corned beef	3 ounces	85	59	185	22	10	5	4	Trace	0	17	3.7	20	.01	.20	2.9	---
91	Corned beef hash	3 ounces	85	67	155	7	10	5	4	Trace	9	11	1.7	---	.01	.08	1.8	---
92	Beef, dried or chipped	2 ounces	57	48	115	19	4	2	2	Trace	0	11	2.9	---	.04	.18	2.2	---
93	Beef and vegetable stew	1 cup	235	82	210	15	10	5	4	Trace	15	28	2.8	2,310	.13	.17	4.4	15

2 Contributed largely from beta-carotene used for coloring.

3 Outer layer of fat on the cut was removed to within approximately ½-inch of the lean. Deposits of fat within the cut were not removed.

TABLE A-6 NUTRITIVE VALUES OF THE EDIBLE PART OF FOODS — Continued

[Dashes in the columns for nutrients show that no suitable value could be found although there is reason to believe that a measurable amount of the nutrient may be present]

	Food, approximate measure, and weight (in grams)	Water	Food energy	Protein	Fat	Fatty acids — Saturated (total)	Fatty acids — Unsaturated Oleic	Fatty acids — Unsaturated Linoleic	Carbohydrate	Calcium	Iron	Vitamin A value	Thiamin	Riboflavin	Niacin	Ascorbic acid
		Percent	Calories	Grams	Grams	Grams	Grams	Grams	Grams	Milligrams	Milligrams	International units	Milligrams	Milligrams	Milligrams	Milligrams
	MEAT, POULTRY, FISH, SHELLFISH; RELATED PRODUCTS—Continued															
94	Beef potpie, baked, 4¼-inch diam., weight before baking about 8 ounces. 1 pie — 227 Grams	55	560	23	33	9	20	2	43	32	4.1	1,860	0.25	0.27	4.5	7
	Chicken, cooked:															
95	Flesh only, broiled — 3 ounces — 85	71	115	20	3	1	1	1	0	8	1.4	80	.05	.16	7.4	---
	Breast, fried, ½ breast:															
96	With bone — 3.3 ounces — 94	58	155	25	5	1	2	1	1	9	1.3	70	.04	.17	11.2	---
97	Flesh and skin only — 2.7 ounces — 76	58	155	25	5	1	2	1	1	9	1.3	70	.04	.17	11.2	---
	Drumstick, fried:															
98	With bone — 2.1 ounces — 59	55	90	12	4	1	2	1	Trace	6	.9	50	.03	.15	2.7	---
99	Flesh and skin only — 1.3 ounces — 38	55	90	12	4	1	2	1	Trace	6	.9	50	.03	.15	2.7	---
100	Chicken, canned, boneless 3 ounces — 85	65	170	18	10	3	4	2	0	18	1.3	200	.03	.11	3.7	3
101	Chicken potpie, baked 4¼-inch diam., weight before baking about 8 ounces. 1 pie — 227	57	535	23	31	10	15	3	42	68	3.0	3,020	.25	.26	4.1	5
	Chili con carne, canned:															
102	With beans — 1 cup — 250	72	335	19	15	7	7	Trace	30	80	4.2	150	.08	.18	3.2	---
103	Without beans — 1 cup — 255	67	510	26	38	18	17	1	15	97	3.6	380	.05	.31	5.6	---
104	Heart, beef, lean, braised — 3 ounces — 85	61	160	27	5	---	---	---	1	5	5.0	20	.21	1.04	6.5	1
	Lamb,[3] cooked:															
105	Chop, thick, with bone, 1 chop, broiled. 4.8 ounces — 137	47	400	25	33	18	12	1	0	10	1.5	---	.14	.25	5.6	---
106	Lean and fat — 4.0 ounces — 112	47	400	25	33	18	12	1	0	10	1.5	---	.14	.25	5.6	---
107	Lean only — 2.6 ounces — 74	62	140	21	6	3	2	Trace	0	9	1.5	---	.11	.20	4.5	---
	Leg, roasted:															
108	Lean and fat — 3 ounces — 85	54	235	22	16	9	6	Trace	0	9	1.4	---	.13	.23	4.7	---
109	Lean only — 2.5 ounces — 71	62	130	20	5	3	2	Trace	0	9	1.4	---	.12	.21	4.4	---
	Shoulder, roasted:															
110	Lean and fat — 3 ounces — 85	50	285	18	23	13	8	1	0	9	1.0	---	.11	.20	4.0	---
111	Lean only — 2.3 ounces — 64	61	130	17	6	3	2	Trace	0	8	1.0	---	.10	.18	3.7	---

Item No.	Food, approximate measure	Weight (g)	Water (%)	Food energy (cal.)	Protein (g)	Fat (g)	Saturated (total) (g)	Oleic (g)	Linoleic (g)	Carbohydrate (g)	Calcium (mg)	Iron (mg)	Vitamin A (I.U.)	Thiamine (mg)	Riboflavin (mg)	Niacin (mg)	Ascorbic acid (mg)
112	Liver, beef, fried — 2 ounces	57	57	130	15	6	—	—	—	3	6	5.0	30,280	.15	2.37	9.4	15
	Pork, cured, cooked:																
113	Ham, light cure, lean and fat, roasted — 3 ounces	85	54	245	18	19	7	8	2	0	8	2.2	0	.40	.16	3.1	—
	Luncheon meat:																
114	Boiled ham, sliced — 2 ounces	57	59	135	11	10	4	4	1	0	6	1.6	0	.25	.09	1.5	—
115	Canned, spiced or unspiced — 2 ounces	57	55	165	8	14	5	6	1	1	5	1.2	0	.18	.12	1.6	—
	Pork, fresh,[3] cooked:																
116	Chop, thick, with bone — 1 chop, 3.5 ounces	98	42	260	16	21	8	9	2	0	8	2.2	0	.63	.18	3.8	—
117	Lean and fat — 2.3 ounces	66	42	260	16	21	8	9	2	0	8	2.2	0	.63	.18	3.8	—
118	Lean only — 1.7 ounces	48	53	130	15	7	2	3	1	0	7	1.9	0	.54	.16	3.3	—
	Roast, oven-cooked, no liquid added:																
119	Lean and fat — 3 ounces	85	46	310	21	24	9	10	2	0	9	2.7	0	.78	.22	4.7	—
120	Lean only — 2.4 ounces	68	55	175	20	10	4	4	1	0	9	2.6	0	.73	.21	4.4	—
	Cuts, simmered:																
121	Lean and fat — 3 ounces	85	46	320	20	26	9	11	2	0	8	2.5	0	.46	.21	4.1	—
122	Lean only — 2.2 ounces	63	60	135	18	6	2	3	1	0	8	2.3	0	.42	.19	3.7	—
	Sausage:																
123	Bologna, slice, 3-in. diam. by 1/8 inch — 2 slices	26	56	80	3	7	—	—	—	Trace	2	.5	—	.04	.06	.7	—
124	Braunschweiger, slice 2-in. diam. by 1/4 inch — 2 slices	20	53	65	3	5	—	—	—	Trace	2	1.2	1,310	.03	.29	1.6	—
125	Deviled ham, canned — 1 tbsp.	13	51	45	2	4	2	2	Trace	0	1	.3	0	.02	.01	.2	—
126	Frankfurter, heated (8 per lb. purchased pkg.) — 1 frank	56	57	170	7	15	—	—	—	1	3	.8	—	.08	.11	1.4	—
127	Pork links, cooked (16 links per lb. raw) — 2 links	26	35	125	5	11	4	5	1	Trace	2	.6	0	.21	.09	1.0	—
128	Salami, dry type — 1 oz.	28	30	130	7	11	—	—	—	Trace	4	1.0	—	.10	.07	1.5	—
129	Salami, cooked — 1 oz.	28	51	90	5	7	—	—	—	Trace	3	.7	—	.07	.07	1.2	—
130	Vienna, canned (7 sausages per 5-oz. can) — 1 sausage	16	63	40	2	3	—	—	—	Trace	1	.3	—	.01	.02	.4	—
	Veal, medium fat, cooked, bone removed:																
131	Cutlet — 3 oz.	85	60	185	23	9	5	4	Trace	—	9	2.7	—	.06	.21	4.6	—
132	Roast — 3 oz.	85	55	230	23	14	7	6	Trace	0	10	2.9	0	.11	.26	6.6	—
	Fish and shellfish:																
133	Bluefish, baked with table fat — 3 oz.	85	68	135	22	4	—	—	—	0	25	.6	40	.09	.08	1.6	—
	Clams:																
134	Raw, meat only — 3 oz.	85	82	65	11	1	—	—	—	2	59	5.2	90	.08	.15	1.1	8
135	Canned, solids and liquid — 3 oz.	85	86	45	7	1	—	—	—	2	47	3.5	—	.01	.09	.9	—
136	Crabmeat, canned — 3 oz.	85	77	85	15	2	—	—	—	1	38	.7	—	.07	.07	1.6	—

[3] Outer layer of fat on the cut was removed to within approximately ½-inch of the lean. Deposits of fat within the cut were not removed.

TABLE A-6 NUTRITIVE VALUES OF THE EDIBLE PART OF FOODS – Continued

[Dashes in the columns for nutrients show that no suitable value could be found although there is reason to believe that a measurable amount of the nutrient may be present]

Food, approximate measure, and weight (in grams)	Water	Food energy	Protein	Fat	Fatty acids Saturated (total)	Unsaturated Oleic	Unsaturated Linoleic	Carbohydrate	Calcium	Iron	Vitamin A value	Thiamin	Riboflavin	Niacin	Ascorbic acid
	Percent	Calories	Grams	Grams	Grams	Grams	Grams	Grams	Milligrams	Milligrams	International units	Milligrams	Milligrams	Milligrams	Milligrams
MEAT, POULTRY, FISH, SHELLFISH; RELATED PRODUCTS—Continued															
Fish and shellfish—Continued															
137 Fish sticks, breaded, cooked, frozen; stick 3¾ by 1 by ½ inch. — 10 sticks or 8 oz. pkg. — 227 Grams	66	400	38	20	5	4	10	15	25	0.9	---	0.09	0.16	3.6	---
138 Haddock, breaded, fried — 3 oz — 85	66	140	17	5	1	3	Trace	5	34	1.0	---	.03	.06	2.7	2
139 Ocean perch, breaded, fried. — 3 oz — 85	59	195	16	11	---	---	---	6	28	1.1	---	.08	.09	1.5	---
140 Oysters, raw, meat only (13–19 med. selects). — 1 cup — 240	85	160	20	4	---	---	---	8	226	13.2	740	.33	.43	6.0	---
141 Salmon, pink, canned — 3 oz — 85	71	120	17	5	1	1	Trace	0	[4]167	.7	60	.03	.16	6.8	---
142 Sardines, Atlantic, canned in oil, drained solids. — 3 oz — 85	62	175	20	9	---	---	---	0	372	2.5	190	.02	.17	4.6	---
143 Shad, baked with table fat and bacon. — 3 oz — 85	64	170	20	10	---	---	---	0	20	.5	20	.11	.22	7.3	---
144 Shrimp, canned, meat. — 3 oz — 85	70	100	21	1	---	---	---	1	98	2.6	50	.01	.03	1.5	---
145 Swordfish, broiled with butter or margarine. — 3 oz — 85	65	150	24	5	---	---	---	0	23	1.1	1,750	.03	.04	9.3	---
146 Tuna, canned in oil, drained solids. — 3 oz — 85	61	170	24	7	2	1	1	0	7	1.6	70	.04	.10	10.1	---
MATURE DRY BEANS AND PEAS, NUTS, PEANUTS; RELATED PRODUCTS															
147 Almonds, shelled, whole kernels. — 1 cup — 142	5	850	26	77	6	52	15	28	332	6.7	0	.34	1.31	5.0	Trace
Beans, dry: Common varieties as Great Northern, navy, and others: Cooked, drained:															
148 Great Northern — 1 cup — 180	69	210	14	1	---	---	---	38	90	4.9	0	.25	.13	1.3	0

Item No.	Food, approximate measure	Measure	Grams	Water (pct.)	Food energy (cal.)	Protein (g)	Fat (g)	Saturated fatty acids (g)	Oleic (g)	Linoleic (g)	Carbohydrate (g)	Calcium (mg)	Iron (mg)	Vitamin A (I.U.)	Thiamin (mg)	Riboflavin (mg)	Niacin (mg)	Ascorbic acid (mg)
149	Navy (pea)	1 cup	190	69	225	15	1	—	—	—	40	95	5.1	0	.27	.13	1.3	0
	Canned, solids and liquid: White with—																	
150	Frankfurters (sliced)	1 cup	255	71	365	19	18	—	—	—	32	94	4.8	330	.18	.15	3.3	Trace
151	Pork and tomato sauce	1 cup	255	71	310	16	7	2	3	1	49	138	4.6	330	.20	.08	1.5	5
152	Pork and sweet sauce	1 cup	255	66	385	16	12	4	5	1	54	161	5.9	—	.15	.10	1.3	—
153	Red kidney	1 cup	255	76	230	15	1	—	—	—	42	74	4.6	10	.13	.10	1.5	—
154	Lima, cooked, drained	1 cup	190	64	260	16	1	—	—	—	49	55	5.9	—	.25	.11	1.3	—
155	Cashew nuts, roasted	1 cup	140	5	785	24	64	11	45	4	41	53	5.3	140	.60	.35	2.5	—
	Coconut, fresh, meat only:																	
156	Pieces, approx. 2 by 2 by ½ inch	1 piece	45	51	155	2	16	14	1	Trace	4	6	.8	0	.02	.01	.2	1
157	Shredded or grated, firmly packed	1 cup	130	51	450	5	46	39	3	Trace	12	17	2.2	0	.07	.03	.7	4
158	Cowpeas or blackeye peas, dry, cooked	1 cup	248	80	190	13	1	—	—	—	34	42	3.2	20	.41	.11	1.1	Trace
159	Peanuts, roasted, salted, halves	1 cup	144	2	840	37	72	16	31	21	27	107	3.0	—	.46	.19	24.7	0
160	Peanut butter	1 tbsp	16	2	95	4	8	2	4	2	3	9	.3	—	.02	.02	2.4	0
161	Peas, split, dry, cooked	1 cup	250	70	290	20	1	—	—	—	52	28	4.2	100	.37	.22	2.2	0
162	Pecans, halves	1 cup	108	3	740	10	77	5	48	15	16	79	2.6	140	.93	.14	1.0	2
163	Walnuts, black or native, chopped	1 cup	126	3	790	26	75	4	26	36	19	Trace	7.6	380	.28	.14	.9	—
	VEGETABLES AND VEGETABLE PRODUCTS																	
	Asparagus, green: Cooked, drained:																	
164	Spears, ½-in. diam. at base	4 spears	60	94	10	1	Trace	—	—	—	2	13	.4	540	.10	.11	.8	16
165	Pieces, 1½ to 2-in. lengths	1 cup	145	94	30	3	Trace	—	—	—	5	30	.9	1,310	.23	.26	2.0	38
166	Canned, solids and liquid	1 cup	244	94	45	5	1	—	—	—	7	44	4.1	1,240	.15	.22	2.0	37
	Beans:																	
167	Lima, immature seeds, cooked, drained	1 cup	170	71	190	13	1	—	—	—	34	80	4.3	480	.31	.17	2.2	29
	Snap: Green:																	
168	Cooked, drained	1 cup	125	92	30	2	Trace	—	—	—	7	63	.8	680	.09	.11	.6	15
169	Canned, solids and liquid	1 cup	239	94	45	2	Trace	—	—	—	10	81	2.9	690	.07	.10	.7	10

[4] If bones are discarded, value will be greatly reduced.

TABLE A-6 NUTRITIVE VALUES OF THE EDIBLE PART OF FOODS – Continued

[Dashes in the columns for nutrients show that no suitable value could be found although there is reason to believe that a measurable amount of the nutrient may be present]

Food, approximate measure, and weight (in grams)		Water	Food energy	Protein	Fat	Fatty acids			Carbohydrate	Calcium	Iron	Vitamin A value	Thiamin	Riboflavin	Niacin	Ascorbic acid
						Saturated (total)	Unsaturated									
							Oleic	Linoleic								
	Grams	Percent	Calories	Grams	Grams	Grams	Grams	Grams	Grams	Milligrams	Milligrams	International units	Milligrams	Milligrams	Milligrams	Milligrams
VEGETABLES AND VEGETABLE PRODUCTS—Continued																
Beans—Continued																
Snap—Continued																
Yellow or wax:																
170 Cooked, drained -- 1 cup	125	93	30	2	Trace	---			6	63	0.8	290	0.09	0.11	0.6	16
171 Canned, solids and liquid. 1 cup	239	94	45	2	1	---			10	81	2.9	140	.07	.10	.7	12
172 Sprouted mung beans, cooked, drained. 1 cup	125	91	35	4	Trace				7	21	1.1	30	.11	.13	.9	8
Beets:																
Cooked, drained, peeled:																
173 Whole beets, 2-in. diam. 2 beets	100	91	30	1	Trace				7	14	.5	20	.03	.04	.3	6
174 Diced or sliced 1 cup	170	91	55	2	Trace				12	24	.9	30	.05	.07	.5	10
175 Canned, solids and liquid. 1 cup	246	90	85	2	Trace				19	34	1.5	20	.02	.05	.2	7
176 Beet greens, leaves and stems, cooked, drained. 1 cup	145	94	25	3	Trace				5	144	2.8	7,400	.10	.22	.4	22
Blackeye peas. See Cowpeas.																
Broccoli, cooked, drained:																
177 Whole stalks, medium size. 1 stalk	180	91	45	6	1				8	158	1.4	4,500	.16	.36	1.4	162
178 Stalks cut into ½-in. pieces. 1 cup	155	91	40	5	1				7	136	1.2	3,880	.14	.31	1.2	140
179 Chopped, yield from 10-oz. frozen pkg. 1⅞ cups	250	92	65	7	1				12	135	1.8	6,500	.15	.30	1.3	143
180 Brussels sprouts, 7-8 sprouts (1¼ to 1½ in. diam.) per cup, cooked. 1 cup	155	88	55	7	1				10	50	1.7	810	.12	.22	1.2	135
Cabbage:																
Common varieties:																

No.	Food, approximate measure	Measure	Weight (g)	Water (%)	Food energy	Protein	Fat				Carbohydrate	Calcium	Iron	Vitamin A	Thiamine	Riboflavin	Niacin	Ascorbic acid
181	Raw: Coarsely shredded or sliced.	1 cup	70	92	15	1	Trace	---	---		4	34	.3	90	.04	.04	.2	38
182	Finely shredded or chopped.	1 cup	90	92	20	1	Trace	---	---		5	44	.4	120	.05	.05	.3	42
183	Cooked	1 cup	145	94	30	2	Trace	---	---		6	64	.4	190	.06	.06	.4	48
184	Red, raw, coarsely shredded.	1 cup	70	90	20	1	Trace	---	---		5	29	.6	30	.06	.04	.3	43
185	Savoy, raw, coarsely shredded.	1 cup	70	92	15	2	Trace	---	---		3	47	.6	140	.04	.06	.2	39
186	Cabbage, celery or Chinese, raw, cut in 1-in. pieces.	1 cup	75	95	10	1	Trace	---	---		2	32	.5	110	.04	.03	.5	19
187	Cabbage, spoon (or pakchoy), cooked.	1 cup	170	95	25	2	Trace	---	---		4	252	1.0	5,270	.07	.14	1.2	26
	Carrots: Raw:																	
188	Whole, 5½ by 1 inch, (25 thin strips).	1 carrot	50	88	20	1	Trace	---	---		5	18	.4	5,500	.03	.03	.3	4
189	Grated	1 cup	110	88	45	1	Trace	---	---		11	41	.8	12,100	.06	.06	.7	9
190	Cooked, diced	1 cup	145	91	45	1	Trace	---	---		10	48	.9	15,220	.08	.07	.7	9
191	Canned, strained or chopped (baby food).	1 ounce	28	92	10	Trace	Trace	---	---		2	7	.1	3,690	.01	.01	.1	1
192	Cauliflower, cooked, flowerbuds.	1 cup	120	93	25	3	Trace	---	---		5	25	.8	70	.11	.10	.7	66
	Celery, raw:																	
193	Stalk, large outer, 8 by about 1½ inches, at root end.	1 stalk	40	94	5	Trace	Trace	---	---		2	16	.1	100	.01	.01	.1	4
194	Pieces, diced	1 cup	100	94	15	1	Trace	---	---		4	39	.3	240	.03	.03	.3	9
195	Collards, cooked	1 cup	190	91	55	5	1	---	---		9	289	1.1	10,260	.27	.37	2.4	87
	Corn, sweet:																	
196	Cooked, ear 5 by 1¾ inches.[5]	1 ear	140	74	70	3	1	---	---		16	2	.5	[6]310	.09	.08	1.0	7
197	Canned, solids and liquid.	1 cup	256	81	170	5	2	---	---		40	10	1.0	[6]690	.07	.12	2.3	13
198	Cowpeas, cooked, immature seeds.	1 cup	160	72	175	13	1	---	---		29	38	3.4	560	.49	.18	2.3	28
	Cucumbers, 10-ounce; 7½ by about 2 inches:																	
199	Raw, pared	1 cucumber	207	96	30	1	Trace	---	---		7	35	.6	Trace	.07	.09	.4	23
200	Raw, pared, center slice ⅛-inch thick.	6 slices	50	96	5	Trace	Trace	---	---		2	8	.2	Trace	.02	.02	.1	6
201	Dandelion greens, cooked.	1 cup	180	90	60	4	1	---	---		12	252	3.2	21,060	.24	.29	---	32

[5] Measure and weight apply to entire vegetable or fruit including parts not usually eaten.

[6] Based on yellow varieties; white varieties contain only a trace of cryptoxanthin and carotenes, the pigments in corn that have biological activity.

TABLE A-6 NUTRITIVE VALUES OF THE EDIBLE PART OF FOODS — Continued

[Dashes in the columns for nutrients show that no suitable value could be found although there is reason to believe that a measurable amount of the nutrient may be present]

	Food, approximate measure, and weight (in grams)	Water	Food energy	Protein	Fat	Fatty acids Saturated (total)	Unsaturated Oleic	Unsaturated Linoleic	Carbohydrate	Calcium	Iron	Vitamin A value	Thiamin	Riboflavin	Niacin	Ascorbic acid
		Percent	Calories	Grams	Grams	Grams	Grams	Grams	Grams	Milligrams	Milligrams	International units	Milligrams	Milligrams	Milligrams	Milligrams
	VEGETABLES AND VEGETABLE PRODUCTS—Continued															
202	Endive, curly (including escarole). 2 ounces---- 57	93	10	1	Trace	----	----	----	2	46	1.0	1,870	0.04	0.08	0.3	6
203	Kale, leaves including stems, cooked. 1 cup------ 110	91	30	4	1	----	----	----	4	147	1.3	8,140	----	----	----	68
	Lettuce, raw:															
204	Butterhead, as Boston types; head, 4-inch diameter. 1 head------ 220	95	30	3	Trace	----	----	----	6	77	4.4	2,130	.14	.13	.6	18
205	Crisphead, as Iceberg; head, 4¾-inch diameter. 1 head---- 454	96	60	4	Trace	----	----	----	13	91	2.3	1,500	.29	.27	1.3	29
206	Looseleaf, or bunching varieties, leaves. 2 large------ 50	94	10	1	Trace	----	----	----	2	34	.7	950	.03	.04	.2	9
207	Mushrooms, canned, solids and liquid. 1 cup------ 244	93	40	5	Trace	----	----	----	6	15	1.2	Trace	.04	.60	4.8	4
208	Mustard greens, cooked-- 1 cup------ 140	93	35	3	1	----	----	----	6	193	2.5	8,120	.11	.19	.9	68
209	Okra, cooked, pod 3 by ⅝ inch. 8 pods------ 85	91	25	2	Trace	----	----	----	5	78	.4	420	.11	.15	.8	17
	Onions:															
	Mature:															
210	Raw, onion 2½-inch diameter. 1 onion------ 110	89	40	2	Trace	----	----	----	10	30	.6	40	.04	.04	.2	11
211	Cooked------ 1 cup------ 210	92	60	3	Trace	----	----	----	14	50	.8	80	.06	.06	.4	14
212	Young green, small, without tops. 6 onions------ 50	88	20	1	Trace	----	----	----	5	20	.3	Trace	.02	.02	.2	12
213	Parsley, raw, chopped-- 1 tablespoon_ 4	85	Trace	Trace	Trace	----	----	----	Trace	8	.2	340	Trace	.01	Trace	7
214	Parsnips, cooked------ 1 cup------ 155	82	100	2	1	----	----	----	23	70	.9	50	.11	.12	.2	16
	Peas, green:															
215	Cooked------ 1 cup------ 160	82	115	9	1	----	----	----	19	37	2.9	860	.44	.17	3.7	33
216	Canned, solids and liquid. 1 cup------ 249	83	165	9	1	----	----	----	31	50	4.2	1,120	.23	.13	2.2	22

No.	Food	Measure														
217	Canned, strained (baby food).	1 ounce	28	86	15	1	Trace	--	--	3	3	.4	140	.02	.02	.4	3
218	Peppers, hot, red, without seeds, dried (ground chili powder, added seasonings).	1 tablespoon	15	8	50	2	2	--	--	8	40	2.3	9,750	.03	.17	1.3	2
	Peppers, sweet: Raw, about 5 per pound:																
219	Green pod without stem and seeds.	1 pod	74	93	15	1	Trace	--	--	4	7	.5	310	.06	.06	.4	94
220	Cooked, boiled, drained	1 pod	73	95	15	1	Trace	--	--	3	7	.4	310	.05	.05	.4	70
	Potatoes, medium (about 3 per pound raw):																
221	Baked, peeled after baking.	1 potato	99	75	90	3	Trace	--	--	21	9	.7	Trace	.10	.04	1.7	20
	Boiled:																
222	Peeled after boiling	1 potato	136	80	105	3	Trace	--	--	23	10	.8	Trace	.13	.05	2.0	22
223	Peeled before boiling	1 potato	122	83	80	2	Trace	--	--	18	7	.6	Trace	.11	.04	1.4	20
	French-fried, piece 2 by ½ by ½ inch:																
224	Cooked in deep fat	10 pieces	57	45	155	2	7	2	2	20	9	.7	Trace	.07	.04	1.8	12
225	Frozen, heated	10 pieces	57	53	125	2	5	1	1	19	5	1.0	Trace	.08	.01	1.5	12
	Mashed:																
226	Milk added	1 cup	195	83	125	4	1	--	--	25	47	.8	50	.16	.10	2.0	19
227	Milk and butter added.	1 cup	195	80	185	4	8	4	3	24	47	.8	330	.16	.10	1.9	18
228	Potato chips, medium, 2-inch diameter.	10 chips	20	2	115	1	8	2	4	10	8	.4	Trace	.04	.01	1.0	3
229	Pumpkin, canned	1 cup	228	90	75	2	1	--	--	18	57	.9	14,590	.07	.12	1.3	12
230	Radishes, raw, small, without tops.	4 radishes	40	94	5	Trace	Trace	--	--	1	12	.4	Trace	.01	.01	.1	10
231	Sauerkraut, canned, solids and liquid.	1 cup	235	93	45	2	Trace	--	--	9	85	1.2	120	.07	.09	.4	33
	Spinach:																
232	Cooked	1 cup	180	92	40	5	1	--	--	6	167	4.0	14,580	.13	.25	1.0	50
233	Canned, drained solids	1 cup	180	91	45	5	1	--	--	6	212	4.7	14,400	.03	.21	.6	24
	Squash: Cooked:																
234	Summer, diced	1 cup	210	96	30	2	Trace	--	--	7	52	.8	820	.10	.16	1.6	21
235	Winter, baked, mashed.	1 cup	205	81	130	4	1	--	--	32	57	1.6	8,610	.10	.27	1.4	27
	Sweetpotatoes: Cooked, medium, 5 by 2 inches, weight raw about 6 ounces:																
236	Baked, peeled after baking.	1 sweet-potato	110	64	155	2	1	--	--	36	44	1.0	8,910	.10	.07	.7	24
237	Boiled, peeled after boiling.	1 sweet-potato	147	71	170	2	1	--	--	39	47	1.0	11,610	.13	.09	.9	25

TABLE A-6 NUTRITIVE VALUES OF THE EDIBLE PART OF FOODS — Continued

[Dashes in the columns for nutrients show that no suitable value could be found although there is reason to believe that a measurable amount of the nutrient may be present]

	Food, approximate measure, and weight (in grams)		Water	Food energy	Protein	Fat	Fatty acids			Carbohydrate	Calcium	Iron	Vitamin A value	Thiamin	Riboflavin	Niacin	Ascorbic acid
							Saturated (total)	Unsaturated									
								Oleic	Linoleic								
		Grams	Percent	Calories	Grams	Grams	Grams	Grams	Grams	Grams	Milligrams	Milligrams	International units	Milligrams	Milligrams	Milligrams	Milligrams
	VEGETABLES AND VEGETABLE PRODUCTS—Continued																
	Sweetpotatoes—Continued																
238	Candied, 3½ by 2¼ inches. 1 sweet-potato.	175	60	295	2	6	2	3	1	60	65	1.6	11,030	0.10	0.08	0.8	17
239	Canned, vacuum or solid pack. 1 cup	218	72	235	4	Trace				54	54	1.7	17,000	.10	.10	1.4	30
	Tomatoes:																
240	Raw, approx. 3-in. diam. 2⅛ in. high; wt, 7 oz. 1 tomato	200	94	40	2	Trace				9	24	.9	1,640	.11	.07	1.3	7 42
241	Canned, solids and liquid. 1 cup	241	94	50	2	1				10	14	1.2	2,170	.12	.07	1.7	41
	Tomato catsup:																
242	Cup. 1 cup	273	69	290	6	1				69	60	2.2	3,820	.25	.19	4.4	41
243	Tablespoon. 1 tbsp	15	69	15	Trace	Trace				4	3	.1	210	.01	.01	.2	2
	Tomato juice, canned:																
244	Cup. 1 cup	243	94	45	2	Trace				10	17	2.2	1,940	.12	.07	1.9	39
245	Glass (6 fl. oz.). 1 glass	182	94	35	2	Trace				8	13	1.6	1,460	.09	.05	1.5	29
246	Turnips, cooked, diced. 1 cup	155	94	35	1	Trace				8	54	.6	Trace	.06	.08	.5	34
247	Turnip greens, cooked. 1 cup	145	94	30	3	Trace				5	252	1.5	8,270	.15	.33	.7	68
	FRUITS AND FRUIT PRODUCTS																
248	Apples, raw (about 3 per lb.),5. 1 apple	150	85	70	Trace	Trace				18	8	.4	50	.04	.02	.1	3
249	Apple juice, bottled or canned. 1 cup	248	88	120	Trace	Trace				30	15	1.5		.02	.05	.2	2
	Applesauce, canned:																
250	Sweetened. 1 cup	255	76	230	1	Trace				61	10	1.3	100	.05	.03	.1	8 3
251	Unsweetened or artificially sweetened. 1 cup	244	88	100	1	Trace				26	10	1.2	100	.05	.02	.1	8 2

No.	Food, approximate measure, and weight (in grams)	Grams	Water (%)	Food energy	Protein	Fat	(Sat.)	(Oleic)	(Linoleic)	Carbo-hydrate	Calcium	Iron	Vitamin A	Thiamine	Riboflavin	Niacin	Ascorbic acid
	Apricots:																
252	Raw (about 12 per lb.) [5] 3 apricots----	114	85	55	1	Trace	---	---	---	14	18	.5	2,890	.03	.04	.7	10
253	Canned in heavy sirup-- 1 cup-------	259	77	220	2	Trace	---	---	---	57	28	.8	4,510	.05	.06	.9	10
254	Dried, uncooked (40 halves per cup). 1 cup-------	150	25	390	8	1	---	---	---	100	100	8.2	16,350	.02	.23	4.9	19
255	Cooked, unsweet-ened, fruit and liquid. 1 cup-------	285	76	240	5	1	---	---	---	62	63	5.1	8,550	.01	.13	2.8	8
256	Apricot nectar, canned--- 1 cup-------	251	85	140	1	Trace	---	---	---	37	23	.5	2,380	.03	.03	.5	[8] 8
	Avocados, whole fruit, raw: [5]																
257	California (mid- and late-winter; diam. 3⅛ in.). 1 avocado---	284	74	370	5	37	7	17	5	13	22	1.3	630	.24	.43	3.5	30
258	Florida (late summer, fall; diam. 3⅝ in.). 1 avocado---	454	78	390	4	33	7	15	4	27	30	1.8	880	.33	.61	4.9	43
259	Bananas, raw, medium size.[5] 1 banana---	175	76	100	1	Trace	---	---	---	26	10	.8	230	.06	.07	.8	12
260	Banana flakes-------- 1 cup-------	100	3	340	4	1	---	---	---	89	32	2.8	760	.18	.24	2.8	7
261	Blackberries, raw----- 1 cup-------	144	84	85	2	1	---	---	---	19	46	1.3	290	.05	.06	.5	30
262	Blueberries, raw------ 1 cup-------	140	83	85	1	1	---	---	---	21	21	1.4	140	.04	.08	.6	20
263	Cantaloups, raw; medium, 5-inch diameter about 1⅔ pounds.[5] ½ melon---	385	91	60	1	Trace	---	---	---	14	27	.8	[9] 6,540	.08	.06	1.2	63
264	Cherries, canned, red, sour, pitted, water pack. 1 cup-------	244	88	105	2	Trace	---	---	---	26	37	.7	1,660	.07	.05	.5	12
265	Cranberry juice cocktail, canned. 1 cup-------	250	83	165	Trace	Trace	---	---	---	42	13	.8	Trace	.03	.03	.1	[10] 40
266	Cranberry sauce, sweet-ened, canned, strained. 1 cup-------	277	62	405	Trace	1	---	---	---	104	17	.6	60	.03	.03	.1	6
267	Dates, pitted, cut------ 1 cup-------	178	22	490	4	1	---	---	---	130	105	5.3	90	.16	.17	3.9	0
268	Figs, dried, large, 2 by 1 in. 1 fig-------	21	23	60	1	Trace	---	---	---	15	26	.6	20	.02	.02	.1	0
269	Fruit cocktail, canned, in heavy sirup. 1 cup-------	256	80	195	1	Trace	---	---	---	50	23	1.0	360	.05	.03	1.3	5

[5] Measure and weight apply to entire vegetable or fruit including parts not usually eaten.

[7] Year-round average. Samples marketed from November through May, average 20 milligrams per 200-gram tomato; from June through October, around 52 milli-grams.

[8] This is the amount from the fruit. Additional ascorbic acid may be added by the manufacturer. Refer to the label for this information.

[9] Value for varieties with orange-colored flesh; value for varieties with green flesh would be about 540 I.U.

[10] Value listed is based on products with label stating 30 milligrams per 6 fl. oz. serving.

TABLE A-6   NUTRITIVE VALUES OF THE EDIBLE PART OF FOODS — Continued

[Dashes in the columns for nutrients show that no suitable value could be found although there is reason to believe that a measurable amount of the nutrient may be present]

	Food, approximate measure, and weight (in grams)	Water	Food energy	Protein	Fat	Fatty acids			Carbohydrate	Calcium	Iron	Vitamin A value	Thiamin	Riboflavin	Niacin	Ascorbic acid
						Saturated (total)	Unsaturated									
							Oleic	Linoleic								
		Percent	Calories	Grams	Grams	Grams	Grams	Grams	Grams	Milligrams	Milligrams	International units	Milligrams	Milligrams	Milligrams	Milligrams
		Grams														

FRUITS AND FRUIT PRODUCTS—Con.

Grapefruit:
Raw, medium, 3¾-in. diam.[5]

	Food	Grams	Water	Food energy	Protein	Fat	Saturated	Oleic	Linoleic	Carbohydrate	Calcium	Iron	Vitamin A	Thiamin	Riboflavin	Niacin	Ascorbic acid
270	White -- ½ grapefruit.	241	89	45	1	Trace	---	---	---	12	19	0.5	10	0.05	0.02	0.2	44
271	Pink or red -- ½ grapefruit.	241	89	50	1	Trace	---	---	---	13	20	0.5	540	0.05	0.02	0.2	44
272	Canned, sirup pack -- 1 cup	254	81	180	2	Trace	---	---	---	45	33	.8	30	.08	.05	.5	76
	Grapefruit juice:																
273	Fresh -- 1 cup	246	90	95	1	Trace	---	---	---	23	22	.5	(11)	.09	.04	.4	92
	Canned, white:																
274	Unsweetened -- 1 cup	247	89	100	1	Trace	---	---	---	24	20	1.0	20	.07	.04	.4	84
275	Sweetened -- 1 cup	250	86	130	1	Trace	---	---	---	32	20	1.0	20	.07	.04	.4	78
	Frozen, concentrate, unsweetened:																
276	Undiluted, can, 6 fluid ounces.	207	62	300	4	1	---	---	---	72	70	.8	60	.29	.12	1.4	286
277	Diluted with 3 parts water, by volume.	247	89	100	1	Trace	---	---	---	24	25	.2	20	.10	.04	.5	96
278	Dehydrated crystals -- 4 oz	113	1	410	6	1	---	---	---	102	100	1.2	80	.40	.20	2.0	396
279	Prepared with water 1 cup (1 pound yields about 1 gallon).	247	90	100	1	Trace	---	---	---	24	22	.2	20	.10	.05	.5	91
	Grapes, raw:[5]																
280	American type (slip skin). 1 cup	153	82	65	1	1	---	---	---	15	15	.4	100	.05	.03	.2	3
281	European type (adherent skin). 1 cup	160	81	95	1	Trace	---	---	---	25	17	.6	140	.07	.04	.4	6
	Grapejuice:																
282	Canned or bottled -- 1 cup	253	83	165	1	Trace	---	---	---	42	28	.8	---	.10	.05	.5	Trace
	Frozen concentrate, sweetened:																
283	Undiluted, can, 6 fluid ounces.	216	53	395	1	Trace	---	---	---	100	22	.9	40	.13	.22	1.5	(12)

No.	Food	Measure	Weight (g)	Water (%)	Food energy (Cal.)	Protein (g)	Fat (g)	Saturated fatty acids (g)	Unsat. oleic (g)	Unsat. linoleic (g)	Carbohydrate (g)	Calcium (mg)	Iron (mg)	Vitamin A (I.U.)	Thiamine (mg)	Riboflavin (mg)	Niacin (mg)	Ascorbic acid (mg)
284	Diluted with 3 parts water, by volume.	1 cup	250	86	135	1	Trace	---	---	---	33	8	.3	10	.05	.08	.5	(12)
285	Grapejuice drink, canned.	1 cup	250	86	135	Trace	Trace	---	---	---	35	8	.3	---	.03	.03	.3	(12)
286	Lemons, raw, 2⅛-in. diam., size 165.⁵ Used for juice.	1 lemon	110	90	20	1	Trace	---	---	---	6	19	.4	10	.03	.01	.1	39
287	Lemon juice, raw.	1 cup	244	91	60	1	Trace	---	---	---	20	17	.5	50	.07	.02	.2	112
	Lemonade concentrate:																	
288	Frozen, 6 fl. oz. per can.	1 can	219	48	430	Trace	Trace	---	---	---	112	9	.4	40	.04	.07	.7	66
289	Diluted with 4⅓ parts water, by volume.	1 cup	248	88	110	Trace	Trace	---	---	---	28	2	Trace	Trace	Trace	.02	.2	17
	Lime juice:																	
290	Fresh.	1 cup	246	90	65	1	Trace	---	---	---	22	22	.5	20	.05	.02	.2	79
291	Canned, unsweetened.	1 cup	246	90	65	1	Trace	---	---	---	22	22	.5	20	.05	.02	.2	52
	Limeade concentrate, frozen:																	
292	Undiluted, can, 6 fluid ounces.	1 can	218	50	410	Trace	Trace	---	---	---	108	11	.2	Trace	.02	.02	.2	26
293	Diluted with 4⅓ parts water, by volume.	1 cup	247	90	100	Trace	Trace	---	---	---	27	2	Trace	Trace	Trace	Trace	Trace	5
294	Oranges, raw, 2⅝-in. diam., all commercial varieties.⁵	1 orange	180	86	65	1	Trace	---	---	---	16	54	.5	260	.13	.05	.5	66
295	Orange juice, fresh, all varieties.	1 cup	248	88	110	2	1	---	---	---	26	27	.5	500	.22	.07	1.0	124
296	Canned, unsweetened.	1 cup	249	87	120	2	Trace	---	---	---	28	25	1.0	500	.17	.05	.7	100
	Frozen concentrate:																	
297	Undiluted, can, 6 fluid ounces.	1 can	213	55	360	5	Trace	---	---	---	87	75	.9	1,620	.68	.11	2.8	360
298	Diluted with 3 parts water, by volume.	1 cup	249	87	120	2	Trace	---	---	---	29	25	.2	550	.22	.02	1.0	120
299	Dehydrated crystals.	4 oz.	113	1	430	6	2	---	---	---	100	95	1.9	1,900	.76	.24	3.3	408
300	Prepared with water (1 pound yields about 1 gallon).	1 cup	248	88	115	2	1	---	---	---	27	25	.5	500	.20	.07	1.0	109
301	Orange-apricot juice drink.	1 cup	249	87	125	1	Trace	---	---	---	32	12	.2	1,440	.05	.02	.5	¹⁰ 40

⁵ Measure and weight apply to entire vegetable or fruit including parts not usually eaten.

¹⁰ Value listed is based on product with label stating 30 milligrams per 6 fl. oz. serving.

¹¹ For white-fleshed varieties value is about 20 I.U. per cup; for red-fleshed varieties, 1,080 I.U. per cup.

¹² Present only if added by the manufacturer. Refer to the label for this information.

TABLE A-6   NUTRITIVE VALUES OF THE EDIBLE PART OF FOODS — Continued

[Dashes in the columns for nutrients show that no suitable value could be found although there is reason to believe that a measurable amount of the nutrient may be present]

	Food, approximate measure, and weight (in grams)		Water	Food energy	Protein	Fat	Fatty acids			Carbohydrate	Calcium	Iron	Vitamin A value	Thiamin	Riboflavin	Niacin	Ascorbic acid
							Saturated (total)	Unsaturated									
								Oleic	Linoleic								
		Grams	Percent	Calories	Grams	Grams	Grams	Grams	Grams	Grams	Milligrams	Milligrams	International units	Milligrams	Milligrams	Milligrams	Milligrams
	FRUITS AND FRUIT PRODUCTS—Con.																
	Orange and grapefruit juice:																
	Frozen concentrate:																
302	Undiluted, can, 6 fluid ounces. 1 can------	210	59	330	4	1				78	61	0.8	800	0.48	0.06	2.3	302
303	Diluted with 3 parts water, by volume. 1 cup------	248	88	110	1	Trace				26	20	.2	270	.16	.02	.8	102
304	Papayas, raw, ½-inch cubes. 1 cup------	182	89	70	1	Trace				18	36	.5	3,190	.07	.08	.5	102
	Peaches:																
	Raw:																
305	Whole, medium, 2-inch diameter, about 4 per pound.[5] 1 peach-----	114	89	35	1	Trace				10	9	.5	[11]1,320	.02	.05	1.0	7
306	Sliced------------- 1 cup------	168	89	65	1	Trace				16	15	.8	[12]2,230	.03	.08	1.6	12
	Canned, yellow-fleshed, solids and liquid:																
	Sirup pack, heavy:																
307	Halves or slices--- 1 cup------	257	79	200	1	Trace				52	10	.8	1,100	.02	.06	1.4	7
308	Water pack-------- 1 cup------	245	91	75	1	Trace				20	10	.7	1,100	.02	.06	1.4	7
309	Dried, uncooked---- 1 cup------	160	25	420	5	1				109	77	9.6	6,240	.02	.31	8.5	28
310	Cooked, unsweetened, 10-12 halves and juice. 1 cup------	270	77	220	3	1				58	41	5.1	3,290	.01	.15	4.2	6
	Frozen:																
311	Carton, 12 ounces, not thawed. 1 carton----	340	76	300	1	Trace				77	14	1.7	2,210	.03	.14	2.4	[14]135
	Pears:																
312	Raw, 3 by 2½-inch diameter.[5] 1 pear------	182	83	100	1	1				25	13	.5	30	.04	.07	.2	7
	Canned, solids and liquid:																
	Sirup pack, heavy:																
313	Halves or slices---- 1 cup------	255	80	195	1	1				50	13	.5	Trace	.03	.05	.3	4

No.	Food	Measure	Weight (g)	Water (%)	Food energy	Protein	Fat		Carbohydrate	Calcium	Iron	Vitamin A (I.U.)	Thiamine	Riboflavin	Niacin	Ascorbic acid
314	Pineapple: Raw, diced	1 cup	140	85	75	1	Trace	---	19	24	.7	100	.12	.04	.3	24
	Canned, heavy sirup pack, solids and liquid:															
315	Crushed	1 cup	260	80	195	1	Trace	---	50	29	.8	120	.20	.06	.5	17
316	Sliced, slices and juice	2 small or 1 large	122	80	90	Trace	Trace	---	24	13	.4	50	.09	.03	.2	8
317	Pineapple juice, canned	1 cup	249	86	135	1	Trace	---	34	37	.7	120	.12	.04	.5	[8]22
	Plums, all except prunes:															
318	Raw, 2-inch diameter, 1 plum about 2 ounces.[5]	1 plum	60	87	25	Trace	Trace	---	7	7	.3	140	.02	.02	.3	3
	Canned, sirup pack (Italian prunes):															
319	Plums (with pits) and juice.[5]	1 cup	256	77	205	1	Trace	---	53	22	2.2	2,970	.05	.05	.9	4
	Prunes, dried, "softenized", medium:															
320	Uncooked[5]	4 prunes	32	28	70	1	Trace	---	18	14	1.1	440	.02	.04	.4	1
321	Cooked, unsweetened, 17–18 prunes and ⅓ cup liquid.[5]	1 cup	270	66	295	2	1	---	78	60	4.5	1,860	.08	.18	1.7	2
322	Prune juice, canned or bottled.	1 cup	256	80	200	1	Trace	---	49	36	10.5	---	.03	.03	1.0	[8]5
	Raisins, seedless:															
323	Packaged, ½ oz. or 1½ tbsp. per pkg.	1 pkg	14	18	40	Trace	Trace	---	11	9	.5	Trace	.02	.01	.1	Trace
324	Cup, pressed down	1 cup	165	18	480	4	Trace	---	128	102	5.8	30	.18	.13	.8	2
	Raspberries, red:															
325	Raw	1 cup	123	84	70	1	1	---	17	27	1.1	160	.04	.11	1.1	31
326	Frozen, 10-ounce carton, not thawed.	1 carton	284	74	275	2	1	---	70	37	1.7	200	.06	.17	1.7	59
327	Rhubarb, cooked, sugar added.	1 cup	272	63	385	1	Trace	---	98	212	1.6	220	.06	.15	.7	17
	Strawberries:															
328	Raw, capped	1 cup	149	90	55	1	1	---	13	31	1.5	90	.04	.10	1.0	88
329	Frozen, 10-ounce carton, not thawed.	1 carton	284	71	310	1	1	---	79	40	2.0	90	.06	.17	1.5	150
330	Tangerines, raw, medium, 2⅜-in. diam., size 176.[5]	1 tangerine	116	87	40	1	Trace	---	10	34	.3	360	.05	.02	.1	27
331	Tangerine juice, canned, sweetened.	1 cup	249	87	125	1	1	---	30	45	.5	1,050	.15	.05	.2	55
332	Watermelon, raw, wedge, 4 by 8 inches (1/16 of 10 by 16-inch melon, about 2 pounds with rind).[5]	1 wedge	925	93	115	2	1	---	27	30	2.1	2,510	.13	.13	.7	30

[5] Measure and weight apply to entire vegetable or fruit including parts not usually eaten.

[8] This is the amount from the fruit. Additional ascorbic acid may be added by the manufacturer. Refer to the label for this information.

[13] Based on yellow-fleshed varieties; for white-fleshed varieties value is about 50 I.U. per 114-gram peach and 80 I.U. per cup of sliced peaches.

[14] This value includes ascorbic acid added by manufacturer.

TABLE A-6 NUTRITIVE VALUES OF THE EDIBLE PART OF FOODS — Continued

[Dashes in the columns for nutrients show that no suitable value could be found although there is reason to believe that a measurable amount of the nutrient may be present]

	Food, approximate measure, and weight (in grams)		Water	Food energy	Protein	Fat	Fatty acids			Carbo-hy-drate	Cal-cium	Iron	Vita-min A value	Thia-min	Ribo-flavin	Niacin	Ascor-bic acid
							Satu-rated (total)	Unsaturated									
								Oleic	Lin-oleic								
		Grams	Percent	Calories	Grams	Grams	Grams	Grams	Grams	Grams	Milligrams	Milligrams	International units	Milligrams	Milligrams	Milligrams	Milligrams
	GRAIN PRODUCTS																
	Bagel, 3-in. diam.:																
333	Egg ------- 1 bagel -------	55	32	165	6	2	---	---	---	28	9	1.2	30	0.14	0.10	1.2	0
334	Water ------- 1 bagel -------	55	29	165	6	2	---	---	---	30	8	1.2	0	.15	.11	1.4	0
335	Barley, pearled, light, uncooked. 1 cup -------	200	11	700	16	2	Trace	1	1	158	32	4.0	0	.24	.10	6.2	0
336	Biscuits, baking powder from home recipe with enriched flour, 2-in. diam. 1 biscuit -------	28	27	105	2	5	1	2	1	13	34	.4	Trace	.06	.06	.1	Trace
337	Biscuits, baking powder from mix, 2-in. diam. 1 biscuit -------	28	28	90	2	3	1	1	1	15	19	.6	Trace	.08	.07	.6	Trace
338	Bran flakes (40% bran), added thiamin and iron. 1 cup -------	35	3	105	4	1	---	---	---	28	25	12.3	0	.14	.06	2.2	0
339	Bran flakes with raisins, added thiamin and iron. 1 cup -------	50	7	145	4	1	---	---	---	40	28	13.5	Trace	.16	.07	2.7	0
	Breads:																
340	Boston brown bread, slice 3 by ¾ in. 1 slice -------	48	45	100	3	1	---	---	---	22	43	.9	0	.05	.03	.6	0
	Cracked-wheat bread:																
341	Loaf, 1 lb. ------- 1 loaf -------	454	35	1,190	40	10	2	5	2	236	399	5.0	Trace	.53	.41	5.9	Trace
342	Slice, 18 slices per loaf. 1 slice -------	25	35	65	2	1	---	---	---	13	22	.3	Trace	.03	.02	.3	Trace
	French or vienna bread:																
343	Enriched, 1 lb. loaf. 1 loaf -------	454	31	1,315	41	14	3	8	2	251	195	10.0	Trace	1.27	1.00	11.3	Trace
344	Unenriched, 1 lb. loaf. 1 loaf -------	454	31	1,315	41	14	3	8	2	251	195	3.2	Trace	.36	.36	3.6	Trace
	Italian bread:																
345	Enriched, 1 lb. loaf. 1 loaf -------	454	32	1,250	41	4	Trace	1	2	256	77	10.0	0	1.32	.91	11.8	0
346	Unenriched, 1 lb. loaf. 1 loaf -------	454	32	1,250	41	4	Trace	1	2	256	77	3.2	0	.41	.27	3.6	0
	Raisin bread:																
347	Loaf, 1 lb. ------- 1 loaf -------	454	35	1,190	30	13	3	8	2	243	322	5.9	Trace	.23	.41	3.2	Trace

No.	Food	Measure																	
348	Slice, 18 slices per loaf.	1 slice	25	35	65	2	1				13	18	.3	Trace	.01	.02	.2	Trace
	Rye bread:																	
	American, light (⅓ rye, ⅔ wheat):																	
349	Loaf, 1 lb.	1 loaf	454	36	1,100	41	5				236	340	7.3	0	.82	.32	6.4	0
350	Slice, 18 slices per loaf.	1 slice	25	36	60	2	Trace				13	19	.4	0	.05	.02	.4	0
351	Pumpernickel, loaf, 1 lb.	1 loaf	454	34	1,115	41	5				241	381	10.9	0	1.04	.64	5.4	0
	White bread, enriched:[15]																	
	Soft-crumb type:																	
352	Loaf, 1 lb.	1 loaf	454	36	1,225	39	15	3	8	2	229	381	11.3	Trace	1.13	.95	10.9	Trace
353	Slice, 18 slices per loaf.	1 slice	25	36	70	2	1				13	21	.6	Trace	.06	.05	.6	Trace
354	Slice, toasted.	1 slice	22	25	70	2	1				13	21	.6	Trace	.06	.05	.6	Trace
355	Slice, 22 slices per loaf.	1 slice	20	36	55	2	1				10	17	.5	Trace	.05	.04	.5	Trace
356	Slice, toasted.	1 slice	17	25	55	2	1				10	17	.5	Trace	.05	.04	.5	Trace
357	Loaf, 1½ lbs.	1 loaf	680	36	1,835	59	22	5	12	3	343	571	17.0	Trace	1.70	1.43	16.3	Trace
358	Slice, 24 slices per loaf.	1 slice	28	36	75	2	1				14	24	.7	Trace	.07	.06	.7	Trace
359	Slice, toasted.	1 slice	24	25	75	2	1				14	24	.7	Trace	.07	.06	.7	Trace
360	Slice, 28 slices per loaf.	1 slice	24	36	65	2	1				12	20	.6	Trace	.06	.05	.6	Trace
361	Slice, toasted.	1 slice	21	25	65	2	1				12	20	.6	Trace	.06	.05	.6	Trace
	Firm-crumb type:																	
362	Loaf, 1 lb.	1 loaf	454	35	1,245	41	17	4	10	2	228	435	11.3	Trace	1.22	.91	10.9	Trace
363	Slice, 20 slices per loaf.	1 slice	23	35	65	2	1				12	22	.6	Trace	.06	.05	.6	Trace
364	Slice, toasted.	1 slice	20	24	65	2	1				12	22	.6	Trace	.06	.05	.6	Trace
365	Loaf, 2 lbs.	1 loaf	907	35	2,495	82	34	8	20	4	455	871	22.7	Trace	2.45	1.81	21.8	Trace
366	Slice, 34 slices per loaf.	1 slice	27	35	75	2	1				14	26	.7	Trace	.07	.05	.6	Trace
367	Slice, toasted.	1 slice	23	35	75	2	1				14	26	.7	Trace	.07	.05	.6	Trace
	Whole-wheat bread, soft-crumb type:																	
368	Loaf, 1 lb.	1 loaf	454	36	1,095	41	12	2	6	2	224	381	13.6	Trace	1.36	.45	12.7	Trace
369	Slice, 16 slices per loaf.	1 slice	28	36	65	3	1				14	24	.8	Trace	.09	.03	.8	Trace
370	Slice, toasted.	1 slice	24	24	65	3	1				14	24	.8	Trace	.09	.03	.8	Trace

[15] Values for iron, thiamin, riboflavin, and niacin per pound of unenriched white bread would be as follows:

	Iron Milligrams	Thiamin Milligrams	Riboflavin Milligrams	Niacin Milligrams
Soft crumb	3.2	.31	.39	5.0
Firm crumb	3.2	.32	.59	4.1

TABLE A-6 NUTRITIVE VALUES OF THE EDIBLE PART OF FOODS – Continued

[Dashes in the columns for nutrients show that no suitable value could be found although there is reason to believe that a measurable amount of the nutrient may be present]

	Food, approximate measure, and weight (in grams)		Water	Food energy	Pro-tein	Fat	Fatty acids			Carbo-hy-drate	Cal-cium	Iron	Vita-min A value	Thia-min	Ribo-flavin	Niacin	Ascor-bic acid
							Satu-rated (total)	Unsaturated									
								Oleic	Lin-oleic								
		Grams	Per-cent	Calo-ries	Grams	Grams	Grams	Grams	Grams	Grams	Milli-grams	Milli-grams	Inter-national units	Milli-grams	Milli-grams	Milli-grams	Milli-grams
	GRAIN PRODUCTS—Continued																
	Bread—Continued																
	Whole-wheat bread, firm-crumb type:																
371	Loaf, 1 lb._____ 1 loaf____	454	36	1,100	48	14	3	6	3	216	449	13.6	Trace	1.18	0.54	12.7	Trace
372	Slice, 18 slices per loaf. 1 slice_____	25	36	60	3	1	—	—	—	12	25	.8	Trace	.06	.03	.7	Trace
373	Slice, toasted_____ 1 slice_____	21	24	60	3	1	—	—	—	12	25	.8	Trace	.06	.03	.7	Trace
374	Breadcrumbs, dry, grated_ 1 cup_____	100	6	390	13	5	1	2	1	73	122	3.6	Trace	.22	.30	3.5	Trace
375	Buckwheat flour, light, sifted. 1 cup_____	98	12	340	6	1	—	—	—	78	11	1.0	0	.08	.04	.4	0
376	Bulgur, canned, seasoned_ 1 cup____	135	56	245	8	4				44	27	1.9	0	.08	.05	4.1	0
	Cakes made from cake mixes:																
	Angelfood:																
377	Whole cake_____ 1 cake_____	635	34	1,645	36	1	—	—	—	377	603	1.9	0	.03	.70	.6	0
378	Piece, ½ of 10-in. diam. cake. 1 piece_____	53	34	135	3	Trace	—	—	—	32	50	.2	0	Trace	.06	.1	0
	Cupcakes, small, 2½ in. diam.:																
379	Without icing_____ 1 cupcake__	25	26	90	1	3	1	1	1	14	40	.1	40	.01	.03	.1	Trace
380	With chocolate icing_ 1 cupcake__	36	22	130	2	5	2	2	1	21	47	.3	60	.01	.04	.1	Trace
	Devil's food, 2-layer, with chocolate icing:																
381	Whole cake_____1 cake_____	1,107	24	3,755	49	136	54	58	16	645	653	8.9	1,660	.33	.89	3.3	1
382	Piece, ⅟16 of 9-in. diam. cake. 1 piece_____	69	24	235	3	9	3	4	1	40	41	.6	100	.02	.06	.2	Trace
383	Cupcake, small, 2½ in. diam. 1 cupcake___	35	24	120	2	4	1	2	Trace	20	21	.3	50	.01	.03	.1	Trace
	Gingerbread:																
384	Whole cake_____ 1 cake_____	570	37	1,575	18	39	10	19	9	291	513	9.1	Trace	.17	.51	4.6	2
385	Piece, ⅑ of 8-in. square cake. 1 piece_____	63	37	175	2	4	1	2	1	32	57	1.0	Trace	.02	.06	.5	Trace
	White, 2-layer, with chocolate icing:																
386	Whole cake_____1 cake_____	1,140	21	4,000	45	122	45	54	17	716	1,129	5.7	680	.23	.91	2.3	2

No.	Food	Measure																
387	Piece, 1/6 of 9-in. diam. cake.	1 piece	71	21	250	3	8	3	3	1	45	70	.4	40	.01	.06	.1	Trace
	Cakes made from home recipes:[16]																	
388	Boston cream pie; piece 1/12 of 8-in. diam.	1 piece	69	35	210	4	6	2	2	1	34	46	.3	140	.02	.08	.1	Trace
	Fruitcake, dark, made with enriched flour:																	
389	Loaf, 1-lb.	1 loaf	454	18	1,720	22	69	15	37	13	271	327	11.8	540	.59	.64	3.6	2
390	Slice, 1/30 of 8-in. loaf.	1 slice	15	18	55	1	2	Trace	1	Trace	9	11	.4	20	.02	.02	.1	Trace
	Plain sheet cake: Without icing:																	
391	Whole cake.	1 cake	777	25	2,830	35	108	30	52	21	434	497	3.1	1,320	.16	.70	1.6	2
392	Piece, 1/9 of 9-in. square cake.	1 piece	86	25	315	4	12	3	6	2	48	55	.3	150	.02	.08	.2	Trace
393	With boiled white icing, piece, 1/9 of 9-in. square cake.	1 piece	114	23	400	4	12	3	6	2	71	56	.3	150	.02	.08	.2	Trace
	Pound:																	
394	Loaf, 8½ by 3½ by 3 in.	1 loaf	514	17	2,430	29	152	34	68	17	242	108	4.1	1,440	.15	.46	1.0	0
395	Slice, ½-in. thick.	1 slice	30	17	140	2	9	2	4	1	14	6	.2	80	.01	.03	.1	0
	Sponge:																	
396	Whole cake.	1 cake	790	32	2,345	60	45	14	20	4	427	237	9.5	3,560	.40	1.11	1.6	Trace
397	Piece, 1/12 of 10-in. diam. cake.	1 piece	66	32	195	5	4	1	2	Trace	36	20	.8	300	.03	.09	.1	Trace
	Yellow, 2-layer, without icing:																	
398	Whole cake.	1 cake	870	24	3,160	39	111	31	53	22	506	618	3.5	1,310	.17	.70	1.7	2
399	Piece, 1/16 of 9-in. diam. cake.	1 piece	54	24	200	2	7	2	3	1	32	39	.2	80	.01	.04	.1	Trace
	Yellow, 2-layer, with chocolate icing:																	
400	Whole cake.	1 cake	1,203	21	4,390	51	156	55	69	23	727	818	7.2	1,920	.24	.96	2.4	Trace
401	Piece, 1/16 of 9-in. diam. cake.	1 piece	75	21	275	3	10	3	4	1	45	51	.5	120	.02	.06	.2	Trace
	Cake icings. See Sugars, Sweets.																	
	Cookies: Brownies with nuts:																	
402	Made from home recipe with enriched flour.	1 brownie	20	10	95	1	6	1	3	1	10	8	.4	40	.04	.02	.1	Trace
403	Made from mix.	1 brownie	20	11	85	1	4	1	2	1	13	9	.4	20	.03	.02	.1	Trace

[16] Unenriched cake flour used unless otherwise specified.

TABLE A-6   NUTRITIVE VALUES OF THE EDIBLE PART OF FOODS — Continued

[Dashes in the columns for nutrients show that no suitable value could be found although there is reason to believe that a measurable amount of the nutrient may be present]

	Food, approximate measure, and weight (in grams)		Water	Food energy	Protein	Fat	Fatty acids			Carbohydrate	Calcium	Iron	Vitamin A value	Thiamin	Riboflavin	Niacin	Ascorbic acid
							Saturated (total)	Unsaturated									
								Oleic	Linoleic								
		Grams	Percent	Calories	Grams	Grams	Grams	Grams	Grams	Grams	Milligrams	Milligrams	International units	Milligrams	Milligrams	Milligrams	Milligrams
	GRAIN PRODUCTS—Continued																
	Cookies—Continued																
	Chocolate chip:																
404	Made from home recipe with enriched flour. 1 cookie	10	3	50	1	3	1	1	1	6	4	0.2	10	0.01	0.01	0.1	Trace
405	Commercial. 1 cookie	10	3	50	1	2	1	1	Trace	7	4	.2	10	Trace	Trace	Trace	Trace
406	Fig bars, commercial. 1 cookie	14	14	50	1	1				11	11	.2	20	Trace	.01	.1	Trace
407	Sandwich, chocolate or vanilla, commercial. 1 cookie	10	2	50	1	2	1	1	Trace	7	2	.1	0	Trace	Trace	.1	0
	Corn flakes, added nutrients:																
408	Plain. 1 cup	25	4	100	2	Trace				21	4	.4	0	.11	.02	.5	0
409	Sugar-covered. 1 cup	40	2	155	2	Trace				36	5	.4	0	.16	.02	.8	0
	Corn (hominy) grits, degermed, cooked:																
410	Enriched. 1 cup	245	87	125	3	Trace				27	2	.7	[17]150	.10	.07	1.0	0
411	Unenriched. 1 cup	245	87	125	3	Trace				27	2	.2	[17]150	.05	.02	.5	0
	Cornmeal:																
412	Whole-ground, unbolted, dry. 1 cup	122	12	435	11	5	1	2	2	90	24	2.9	[17]620	.46	.13	2.4	0
413	Bolted (nearly whole-grain) dry. 1 cup	122	12	440	11	4	Trace	1	2	91	21	2.2	[17]590	.37	.10	2.3	0
	Degermed, enriched:																
414	Dry form. 1 cup	138	12	500	11	2				108	8	4.0	[17]610	.61	.36	4.8	0
415	Cooked. 1 cup	240	88	120	3	1				26	2	1.0	[17]140	.14	.10	1.2	0
	Degermed, unenriched:																
416	Dry form. 1 cup	138	12	500	11	2				108	8	1.5	[17]610	.19	.07	1.4	0
417	Cooked. 1 cup	240	88	120	3	1				26	2	.5	[17]140	.05	.02	.2	0
418	Corn muffins, made with enriched degermed cornmeal and enriched flour; muffin 2⅜-in. diam. 1 muffin	40	33	125	3	4	2	2	Trace	19	42	.7	[17]120	.08	.09	.6	Trace

No.	Food, approximate measure, and weight (in grams)	Measure	Grams	Water (%)	Food energy (cal.)	Protein (g)	Fat (g)	Saturated fat (g)	Oleic (g)	Linoleic (g)	Carbohydrate (g)	Calcium (mg)	Iron (mg)	Vitamin A (I.U.)	Thiamin (mg)	Riboflavin (mg)	Niacin (mg)	Ascorbic acid (mg)
419	Corn muffins, made with mix, egg, and milk; muffin 2⅜-in. diam.	1 muffin-----	40	30	130	3	4	1	2	1	20	96	.6	100	.07	.08	.6	Trace
420	Corn, puffed, presweetened, added nutrients.	1 cup-------	30	2	115	1	Trace	-----	-----	27	3	.5	0	.13	.05	.6	0
421	Corn, shredded, added nutrients.	1 cup-------	25	3	100	2	Trace	-----	-----	22	1	.6	0	.11	.05	.5	0
	Crackers:																	
422	Graham, 2½-in. square.	4 crackers---	28	6	110	2	3	-----	-----	21	11	.4	0	.01	.06	.4	0
423	Saltines.	4 crackers---	11	4	50	1	1	-----	-----	8	2	.1	0	Trace	Trace	.1	0
	Danish pastry, plain (without fruit or nuts):																	
424	Packaged ring, 12 ounces.	1 ring-------	340	22	1,435	25	80	24	37	15	155	170	3.1	1,050	.24	.51	2.7	Trace
425	Round piece, approx. 4¼-in. diam. by 1 in.	1 pastry-----	65	22	275	5	15	5	7	3	30	33	.6	200	.05	.10	.5	Trace
426	Ounce.	1 oz-------	28	22	120	2	7	2	3	1	13	14	.3	90	.02	.04	.3	Trace
427	Doughnuts, cake type.	1 doughnut---	32	24	125	1	6	1	4	Trace	16	13	18.4	30	18.05	18.05	18.4	Trace
428	Farina, quick-cooking, enriched, cooked.	1 cup-------	245	89	105	3	Trace	-----	-----	22	147	19.7	0	19.12	19.07	191.0	0
	Macaroni, cooked:																	
	Enriched:																	
429	Cooked, firm stage (undergoes additional cooking in a food mixture).	1 cup-------	130	64	190	6	1	-----	-----	39	14	191.4	0	19.23	19.14	191.8	0
430	Cooked until tender.	1 cup-------	140	72	155	5	1	-----	-----	32	8	191.3	0	19.20	19.11	191.5	0
	Unenriched:																	
431	Cooked, firm stage (undergoes additional cooking in a food mixture).	1 cup-------	130	64	190	6	1	-----	-----	39	14	.7	0	.03	.03	.5	0
432	Cooked until tender.	1 cup-------	140	72	155	5	1	-----	-----	32	11	.6	0	.01	.01	.4	0
433	Macaroni (enriched) and cheese, baked.	1 cup-------	200	58	430	17	22	10	9	2	40	362	1.8	860	.20	.40	1.8	Trace
434	Canned.	1 cup-------	240	80	230	9	10	4	3	1	26	199	1.0	260	.12	.24	1.0	Trace
435	Muffins, with enriched white flour; muffin, 3-inch diam.	1 muffin ----	40	38	120	3	4	1	2	1	17	42	.6	40	.07	.09	.6	Trace
	Noodles (egg noodles), cooked:																	
436	Enriched.	1 cup-------	160	70	200	7	2	1	1	Trace	37	16	191.4	110	19.22	19.13	191.9	0
437	Unenriched.	1 cup-------	160	70	200	7	2	1	1	Trace	37	16	1.0	110	.05	.03	.6	0

[17] This value is based on product made from yellow varieties of corn; white varieties contain only a trace.

[18] Based on product made with enriched flour. With unenriched flour, approximate values per doughnut are: Iron, 0.2 milligram; thiamin, 0.01 milligram; riboflavin, 0.03 milligram; niacin, 0.2 milligram.

[19] Iron, thiamin, riboflavin, and niacin are based on the minimum levels of enrichment specified in standards of identity promulgated under the Federal Food, Drug, and Cosmetic Act.

TABLE A-6 NUTRITIVE VALUES OF THE EDIBLE PART OF FOODS — Continued

[Dashes in the columns for nutrients show that no suitable value could be found although there is reason to believe that a measurable amount of the nutrient may be present]

	Food, approximate measure, and weight (in grams)	Water	Food energy	Protein	Fat	Fatty acids Saturated (total)	Unsaturated Oleic	Unsaturated Linoleic	Carbohydrate	Calcium	Iron	Vitamin A value	Thiamin	Riboflavin	Niacin	Ascorbic acid
		Percent	Calories	Grams	Grams	Grams	Grams	Grams	Grams	Milligrams	Milligrams	International units	Milligrams	Milligrams	Milligrams	Milligrams
	GRAIN PRODUCTS—Continued															
438	Oats (with or without corn) puffed, added nutrients. 1 cup —— 25 Grams	3	100	3	1	—			19	44	1.2	0	0.24	0.04	0.5	0
439	Oatmeal or rolled oats, cooked. 1 cup —— 240	87	130	5	2	—		1	23	22	1.4	0	.19	.05	.2	0
	Pancakes, 4-inch diam.:															
440	Wheat, enriched flour (home recipe). 1 cake —— 27	50	60	2	2	Trace	1	Trace	9	27	.4	30	.05	.06	.4	Trace
441	Buckwheat (made from mix with egg and milk). 1 cake —— 27	58	55	2	2	1	1	Trace	6	59	.4	60	.03	.04	.2	Trace
442	Plain or buttermilk (made from mix with egg and milk). 1 cake —— 27	51	60	2	2	1	1	Trace	9	58	.3	70	.04	.06	.2	Trace
	Pie (piecrust made with unenriched flour): Sector, 4-in., ⅐ of 9-in. diam. pie:															
443	Apple (2-crust) —— 1 sector —— 135	48	350	3	15	4	7	3	51	11	.4	40	.03	.03	.5	1
444	Butterscotch (1-crust) —— 1 sector —— 130	45	350	6	14	5	6	2	50	98	1.2	340	.04	.13	.3	Trace
445	Cherry (2-crust) —— 1 sector —— 135	47	350	4	15	4	7	3	52	19	.4	590	.03	.03	.7	Trace
446	Custard (1-crust) —— 1 sector —— 130	58	285	8	14	5	6	2	30	125	.8	300	.07	.21	.4	0
447	Lemon meringue (1-crust). 1 sector —— 120	47	305	4	12	4	6	2	45	17	.6	200	.04	.10	.2	4
448	Mince (2-crust) —— 1 sector —— 135	43	365	3	16	4	8	3	56	38	1.4	Trace	.09	.05	.5	1
449	Pecan (1-crust) —— 1 sector —— 118	20	490	6	27	4	16	5	60	55	3.3	190	.19	.08	.4	Trace
450	Pineapple chiffon (1-crust). 1 sector —— 93	41	265	6	11	3	5	2	36	22	.8	320	.04	.08	.4	1
451	Pumpkin (1-crust) —— 1 sector —— 130	59	275	5	15	5	6	2	32	66	.7	3,210	.04	.13	.7	Trace
	Piecrust, baked shell for pie made with:															
452	Enriched flour —— 1 shell —— 180	15	900	11	60	16	28	12	79	25	3.1	0	.36	.25	3.2	0
453	Unenriched flour —— 1 shell —— 180	15	900	11	60	16	28	12	79	25	.9	0	.05	.05	.9	0

No.	Food	Measure	Grams	Water	Food energy	Protein	Fat	Saturated	Oleic	Linoleic	Carbohydrate	Calcium	Iron	Vitamin A	Thiamin	Riboflavin	Niacin	Ascorbic acid
454	Piecrust mix including stick form: Package, 10-oz., for double crust.	1 pkg.	284	9	1,480	20	93	23	46	21	141	131	1.4	0	.11	.11	2.0	0
455	Pizza (cheese) 5½-in. sector; ⅛ of 14-in. diam. pie.	1 sector	75	45	185	7	6	2	3	Trace	27	107	.7	290	.04	.12	.7	4
	Popcorn, popped:																	
456	Plain, large kernel	1 cup	6	4	25	1	Trace				5	1	.2		----	.01	.1	0
457	With oil and salt	1 cup	9	3	40	1	2	Trace	Trace		5	1	.2		----	.01	.2	0
458	Sugar coated	1 cup	35	4	135	2	1	1	Trace		30	2	.5		----	.02	.4	0
	Pretzels:																	
459	Dutch, twisted	1 pretzel	16	5	60	2	1				12	4	.2	0	Trace	Trace	.1	0
460	Thin, twisted	1 pretzel	6	5	25	1	Trace				5	1	.1	0	Trace	Trace	Trace	0
461	Stick, small, 2¼ inches	10 sticks	3	5	10	Trace	Trace				2	1	Trace	0	Trace	Trace	Trace	0
462	Stick, regular, 3⅛ inches	5 sticks	3	5	10	Trace	Trace				2	1	Trace	0	Trace	Trace	Trace	0
	Rice, white: Enriched:																	
463	Raw	1 cup	185	12	670	12	1				149	44	[20]5.4	0	[20].81	[20].06	[20]6.5	0
464	Cooked	1 cup	205	73	225	4	Trace				50	21	[20]1.8	0	[20].23	[20].02	[20]2.1	0
465	Instant, ready-to-serve	1 cup	165	73	180	4	Trace				40	5	[20]1.3	0	[20].21	[20]---	[20]1.7	0
466	Unenriched, cooked	1 cup	205	73	225	4	Trace				50	21	.4	0	.04	.02	.8	0
467	Parboiled, cooked	1 cup	175	73	185	4	Trace				41	33	[20]1.4	0	[20].19	[20]---	[20]2.1	0
468	Rice, puffed, added nutrients.	1 cup	15	4	60	1	Trace				13	3	.3	0	.07	.01	.7	0
	Rolls, enriched: Cloverleaf or pan:																	
469	Home recipe	1 roll	35	26	120	3	3	1	1	1	20	16	.7	30	.09	.09	.8	Trace
470	Commercial	1 roll	28	31	85	2	2	Trace	1	1	15	21	.5	Trace	.08	.05	.6	Trace
471	Frankfurter or hamburger.	1 roll	40	31	120	3	2	1	1	1	21	30	.8	Trace	.11	.07	.9	Trace
472	Hard, round or rectangular.	1 roll	50	25	155	5	2	Trace	1	Trace	30	24	1.2	Trace	.13	.12	1.4	Trace
473	Rye wafers, whole-grain, 1⅞ by 3½ inches.	2 wafers	13	6	45	2	Trace				10	7	.5	0	.04	.03	.2	0
474	Spaghetti, cooked, tender stage, enriched.	1 cup	140	72	155	5	1				32	11	[19]1.3	0	[19].20	[19].11	[19]1.5	0

[19] Iron, thiamin, riboflavin, and niacin are based on the minimum levels of enrichment specified in standards of identity promulgated under the Federal Food, Drug, and Cosmetic Act.

[20] Iron, thiamin, and niacin are based on the minimum levels of enrichment specified in standards of identity promulgated under the Federal Food, Drug, and Cosmetic Act. Riboflavin is based on unenriched rice. When the minimum level of enrichment for riboflavin specified in the standards of identity becomes effective the value will be 0.12 milligram per cup of parboiled rice and of white rice.

TABLE A-6 NUTRITIVE VALUES OF THE EDIBLE PART OF FOODS — Continued

[Dashes in the columns for nutrients show that no suitable value could be found although there is reason to believe that a measurable amount of the nutrient may be present]

	Food, approximate measure, and weight (in grams)	Water	Food energy	Protein	Fat	Fatty acids			Carbohydrate	Calcium	Iron	Vitamin A value	Thiamin	Riboflavin	Niacin	Ascorbic acid
						Saturated (total)	Unsaturated Oleic	Unsaturated Linoleic								
	Grams	*Percent*	*Calories*	*Grams*	*Grams*	*Grams*	*Grams*	*Grams*	*Grams*	*Milligrams*	*Milligrams*	*International units*	*Milligrams*	*Milligrams*	*Milligrams*	*Milligrams*
	GRAIN PRODUCTS—Continued															
	Spaghetti with meat balls, and tomato sauce:															
475	Home recipe — 1 cup — 248	70	330	19	12	4	6	1	39	124	3.7	1,590	0.25	0.30	4.0	22
476	Canned — 1 cup — 250	78	260	12	10	2	3	4	28	53	3.3	1,000	.15	.18	2.3	5
	Spaghetti in tomato sauce with cheese:															
477	Home recipe — 1 cup — 250	77	260	9	9	2	5	1	37	80	2.3	1,080	.25	.18	2.3	13
478	Canned — 1 cup — 250	80	190	6	2	1	1	1	38	40	2.8	930	.35	.28	4.5	10
479	Waffles, with enriched flour, 7-in. diam. — 1 waffle — 75	41	210	7	7	2	4	1	28	85	1.3	250	.13	.19	1.0	Trace
480	Waffles, made from mix, enriched, egg and milk added, 7-in. diam. — 1 waffle — 75	42	205	7	8	3	3	1	27	179	1.0	170	.11	.17	.7	Trace
481	Wheat, puffed, added nutrients. — 1 cup — 15	3	55	2	Trace	---	---	---	12	4	.6	0	.08	.03	1.2	0
482	Wheat, shredded, plain — 1 biscuit — 25	7	90	2	1	---	---	---	20	11	.9	0	.06	.03	1.1	0
483	Wheat flakes, added nutrients. — 1 cup — 30	4	105	3	Trace	---	---	---	24	12	1.3	0	.19	.04	1.5	0
	Wheat flours:															
484	Whole-wheat, from hard wheats, stirred. — 1 cup — 120	12	400	16	2	Trace	1	1	85	49	4.0	0	.66	.14	5.2	0
	All-purpose or family flour, enriched:															
485	Sifted — 1 cup — 115	12	420	12	1	---	---	---	88	18	[19]3.3	0	[19].51	[19].30	[19]4.0	0
486	Unsifted — 1 cup — 125	12	455	13	1	---	---	---	95	20	[19]3.6	0	[19].55	[19].33	[19]4.4	0
487	Self-rising, enriched — 1 cup — 125	12	440	12	1	---	---	---	93	331	[19]3.6	0	[19].55	[19].33	[19]4.4	0
488	Cake or pastry flour, sifted. — 1 cup — 96	12	350	7	1	---	---	---	76	16	.5	0	.03	.03	.7	0
	FATS, OILS															
	Butter:															
	Regular, 4 sticks per pound:															
489	Stick — ½ cup — 113	16	810	1	92	51	30	3	1	23	0	[21]3,750	---	---	---	0

No.	Food	Measure																	
490	Tablespoon (approx. ⅛ stick).	1 tbsp.	14	16	100	Trace	12	6	4	Trace	Trace	3	0	[22]470	--	--	--	0
491	Pat (1-in. sq. ⅓-in. high; 90 per lb.).	1 pat	5	16	35	Trace	4	2	1	Trace	Trace	1	0	[22]170	--	--	--	0
	Whipped, 6 sticks or 2, 8-oz. containers per pound:																	
492	Stick	½ cup	76	16	540	1	61	34	20	2	Trace	15	0	[22]2,500	--	--	--	0
493	Tablespoon (approx. ⅛ stick).	1 tbsp.	9	16	65	Trace	8	4	3	Trace	Trace	2	0	[22]310	--	--	--	0
494	Pat (1¼-in. sq. ⅓-in. high; 120 per lb.).	1 pat	4	16	25	Trace	3	2	1	Trace	Trace	1	0	[22]130	--	--	--	0
	Fats, cooking:																	
495	Lard	1 cup	205	0	1,850	0	205	78	94	20	0	0	0	0	0	0	0	0
496		1 tbsp.	13	0	115	0	13	5	6	1	0	0	0	0	0	0	0	0
497	Vegetable fats	1 cup	200	0	1,770	0	200	50	100	44	0	0	0	--	0	0	0	0
498		1 tbsp.	13	0	110	0	13	3	6	3	0	0	0	--	0	0	0	0
	Margarine: Regular, 4 sticks per pound:																	
499	Stick	½ cup	113	16	815	1	92	17	46	25	1	23	0	[22]3,750	0	0	0	0
500	Tablespoon (approx. ⅛ stick).	1 tbsp.	14	16	100	Trace	12	2	6	3	Trace	3	0	[22]470	0	0	0	0
501	Pat (1-in. sq. ⅓-in. high; 90 per lb.).	1 pat	5	16	35	Trace	4	1	2	1	Trace	1	0	[22]170	0	0	0	0
	Whipped, 6 sticks per pound:																	
502	Stick	½ cup	76	16	545	1	61	11	31	17	Trace	15	0	[22]2,500	0	0	0	0
	Soft, 2 8-oz. tubs per pound:																	
503	Tub	1 tub	227	16	1,635	1	184	34	68	68	1	45	0	[22]7,500	0	0	0	0
504	Tablespoon	1 tbsp.	14	16	100	Trace	11	2	4	4	Trace	3	0	[22]470	0	0	0	0
	Oils, salad or cooking:																	
505	Corn	1 cup	220	0	1,945	0	220	22	62	117	0	0	0	--	0	0	0	0
506		1 tbsp.	14	0	125	0	14	1	4	7	0	0	0	--	0	0	0	0
507	Cottonseed	1 cup	220	0	1,945	0	220	55	46	110	0	0	0	--	0	0	0	0
508		1 tbsp.	14	0	125	0	14	4	3	7	0	0	0	--	0	0	0	0
509	Olive	1 cup	220	0	1,945	0	220	24	167	15	0	0	0	--	0	0	0	0
510		1 tbsp.	14	0	125	0	14	2	11	1	0	0	0	--	0	0	0	0
511	Peanut	1 cup	220	0	1,945	0	220	40	103	64	0	0	0	--	0	0	0	0
512		1 tbsp.	14	0	125	0	14	3	7	4	0	0	0	--	0	0	0	0
513	Safflower	1 cup	220	0	1,945	0	220	18	37	165	0	0	0	--	0	0	0	0
514		1 tbsp.	14	0	125	0	14	1	2	10	0	0	0	--	0	0	0	0
515	Soybean	1 cup	220	0	1,945	0	220	33	44	114	0	0	0	--	0	0	0	0
516		1 tbsp.	14	0	125	0	14	2	3	7	0	0	0	--	0	0	0	0

[19] Iron, thiamin, riboflavin, and niacin are based on the minimum levels of enrichment specified in standards of identity promulgated under the Federal Food, Drug, and Cosmetic Act.

[21] Year-round average.

[22] Based on the average vitamin A content of fortified margarine. Federal specifications for fortified margarine require a minimum of 15,000 I.U. of vitamin A per pound.

TABLE A-6 NUTRITIVE VALUES OF THE EDIBLE PART OF FOODS — Continued

[Dashes in the columns for nutrients show that no suitable value could be found although there is reason to believe that a measurable amount of the nutrient may be present]

	Food, approximate measure, and weight (in grams)	Water	Food energy	Protein	Fat	Fatty acids Saturated (total)	Unsaturated Oleic	Unsaturated Linoleic	Carbohydrate	Calcium	Iron	Vitamin A value	Thiamin	Riboflavin	Niacin	Ascorbic acid
		Percent	Calories	Grams	Grams	Grams	Grams	Grams	Grams	Milligrams	Milligrams	International units	Milligrams	Milligrams	Milligrams	Milligrams
	FATS, OILS—Continued															
	Salad dressings:															
517	Blue cheese 1 tbsp. — 15 g	32	75	1	8	2	2	4	1	12	Trace	30	Trace	0.02	Trace	Trace
	Commercial, mayonnaise type:															
518	Regular 1 tbsp. — 15 g	41	65	Trace	6	1	1	3	2	2	Trace	30	Trace	Trace	Trace	------
519	Special dietary, low-calorie. 1 tbsp. — 16 g	81	20	Trace	2	Trace	Trace	1	1	3	Trace	40	Trace	Trace	Trace	------
	French:															
520	Regular 1 tbsp. — 16 g	39	65	Trace	6	1	1	3	3	2	.1	------	Trace	------	Trace	------
521	Special dietary, low-fat with artificial sweeteners. 1 tbsp. — 15 g	95	Trace	Trace	Trace	------	------	------	Trace	2	.1	------	------	------	------	------
522	Home cooked, boiled 1 tbsp. — 16 g	68	25	1	2	1	1	Trace	2	14	.1	80	.01	.03	Trace	Trace
523	Mayonnaise 1 tbsp. — 14 g	15	100	Trace	11	2	2	6	Trace	3	.1	40	Trace	.01	Trace	Trace
524	Thousand island 1 tbsp. — 16 g	32	80	Trace	8	1	2	4	3	2	.1	50	Trace	Trace	Trace	Trace
	SUGARS, SWEETS															
	Cake icings:															
525	Chocolate made with milk and table fat. 1 cup — 275 g	14	1,035	9	38	21	14	1	185	165	3.3	580	.06	.28	.6	1
526	Coconut (with boiled icing). 1 cup — 166 g	15	605	3	13	11	1	Trace	124	10	.8	0	.02	.07	.3	0
527	Creamy fudge from mix with water only. 1 cup — 245 g	15	830	7	16	5	8	3	183	96	2.7	Trace	.05	.20	.7	Trace
528	White, boiled 1 cup — 94 g	18	300	1	0	------	------	------	76	2	Trace	0	Trace	.03	Trace	0
	Candy:															
529	Caramels, plain or chocolate. 1 oz — 28 g	8	115	1	3	2	1	Trace	22	42	.4	Trace	.01	.05	.1	Trace
530	Chocolate, milk, plain 1 oz — 28 g	1	145	2	9	5	3	Trace	16	65	.3	80	.02	.10	.1	Trace
531	Chocolate-coated peanuts. 1 oz — 28 g	1	160	5	12	3	6	2	11	33	.4	Trace	.10	.05	2.1	Trace

No.	Food	Measure	Grams	Water (%)	Food energy (Cal.)	Protein (g)	Fat (g)	Saturated (g)	Oleic (g)	Linoleic (g)	Carbohydrate (g)	Calcium (mg)	Iron (mg)	Vitamin A (I.U.)	Thiamin (mg)	Riboflavin (mg)	Niacin (mg)	Ascorbic acid (mg)
532	Fondant; mints, uncoated; candy corn.	1 oz.	28	8	105	Trace	1				25	4	.3	0	0	Trace	Trace	0
533	Fudge, plain.	1 oz.	28	8	115	1	3	1	2	Trace	21	22	.3	Trace	.01	.03	.1	Trace
534	Gum drops.	1 oz.	28	12	100	Trace	Trace				25	2	.1	0	0	Trace	Trace	0
535	Hard.	1 oz.	28	1	110	0	Trace				28	6	.5	0	0	0	0	0
536	Marshmallows.	1 oz.	28	17	90	1	Trace				23	5	.5	0	0	Trace	Trace	0
	Chocolate-flavored sirup or topping:																	
537	Thin type.	1 fl. oz.	38	32	90	1	1	Trace	Trace	Trace	24	6	.6	Trace	.01	.03	.2	0
538	Fudge type.	1 fl. oz.	38	25	125	2	5	3	1	Trace	20	48	.5	60	.02	.08	.2	Trace
	Chocolate-flavored beverage powder (approx. 4 heaping teaspoons per oz.):																	
539	With nonfat dry milk.	1 oz.	28	2	100	1	1				20	167	.5	10	.04	.21	.2	1
540	Without nonfat dry milk.	1 oz.	28	1	100	1	1				25	9	.6	0	.01	.03	.1	0
541	Honey, strained or extracted.	1 tbsp.	21	17	65	0	0				17	1	.1	0	Trace	.01	.1	Trace
542	Jams and preserves.	1 tbsp.	20	29	55	Trace	Trace				14	4	.2	Trace	Trace	.01	Trace	Trace
543	Jellies.	1 tbsp.	18	29	50	Trace	Trace				13	4	.3	Trace	Trace	.01	Trace	1
	Molasses, cane:																	
544	Light (first extraction).	1 tbsp.	20	24	50	—	—				13	33	.9	—	.01	.01	Trace	—
545	Blackstrap (third extraction).	1 tbsp.	20	24	45	—	—				11	137	3.2	—	.02	.04	.4	—
	Sirups:																	
546	Sorghum.	1 tbsp.	21	23	55	—	—				14	35	2.6	—	0	.02	Trace	—
547	Table blends, chiefly corn, light and dark.	1 tbsp.	21	24	60	0	0				15	9	.8	0	0	0	0	0
	Sugars:																	
548	Brown, firm packed.	1 cup	220	2	820	0	0				212	187	7.5	0	.02	.07	.4	0
	White:																	
549	Granulated.	1 cup	200	Trace	770	0	0				199	0	.2	0	0	0	0	0
550		1 tbsp.	11	Trace	40	0	0				11	0	Trace	0	0	0	0	0
551	Powdered, stirred before measuring.	1 cup	120	Trace	460	0	0				119	0	.1	0	0	0	0	0
	MISCELLANEOUS ITEMS																	
552	Barbecue sauce.	1 cup	250	81	230	4	17	2	5	9	20	53	2.0	900	.03	.03	.8	13
	Beverages, alcoholic:																	
553	Beer.	12 fl. oz.	360	92	150	1	0				14	18	Trace	—	.01	.11	2.2	—
	Gin, rum, vodka, whiskey:																	
554	80-proof.	1½ fl. oz. jigger.	42	67	100	—	—				Trace	—	—	—	—	—	—	—
555	86-proof.	1½ fl. oz. jigger.	42	64	105	—	—				Trace	—	—	—	—	—	—	—
556	90-proof.	1½ fl. oz. jigger.	42	62	110	—	—				Trace	—	—	—	—	—	—	—

TABLE A-6 NUTRITIVE VALUES OF THE EDIBLE PART OF FOODS — Continued

[Dashes in the columns for nutrients show that no suitable value could be found although there is reason to believe that a measurable amount of the nutrient may be present]

	Food, approximate measure, and weight (in grams)		Water	Food energy	Pro-tein	Fat	Fatty acids			Carbo-hy-drate	Cal-cium	Iron	Vita-min A value	Thia-min	Ribo-flavin	Niacin	Ascor-bic acid
							Satu-rated (total)	Unsaturated									
								Oleic	Lin-oleic								
		Grams	Per-cent	Calo-ries	Grams	Grams	Grams	Grams	Grams	Grams	Milli-grams	Milli-grams	Inter-national units	Milli-grams	Milli-grams	Milli-grams	Milli-grams
	MISCELLANEOUS ITEMS—Continued																
	Beverages, alcoholic—Continued																
	Gin, rum, vodka, whiskey—Con.																
557	94-proof, 1½ fl. oz. jigger.	42	60	115	—	0				Trace	—	—		—	—	—	
558	100-proof, 1½ fl. oz. jigger.	42	58	125	—	0				Trace	—	—		—	—	—	
	Wines:																
559	Dessert, 3½ fl. oz. glass.	103	77	140	Trace	0				8	8	—		.01	.02	.2	
560	Table, 3½ fl. oz. glass.	102	86	85	Trace	0				4	9	.4		Trace	.01	.1	
	Beverages, carbonated, sweetened, nonalcoholic:																
561	Carbonated water, 12 fl. oz.	366	92	115	0	0				29	—	—	0	0	0	0	0
562	Cola type, 12 fl. oz.	369	90	145	0	0				37	—	—	0	0	0	0	0
563	Fruit-flavored sodas and Tom Collins mixes, 12 fl. oz.	372	88	170	0	0				45	—	—	0	0	0	0	0
564	Ginger ale, 12 fl. oz.	366	92	115	0	0				29	—	—	0	0	0	0	0
565	Root beer, 12 fl. oz.	370	90	150	0	0				39	—	—	0	0	0	0	0
566	Bouillon cubes, approx. ½ in., 1 cube.	4	4	5	1	Trace				Trace	—	—					
	Chocolate:																
567	Bitter or baking, 1 oz.	28	2	145	3	15	8	6	Trace	8	22	1.9	20	.01	.07	.4	0
568	Semi-sweet, small pieces, 1 cup.	170	1	860	7	61	34	22	1	97	51	4.4	30	.02	.14	.9	0
	Gelatin:																
569	Plain, dry powder in envelope, 1 envelope.	7	13	25	6	Trace				0	—	—					
570	Dessert powder, 3-oz. package, 1 pkg.	85	2	315	8	0				75	—	—					
571	Gelatin dessert, prepared with water, 1 cup.	240	84	140	4	0				34	—	—					

Item No.	Food, approximate measure, and description	Measure	Grams	Water (%)	Food energy (Cal.)	Protein (g)	Fat (g)	Fatty acids — Saturated (total) (g)	Unsaturated Oleic (g)	Unsaturated Linoleic (g)	Carbohydrate (g)	Calcium (mg)	Iron (mg)	Vitamin A value (I.U.)	Thiamin (mg)	Riboflavin (mg)	Niacin (mg)	Ascorbic acid (mg)
	Olives, pickled:																	
572	Green	4 medium or 3 extra large or 2 giant.	16	78	15	Trace	2	Trace	2	Trace	Trace	8	.2	40	—	Trace	—	—
573	Ripe: Mission	3 small or 2 large.	10	73	15	Trace	2	Trace	2	Trace	Trace	9	.1	10	Trace	Trace	—	—
	Pickles, cucumber:																	
574	Dill, medium, whole, 3¾ in. long, 1¼ in. diam.	1 pickle	65	93	10	1	Trace	—	—	—	1	17	.7	70	Trace	.01	Trace	4
575	Fresh, sliced, 1½ in. diam., ¼ in. thick.	2 slices	15	79	10	Trace	Trace	—	—	—	3	5	.3	20	Trace	Trace	Trace	1
576	Sweet, gherkin, small, whole, approx. 2½ in. long, ¾ in. diam.	1 pickle	15	61	20	Trace	Trace	—	—	—	6	2	.2	10	Trace	Trace	Trace	1
577	Relish, finely chopped, sweet.	1 tbsp.	15	63	20	Trace	Trace	—	—	—	5	3	.1	—	Trace	Trace	Trace	—
	Popcorn. See Grain Products.																	
578	Popsicle, 3 fl. oz. size	1 popsicle	95	80	70	0	0	0	0	0	18	0	Trace	0	0	0	0	0
	Pudding, home recipe with starch base:																	
579	Chocolate	1 cup	260	66	385	8	12	7	4	Trace	67	250	1.3	390	.05	.36	.3	1
580	Vanilla (blanc mange)	1 cup	255	76	285	9	10	5	3	Trace	41	298	Trace	410	.08	.41	.3	2
581	Pudding mix, dry form, 4-oz. package.	1 pkg.	113	2	410	3	2	1	1	Trace	103	23	1.8	Trace	.02	.08	.5	0
582	Sherbet	1 cup	193	67	260	2	2	—	—	—	59	31	Trace	120	.02	.06	Trace	4
	Soups: Canned, condensed, ready-to-serve: Prepared with an equal volume of milk:																	
583	Cream of chicken	1 cup	245	85	180	7	10	3	3	3	15	172	.5	610	.05	.27	.7	2
584	Cream of mushroom	1 cup	245	83	215	7	14	4	4	5	16	191	.5	250	.05	.34	.7	1
585	Tomato	1 cup	250	84	175	7	7	3	2	1	23	168	.8	1,200	.10	.25	1.3	15
	Prepared with an equal volume of water:																	
586	Bean with pork	1 cup	250	84	170	8	6	1	2	2	22	63	2.3	650	.13	.08	1.0	3
587	Beef broth, bouillon consomme.	1 cup	240	96	30	5	0	—	—	—	3	Trace	.5	Trace	Trace	.02	1.2	—
588	Beef noodle	1 cup	240	93	70	4	3	1	1	1	7	7	1.0	50	.05	.07	1.0	Trace
589	Clam chowder, Manhattan type (with tomatoes, without milk).	1 cup	245	92	80	2	3	—	—	—	12	34	1.0	880	.02	.02	1.0	—
590	Cream of chicken	1 cup	240	92	95	3	6	1	2	3	8	24	.5	410	.02	.05	.7	Trace
591	Cream of mushroom	1 cup	240	90	135	2	10	1	3	5	10	41	.5	70	.02	.12	.7	Trace
592	Minestrone	1 cup	245	90	105	5	3	—	—	—	14	37	1.0	2,350	.07	.05	1.0	—

TABLE A-6 NUTRITIVE VALUES OF THE EDIBLE PART OF FOODS — Continued

[Dashes in the columns for nutrients show that no suitable value could be found although there is reason to believe that a measurable amount of the nutrient may be present]

	Food, approximate measure, and weight (in grams)	Water	Food energy	Protein	Fat	Fatty acids Saturated (total)	Unsaturated Oleic	Unsaturated Linoleic	Carbohydrate	Calcium	Iron	Vitamin A value	Thiamin	Riboflavin	Niacin	Ascorbic acid
		Percent	Calories	Grams	Grams	Grams	Grams	Grams	Grams	Milligrams	Milligrams	International units	Milligrams	Milligrams	Milligrams	Milligrams
	MISCELLANEOUS ITEMS—Continued															
	Soups—Continued															
	Canned, condensed, ready-to-serve—Con.															
	Prepared with an equal volume of water—Con.															
593	Split pea 1 cup ... 245	85	145	9	3	1	2	Trace	21	29	1.5	440	0.25	0.15	1.5	1
594	Tomato 1 cup ... 245	90	90	2	3	Trace	1	1	16	15	.7	1,000	.05	.05	1.2	12
595	Vegetable beef 1 cup ... 245	92	80	5	2	---	---	---	10	12	.7	2,700	.05	.05	1.0	---
596	Vegetarian 1 cup ... 245	92	80	2	2	---	---	---	13	20	1.0	2,940	.05	.05	1.0	---
	Dehydrated, dry form:															
597	Chicken noodle (2-oz. package). 1 pkg ... 57	6	220	8	6	2	3	1	33	34	1.4	190	.30	.15	2.4	3
598	Onion mix (1½-oz. package). 1 pkg ... 43	3	150	6	5	1	2	1	23	42	.6	30	.05	.03	.3	6
599	Tomato vegetable with noodles (2½-oz. pkg.). 1 pkg ... 71	4	245	6	6	2	3	1	45	33	1.4	1,700	.21	.13	1.8	18
	Frozen, condensed:															
	Clam chowder, New England type (with milk, without tomatoes):															
600	Prepared with equal volume of milk. 1 cup ... 245	83	210	9	12	---	---	---	16	240	1.0	250	.07	.29	.5	Trace
601	Prepared with equal volume of water. 1 cup ... 240	89	130	4	8	---	---	---	11	91	1.0	50	.05	.10	.5	---
	Cream of potato:															
602	Prepared with equal volume of milk. 1 cup ... 245	83	185	8	10	5	3	Trace	18	208	1.0	590	.10	.27	.5	Trace
603	Prepared with equal volume of water. 1 cup ... 240	90	105	3	5	3	2	Trace	12	58	1.0	410	.05	.05	.5	---

No.	Food and description	Measure																
	Cream of shrimp:																	
604	Prepared with equal volume of milk.	1 cup	245	82	245	9	16	---	---	---	15	189	.5	290	.07	.27	.5	Trace
605	Prepared with equal volume of water.	1 cup	240	88	160	5	12	---	---	---	8	38	.5	120	.05	.05	.5	---
	Oyster stew:																	
606	Prepared with equal volume of milk.	1 cup	240	83	200	10	12	---	---	---	14	305	1.4	410	.12	.41	.5	Trace
607	Prepared with equal volume of water.	1 cup	240	90	120	6	8	---	---	---	8	158	1.4	240	.07	.19	.5	---
608	Tapioca, dry, quick-cooking.	1 cup	152	13	535	1	Trace	---	---	---	131	15	.6	0	0	0	0	0
	Tapioca desserts:																	
609	Apple.	1 cup	250	70	295	1	Trace	---	---	---	74	8	.5	30	Trace	Trace	Trace	Trace
610	Cream pudding.	1 cup	165	72	220	8	8	4	3	Trace	28	173	.7	480	.07	.30	.2	2
611	Tartar sauce.	1 tbsp.	14	34	75	Trace	8	1	4	3	1	3	.1	30	Trace	Trace	Trace	Trace
612	Vinegar.	1 tbsp.	15	94	Trace	Trace	0	---	---	---	1	1	.1	---	---	---	---	---
613	White sauce, medium.	1 cup	250	73	405	10	31	16	10	1	22	288	.5	1,150	.10	.43	.5	2
	Yeast:																	
614	Baker's, dry, active.	1 pkg.	7	5	20	3	Trace	---	---	---	3	3	1.1	Trace	.16	.38	2.6	Trace
615	Brewer's, dry.	1 tbsp.	8	5	25	3	Trace	---	---	---	3	17	1.4	Trace	1.25	.34	3.0	Trace
	Yoghurt. See Milk, Cheese, Cream, Imitation Cream.																	

Source: United States Department of Agriculture Home and Garden Bulletin No. 72

BIBLIOGRAPHY

BOOKS

American Home Economics Association. *Handbook of Food Preparation.* Washington, D. C., 1975.

Berland, Theodore. *Rating the Diets.* Skokie, Illinois: Publications International, Ltd., 1975.

Farmer, Fannie M. *Fannie Farmer Cookbook.* Edited by Wilma L. Perkins. Boston: Little, Brown & Co., 1965.

Kansas State University. *Practical Cookery.* New York: John Wiley & Sons, Inc., 1975.

Margolius, Sidney. *Health Foods: Facts or Fakes.* New York: Walker and Co., 1975.

Mayo Clinic Diet Manual. Philadelphia: W.B. Saunders Co., 1971.

McWilliams, Margaret. *Nutrition for the Growing Years.* New York: John Wiley & Sons, Inc., 1975.

Mitchell, Helen S., et al. *Nutrition in Health and Disease.* New York: J. B. Lippincott Company, 1976.

National Academy of Sciences. *Recommended Dietary Allowances.* 8th ed. Washington, D. C., 1974.

Robinson, Corinne H. *Basic Nutrition and Diet Therapy.* New York: Macmillan Publishing Co., Inc., 1975.

Spock, Dr. Benjamin. *Baby and Child Care.* New York: Pocket Books, 1977.

Turner, Dorothea. *Handbook of Diet Therapy.* Chicago: The University of Chicago Press, 1970.

Williams, Sue Rodwell. *Essentials of Nutrition and Diet Therapy.* St. Louis: The C. V. Mosby Company, 1974.

Williams, Sue Rodwell. *Mowry's Basic Nutrition and Diet Therapy.* 5th ed. St. Louis: The C. V. Mosby Company, 1975.

Wilson, Eva D., et al. *Principles of Nutrition.* 3d ed. New York: John Wiley & Sons, Inc., 1975.

PUBLICATIONS AND PERIODICALS

Agency for International Development. *Malnutrition and Infection During Pregnancy.* Copyright 1975 by the American Medical Association. Washington, D. C.

American Heart Association. 1969. *Your Mild Sodium-Restricted Diet* (revised). Dallas, Texas.

American Heart Association. 1969. *Your 1000 Milligram Sodium Diet* (revised). Dallas, Texas.

American Heart Association. 1968. *Your 500 Milligram Sodium Diet* (revised). Dallas, Texas.

American Heart Association. 1968. *The Way to a Man's Heart.* Dallas, Texas.

American Diabetes Association, Inc., and the American Dietetic Association. 1976. *Exchange Lists for Meal Planning.* New York, New York.

Committee on Food and Nutrition. "Principles of Nutrition and Dietary Recommendations for Patients with Diabetes Mellitus: 1971." *Journal of the American Diabetes Association* 20: 633-34, September 1971.

Council on Foods and Nutrition. "Nutritional Therapy for Adults with Renal Disease." *Journal of the American Medical Association* 223:68-72, January 1, 1973.

Council on Foods and Nutrition. "Diet and Coronary Heart Disease, A Council Statement." *Journal of the American Medical Association,* vol. 222, No. 13, December 25, 1972.

Council on Foods and Nutrition. "Malnutrition and Hunger in the U.S." *Journal of the American Medical Association,* vol. 213, No. 2, July 13, 1970.

Council on Foods and Nutrition. "Improvement of the Nutritive Quality of Foods — General Policies." *Journal of the American Medical Association,* vol. 225, August 27, 1973.

Council on Foods and Nutrition. "Iron in Enriched Wheat Flour, Farina, Bread, Buns, and Rolls." *Journal of the American Medical Association,* vol. 220, May 8, 1972.

Council on Foods and Nutrition. "Vitamin A Physiology." by O. A. Roels, Ph.D. *Journal of the American Medical Association,* vol. 214, No. 6, November 9, 1970.

Department of Health, Education and Welfare. 1975. *Textured Plant Protein Products.* Publication No. (FDA) 76-2004. Washington, D. C.

_____ 1976. *What About Vitamin C?* by Margaret Morrison. Publication No. (FDA) 75-2015. Washington, D. C.

_____ 1976. *Vitamin E — Miracle or Myth?* Publication No. (FDA) 76-2011. Washington, D. C.

_____ 1974. *We Want to Know About Nutrition Labels.* Publication No. (FDA) 74-2039. Washington, D. C.

_____ 1976. *Nutrition Labels and U.S. RDA.* Publication No. (FDA) 76-2042. Washington, D. C.

_____ 1976. *Nutrition Labeling — Terms You Should Know.* Publication No. (FDA) 76-2012. Washington, D. C.

_____ 1974. *Enforcing the Food, Drug, and Cosmetic Act.* Publication No. (FDA) 74-1018. Washington, D. C.

_____ 1976. *Food Standards.* Publication No. (FDA) 76-2024. Washington, D. C.

_____ 1974. *We Want You to Know About Salmonella and Food Poisoning.* Publication No. (FDA) 74-2011. Washington, D. C.

_____ 1974. *Safe Handling of Foods in the Home.* by Madean Horner. Publication No. (FDA) 73-2002. Washington, D. C.

_____ 1974. *Facts About Food Poisoning.* Publication No. (FDA) 74-2046. Washington, D. C.

_____ 1976. *Can Your Kitchen Pass the Food Storage Test?* by Jane Heenan. Publication No. (FDA) 74-2052. Washington, D. C.

_____ 1976. *A Primer on Dietary Minerals.* Publication No. (FDA) 75-2013. Washington, D. C.

_____ 1976. *Myths of Vitamins.* by Jane Heenan. Publication No. (FDA) 76-2047. Washington, D. C.

_____ 1974. *Some Questions and Answers About Food Additives.* Publication No. (FDA) 74-2056. Washington, D. C.

Irwin, Michael H. K. *Overweight, A Problem for Millions.* Public Affairs Pamphlet No. 364A. New York, New York, 1973.

National Academy of Sciences, Committee on Nutrition Misinformation. *Hazards of Overuse of Vitamin D.* Washington, D. C., November 1974.

National Live Stock and Meat Board. 1974. *Lessons on Meat.* Chicago.

Singleton, Nan Chachere, et al. "The Diet of Pregnant Teenagers." *Journal of Home Economics,* September 1976, pp. 43–45.

The Prudent Diet. Bureau of Nutrition, Department of Health, City of New York, 1974.

United States Department of Agriculture. 1975. *Nutrition . . . Food at Work for You.* Washington, D. C.

_____ 1974. "Food Shopper Language." *1974 Yearbook of Agriculture.* Washington, D. C.

_____ 1969. *Keeping Food Safe to Eat.* Home and Garden Bulletin No. 162. Washington, D. C.

_____ 1973. *Food and Your Weight.* House and Garden Bulletin No. 74. Washington, D. C.

_____ 1971. *Nutritive Value of Foods.* Home and Garden Bulletin No. 72. Washington, D. C.

_____ 1972. *How to Use USDA Grades in Buying Food.* Home and Garden Bulletin 196. Washington, D. C.

_____ 1975. *Soybeans in Family Meals.* Home and Garden Bulletin 208. Washington, D. C.

_____ 1963. "Composition of Foods." *Agriculture Handbook No. 8.* Washington, D. C.

United States Department of Agriculture. 1976. *Organic, Inorganic: What They Mean.* by Ruth M. Leverton, Washington, D. C.

_____ 1974. *Fats in Food and Diet.* Agricultural Information Bulletin No. 361. Washington, D. C.

_____ 1971. *Textured Vegetable Protein Products.* Agricultural Research Service. Washington, D. C.

_____ 1976. *Edible Soy Protein.* Farmer Cooperative Service, FCS Research Report 33. Washington, D. C.

_____ ·1969. *Diets of Men, Women and Children.* Talk by Daniel A. Swope, Consumer and Food Economics Research Division at the 46th Annual Agricultural Outlook Conference, Washington, D. C.

_____ 1975. *Convenience Foods — 1975 Cost Update — a Preliminary Paper.* Talk by Larry Traub, Economic Research Service, and Dianne Odland, Agricultural Research Service, at the National Agricultural Outlook Conference, Washington, D. C.

United States Department of Commerce, National Bureau of Standards. 1973. *What About Metric.* by Louis E. Barbrow. Washington, D. C.

_____ 1975. *Some References on Metric Information.* National Bureau of Standards Special Publication No. 389. Washington, D. C.

ACKNOWLEDGMENTS

The author wishes to express her appreciation to the members of her family for their patience and understanding during the writing of this revision. Appreciation is also expressed to the following persons and organizations:

Leonard Elliott, Director of Public Information of the American Diabetes Association, for his help with the chapter on Diabetes.

Dorothea Turner, of the Dietetic Association, for review of the chapter on the Diabetic Diet.

Catherine White, RN, for assistance with the chapter on Tube Feeding.

American Dairy Association, for figure 4-1 D

American Heart Association, for tables 29-1, A-2, A-3, and A-4

Black Hawk College, for figure 16-2

Bureau of Nutrition, Department of Health, New York, NY, for table 3-3

Chesebrough-Ponds, Inc., Hospital Products Division, for figure 31-3

Food and Drug Administration, U.S. Department of Health, Education, and Welfare, for figure 11-1

Food and Nutrition Board, National Academy of Sciences, National Research Council, for tables 2-2, 2-3, 4-2, 5-3, 6-1, 7-1, 7-2, 9-2, 17-1, 18-1, and A-1

Gerber Products Company, for figures 18-1, 18-3, and 18-4

Lea and Febiger, for table 30-1

J. B. Lippincott Company, for table 4-3

Manufacturing Chemists Association, for tables 10-1 and 10-2

Metropolitan Life Insurance Company, for table A-2

National Bureau of Standards, U.S. Department of Commerce, for tables 15-3 and 15-4

National Canners Association, for table 11-1

National Dairy Council, for figures 8-1, 10-1, 10-2 and 10-9

National Education Association, for figures 3-1 and 5-1

National Live Stock and Meat Board, for figures 10-3, 10-4, 10-5, 10-6, 10-7 and 12-1

Dr. R. L. Nemir, for figure 5-2

Parent's Magazine, for figure 16-1

Tupperware, for figures 3-2, 10-8, 15-1 and 15-2

Upjohn Company, for figures 5-2 and 6-1

United Nations, for figures 1-1 and 5-4

United States Department of Agriculture, for figure 13-1 and tables 10-4, 11-3, 13-1, 27-3 and A-6

World Health Organization for page viii and figures 1-2, 4-2, 4-3 and 5-3

Contributions by Delmar Staff:
    Series Editor — Angela R. Emmi
    Revision Editors — Ruth Saur, Anne Greatbatch
    Editorial Assistant — Hazel Kozakiewicz

INDEX

A

A la king, 129
Absorption, 10
Abstinence, 224
Accompaniment dishes, 97
Acidosis, 43
Acknowledgments, 287
Agriculture (USDA) United States
    Department of, grade stamps,
    104
Alkaline, 43
Alkalosis, 43
Allergens, 222
Allergy(ies), 126, 222
Allergy diets, 222-226
American Diabetes Association,
    202, 203
American Heart Association, 216,
    218, 219
Amino acids, 30, 31, 32
Anabolism, 11
Anemia, 52
    nutritional, 43
    pernicious, 53
Anorexia, 51
Anorexia nervosa, 194
Antibiotic therapy, 51
Appendix, 236-283
Arthritis, 195
Aspic, 129
Aspiration, 227
Atherosclerosis, 209
Au gratin, 129
Avitaminosis, 48

B

Baby and Child Care (Spock), 160
Bacteria, 87
Bake, 129

Baking powder, 216
Baking soda, 216
Balanced diet, 62
Barbecue, 129
Basal metabolism rate (BMR),
    12
Baste, 129
Beat, 129
Beef cuts, 91
Beriberi, 52
Beverages, 85-87
Bibliography, 284-286
Bile, 10
Biotin, 53
    sources of, 53
Blanch, 129
Bland, definition of, 185
Bland diet, 185-187
    sample menu for, 186
    selecting foods for, 185
Bland foods, 73
Blend, 129
Blind patients, 146-147
Blindness, 50
Blood plasma, 2
Body, 9
Boil, 129
Bomb calorimeter, 12
Bone marrow, 43
Botulism, 123
Braise, 129
Bran, 21
Bread and cereal group, 67, 98
Brine, 216
Broil, 129
Brush, 129
Bubbling, 158
Bulk, 11
Butter, 89

C

Caffeine, 87
Calcium and phosphorus, 41-42
Caloric requirements
    calculating, 12
    during pregnancy, 154
    minimum, 14
Caloric value, 12
Calorie, 12
Canned foods, 105
Capillaries, 11
Carbohydrates, 2, 19-23
    classification of, 20
    and fats, 19-29
    functions of, 19
    sources of, 20
Carboxypeptidases, 10
Cardiac conditions, 195
Cardiovascular conditions, 43
Carotene, 50
Carrier, 122
Casserole, 129
Catabolism, 11
Cellulose, 22
Cheese, 88-89
    natural, classification of, 88
    processed, 88
Cheilosis, 52
Chemical elements in human body,
    38
Choking, 146
Cholesterol, 25, 206
    content in foods, 208
Chop, 129
Chyme, 9
Chymotrypsin, 10
Cleaning equipment and kitchen
    surfaces, 117
Cobalamin. *See* Vitamin B_{12}

Cobalt, 44
Coffee, decaffeinated, 87
Colitis, 188
Collagen, 53
Combine, 129
Compote, 129
Container sizes, 106
Convalescent diet. *See* Light diet
Convenience foods, 74, 105
Cooking
   substitutions, 107
   time-saving techniques, 116
Cream, 88
Cream (to mix), 130
Croquette, 130
Cube, 130
Cyanotic, 229

D

Decaffeinated coffee, 87
Deficiency disease, 3
Dehydrated, 105
Dehydration, 43
Desensitized, 224
Deviled, 130
Dextrin, 22
Diabetes mellitus, 201
Diabetic diet, 201–205
   food usually allowed in, 203
   food usually omitted in, 203
   types of, 201–203
   unweighted, 202
   weighted, 201
Diabetic patients, teaching, 203
Dice, 130
Diet(s)
   allergy, 222–226
   based on exchange lists, 202–203
   bland, 185–187
   convalescent. *See* Diet, light
   crash reducing, 78, 197
   diabetic, 201–205
   elimination, 222–224
   fat controlled, 206–211
   fat restricted. *See* Diet, low fat
   high and low calorie, 194–200
   high fiber, 188
   hospital, 168
   light, 181–184
   liquid, 172–176
   low cholesterol, 206–209
   low fat, 206

modified in residue content,
      188–193
   protein, 212–215
   regular, 168–169
   restricted residue, 188
   sodium restricted, 216–221
   soft, 177–180
   special, 167–235
   therapeutic, 167
   tube feeding, 227–235
   unweighted, 202
   weighted, 201
Diet therapy, 4, 167–171
Dietary allowances
   during pregnancy and lactation,
      153
   recommended daily, 63, 236–237
Dietary requirements, 22–23
Dietitian, 167
Digestion, 8–9
   and absorption, 22
   in the mouth, 9
   in the small intestine, 9–10
   in the stomach, 9
Digestive organs, basic functions of,
      10
Digestive system, 8
Disaccharides, 21
Dishwashing, 115–117
Di-sodium phosphate, 217
Diverticulosis, 188
Dredge, 130
Duodenum, 9
Dust, 130
Dysentery, 123

E

Eating habits, developing good,
      78–84
Economy in purchasing, 106
Edema, 33, 43, 216
Eggs, 89
Elimination diets, 222–224
Endosperm, 21
Energy expenditures in daily
      activities, 13
Energy needs
   by age, 82
   determining, 12
English system, 137
   conversion from metric system,
      139

Enriched, 39, 48
Entree, 97
Enzyme(s), 9
   and foods acted upon, 9
Equipment
   cleaning, 117
   selection of, 117
Esophagus, 9

F

Fats, 2, 23–26
   classification of, 24
   dietary requirements, 26
   digestion and absorption of, 25
   functions of, 23
   invisible, 24
   metabolism and elimination of,
      25–26
   monounsaturated, 24
   polyunsaturated, 24
   saturated, 24, 209
   sources of, 23
   table of, 23
   types of in common foods, 25
   unsaturated, 209
   visible, 24
Fat controlled diets, 206–211
Fat restricted diet. *See* Low fat
      diet
Fatty acids, 11
Fecal matter, 172
Federal Food, Drug and Cosmetics
      Act, 103
Fetus, 152
Fiber, 11, 188
Fish, 95
Flake, 130
Flatulence, 172
Flatware, 117
Fluorine, 44
Folacin, 53
   sources of, 53
Fold, 130
Food(s)
   body's use of, 8–18
   cholesterol content of, 208
   containing sodium, 216–217
   convenience, 74, 105
   customs, 78
   freeze-dried, 105
   frozen, 105
   health, 98

intended use of, 106-107
labeling, 103-104
for mother and baby, 152-166
natural, 38, 98
nutritive values of, 249-283
poisoning, 126
purchasing, 103-114
quality, 85-102
quantities needed, 107
residue, 11
restored, 49
seasonal, 107
storage, 126
supplements, 161
temperature control of bacteria, 125
Food additives, 85, 86
reasons for using, 86
Food and Drug Administration (FDA), U.S., 48, 85, 103
Food and Nutrition Board of the National Research Council, 12, 22, 32, 39, 50, 53, 62, 154
Food contamination, prevention of, 123
Food groups, basic four, 62-71, 72, 80, 103
Food habits, cultural, 79-80
Food residue, 188
Formulas, preparation of, 160-161
aseptic method, 160
terminal method, 160
Fortified, 48
Freeze-dried foods, 105
Freeze-drying, 105
Frozen foods, 105
Fructose, 21
Fruits, 97
Fry, 130
Fundus, 9

G

Galactose, 21
Garnish, 130
Gastric juices, 9
Gastric lipase, 9
Germ, 21
Glossitis, 53
Glucose, 21
oxidation of, 22
Glycogen, 21, 22

Goiter, 44
Grades, 104-105
Grate, 130
Grill, 130

H

Half and half, 88
Hare, 90
Health foods, 98
Heat
dry, 90
moist, 90
Hemoglobin, 43
Hemolysis, 51
Hemorrhage, 51
High caloric diet, 194
sample menu for, 195
High fiber diets, 188
sample menu for, 189
Hollow calorie foods, 3
Hospital diets, 168
Hydrochloric acid, 9
Hydrogenation, 25
Hydrolysis, 9
Hypersensitivity, 222
Hyperthyroidism, 11, 12, 194
Hypervitaminosis, 48
Hypervitaminosis D, 51
Hypervitaminosis K, 51
Hypoglycemic agents, 201

I

Ileitis, 188
Illness
bacterial foodborne, 124
food-related, 122-128
Immunity, 158
Infancy
diet during, 158-166
feeding methods during, 158
feeding schedule during 160
recommended daily dietary requirements during, 158
Infectious organism, 122
Ingredients, measuring and weighing, 137-144
Insulin, 201
Iodine, 43-44
Iodized salt, 43
Iron deficiency, 3
Iron and copper, 43
Irradiated, 51

J

Jewish dietary laws, 81
Joule, 12
Julienne, 130

K

Kitchen equipment, 115-121
Knead, 130
Kwashiorkor, 34
effects of, 34

L

Lactase, 10
Lactation, 155
caloric requirement during, 155
2600 caloric menu during, 155
Lacteals, 11
Lactose, 21, 173
Lamb cuts, 93
Large intestine, absorption in, 11
Leftovers, using, 74
Light diet, 181-184
sample menu for, 182
Lipoproteins, 25
Liquid diets, 172-176
clear liquid, 172
foods allowed in, 172, 173
full liquid, 173
sample menu for, 172, 173
Low calorie diet, 194-197
sample menu for, 196
selecting foods for 196
Low fat diet, 206
sample menu for, 207
selecting foods for, 207

M

Macrominerals, 39
Magnesium, 43
Malnutrition, 2-4
characteristics of, 2
definition of, 2
Maltase, 9, 10
Maltose, 21
Manganese, 44
Marasmus, 33, 34
Margarine, fortified, 25
Marinade, 130
Marinate, 130
Meals
appearance, 72
flavor and aroma, 72-73

Meals (cont.)
  planning, 62–114
  planning appetizing, 72–77
  for patients, 145–151
  preparation, 115–151
  satiety, 73
  texture, 73
  variety, 72
  weekly planning, 74
Measuring devices, 137–141
Meat(s)
  alternates, 67
  basic cuts, 90
  cooked, yield of, 96
Meat group, 67, 90
Meats, poultry and fish, 89–94
  storage and cooking of, 95
Menu pattern, 73–74
  adapting, 74
Menu planning, 106
Metabolism, 8, 11–12
  and elimination, 22
  and thyroid gland, 11–12
Metric equivalents, 138
Metric system, 137
  conversion from English system,
    139
  unit relationships, 138
Microminerals, 39
Microorganisms in food, 122–123
Milk
  butter, 88
  certified, 87
  chocolate, 88
  dried, 88
  evaporated, 88
  homogenized, 88
  low fat, 88
  and milk products group, 66–67,
    87–89
  mothers', 158
  raw, 87
  skim, 88
  sweetened condensed, 88
  synthetic, 160
  whole, 87
Mince, 130
Minerals, 2, 38–47
  cooking foods containing, 44
  food sources of, 40–41
Mineral elements, 38
Mineral needs, recommended daily,
  39

Mocha, 130
Monosaccharides, 20
Monosodium glutamate (MSG), 216
Monosaturated, 24
Morning sickness, 152
Mortality rate, infant, 152
Mucous membranes, 50

N

Natural foods, 38, 98
Nephritic conditions, 43
Niacin, 52
  best sources of, 52
Nicotinic acid. *See* Niacin
Nutrient(s), 1
  essential, 1–2
  provided by sample menu, 65
Nutrition, 1
  basic, 1–61
  introduction to, 1–7
  study of, 4
Nutrition labeling, 103, 104
Nutritional anemia, 43
Nutritional needs, 80–82
  adolescence, 81
  childhood, 80–81
  middle age, 81–82
  old age, 82
Nutritional value, 85
Nutritive value of foods, 249–283

O

Organic food, 98
Osteomalacia, 50
Oxidation, 11

P

Packaging, 105
Pan-broil, 130
Pancreatic amylase, 10
Pancreatic enzymes, 32
Pantothenic acid, 53
  sources of, 53
Parboil, 130
Pasteurization, 87
Patient, ambulatory, 169
Patient's meal
  blind patients, 146–147
  preparation of, 145–151
  serving, 145
Pediatrician, 160
Pellagra, 52

Pepsin, 9
Peptidases, 10
Perfringens poisoning, 123
Peristalsis, 9
Pernicious anemia, 53
Pigmentation, 50
Poach, 130
Polypeptides, 32
Polysaccharides, 21
Polyunsaturated, 24
Pork cuts, 94
Posture, 1
Poultry, 95
  leftover, 95
Pregnancy, 4
  caloric requirement during, 154
  dietary modifications during, 154
  morning sickness during, 152
  nausea during, 152
  2400 calorie menu for, 153
  weight gain during, 154–155
Pregnancy and lactation, diet dur-
    ing, 152–157
Pressure cooker, 123
Proteins, 2, 30–37
  classification of, 31
  complete, 31
  dietary requirements, 32–34
  digestion and absorption of, 32
  functions of, 30
  in an average diet, 33
  incomplete, 31
  metabolism and elimination of,
    32
  requirement, daily, 33
  sources of, 32
  textured, 32
Protein diets, 212–215
  foods included in, 212
  high, 212
  low, 213
  sample menu for, 212, 213
  selecting food for, 213
Protein sparing action, 19
Provitamins, 48
Ptyalin, 9
Puree, 130
Pylorus, 9

R

Reducing diets, crash, 78, 197
Regular diet, 168–169

Recipes, reading, 129-136
Recommended Daily Allowances
        (RDA), 104
Recommended Daily Dietary
        Requirements, 82
Refrigeration and bacteria, 123
Rennin, 9, 32
Residue content, diets modified in,
        188-193
Residue diets, 188-190
    minimum, 190
    restricted, 189
Restored foods, 49
Riboflavin, 52
Riboflavin deficiency, symptoms
        of, 52
Rickets, 41

S

Safety, kitchen, 117
Saliva, 9
Salivary amylase, 9
Salmonellosis, 122
Salt, 85
Saturated, 24
Saute, 130
Scald, 130
Scurvy, 53
Score, 130
Sear, 130
Semi-Fowler's position, 228
Servings per package or per pound,
        108
Shred, 130
Sift, 130
Simmer, 130
Skewer, 133
Skin tests, 222
Small intestine, absorption in, 11
Sodium, 316
    foods containing, 216-217
Sodium, potassium and chloride,
        42-43
Sodium alginate, 217
Sodium benzoate, 217
Sodium hydroxide, 217
Sodium propionate, 217
Sodium restricted diets, 217
    500 milligram, 219
    food lists for, 240-247
    mild, 217-218
    1000 milligram, 218-219

    plan for, 239
    sample menu for, 218
Sodium restriction, adjustment
        to, 219
Sodium sulfite, 217
Soft diet, 177-180
    indications for, 177
    sample menu for, 178
    selecting food in, 177
Souffle, 133
Special diets, 167-235
Stamina, 1
Staphylococcal poisoning, 123
Starch, 21
Steam, 133
Steapsin, 10
Steep, 133
Stew, 133
Stimulants, 87
Stock, 133
Stomach, 9
    parts of, 9
Store or market, selection of,
        107-109
Substitutions, 107
Sucrase, 9, 10
Sucrose, 21
Sulfur, 43
Synthetic, 48

T

Temperature conversions, 248
Tetany, 42
Theine, 87
Therapeutic diets, 167
Thiamine, 52
Thiamine deficiency, symptoms
        of, 52
Thyroid gland, 44
Timbale, 133
Toxemia, 152
Trichinosis, 123
Trypsin, 10
Tryptophan, 52
Tube feeding, 227-235
    administering, 228-231
    drip method, 230-231
    funnel method, 228-230
    reasons for, 227

U

Unweighted or free diet, 202
Utensils, small kitchen, 118

V

Veal cuts, 92
Vegetable and fruit group, 64
Vegetables, 96-97
Venison, 90
Villi, 11
Vitamin drops, 161
Vitamins, 2, 48-61
    fat-soluble, 49
    recommended daily allowances,
        49
    sources of, 54-55
    water-soluble, 51-52
Vitamin A, 50
    food sources of, 50
    fruits and vegetables rich in, 66
Vitamin B complex, 52
Vitamin B_6, 52
    food sources of, 52
Vitamin B_{12}, 53
    food sources of, 53
Vitamin C, 53
    fruits and vegetables rich in, 66
    sources of, 53
Vitamin D, 50-51
    sources of, 51
Vitamin E, 51
    best sources of, 51
Vitamin K, 51
    best sources of, 51
    deficiency, 51
Vitamin supplements, 48
Volume equivalents, 140

W

Water, 2
Weaning, 161
Weight(s), table of desirable, 238
Weight regulation
    chemical method of, 201
    clinical method of, 202
Weighted diet, 201
Weights and measures
    equivalent, 140
    systems of, 137
Whip, 133

X

Xerophthalmia, 50

Z

Zinc, 44